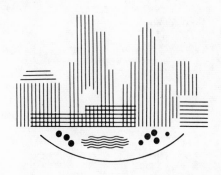

THE RISE OF URBAN AMERICA

A HALF CENTURY
OF PUBLIC HEALTH

Mazyck Porcher Ravenel, editor

ARNO PRESS

&

The New York Times

NEW YORK · 1970

Reprint Edition 1970 by Arno Press Inc.

Reprinted from a copy in The University of Illinois Library

LC# 74-112569
ISBN 0-405-02472-X

THE RISE OF URBAN AMERICA
ISBN for complete set 0-405-02430-4

Manufactured in the United States of America

A HALF CENTURY
OF PUBLIC HEALTH

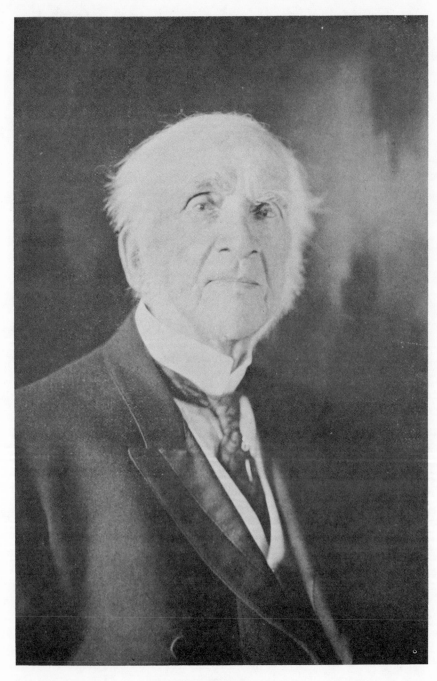

STEPHEN SMITH, M. D.

Founder and First President, American Public Health Association

A HALF CENTURY
OF PUBLIC HEALTH

JUBILEE HISTORICAL VOLUME

OF THE

AMERICAN PUBLIC HEALTH ASSOCIATION

IN COMMEMORATION OF
THE FIFTIETH ANNIVERSARY CELEBRATION
OF ITS FOUNDATION
NEW YORK CITY, NOVEMBER 14-18, 1921

EDITED BY

MAZÿCK P. RAVENEL, M. D.
President

AMERICAN PUBLIC HEALTH ASSOCIATION
NEW YORK
MCMXXI

— FROM —
The Nichols Press
LYNN, MASS.

TO

Stephen Smith, M. D., LL. D.

NOTED SURGEON, PIONEER SANITARIAN, EMINENT CITIZEN

FOUNDER AND FIRST PRESIDENT

OF THE AMERICAN PUBLIC HEALTH ASSOCIATION

AND TO ALL THOSE WHO HAVE AIDED

THE ASSOCIATION TOWARD THE ATTAINMENT OF ITS IDEALS

THIS VOLUME IS AFFECTIONATELY DEDICATED

FOREWORD

"FOR countless generations the prophets and kings of humanity have desired to see the things which men have seen, and to hear the things which men have heard, in the course of this wonderful nineteenth century. To the call of the watchers on the towers of progress there has been the one sad answer — the people sit in darkness and in the shadow of death. Politically, socially, and morally the race has improved, but for the unit, for the individual, there was little hope. Cold philosophy shed a glimmer of light on his path, religion in its various guises illumined his sad heart, but neither availed to lift the curse of suffering from the sin-begotten son of Adam. In the fullness of time, long expected, long delayed, at last science emptied upon him from the horn of Amalthea blessings which cannot be enumerated, blessings which have made the century forever memorable; and which have followed each other with a rapidity so bewildering that we know not what next to expect." (Osler).

The American Public Health Association has been fortunate, not only in having come into existence at an opportune time, but also in having lived during a period made notable for all time by remarkable discoveries in every branch of science. Wonderful in themselves as these discoveries have been, their chief value has lain in their usefulness to man. In no field have more remarkable advances been achieved than in medicine, both curative and preventive. Both have been revolutionized; knowledge has replaced guess-work; experiment has superseded empiricism and superstition; medicine has become a science rather than an art, — all through the brilliant researches begun by Pasteur, and carried on by Koch and a host of earnest workers who followed in their footsteps.

Recognizing that the Association has been privileged to look upon, and through its members to take an active part in, these wonderful discoveries and advances, and that its activities have been largely influenced by them, it has seemed fitting to tell the story in a series of historical articles at this time, in commemoration of our Fiftieth Anniversary Celebration.

THE EDITOR

CONTENTS

LIST OF CONTRIBUTORS

CARL L. ALSBERG, M. A., M. D.,

Director, Food Research Institute, Leland Stanford Jr. University; Chemical Biologist, Bureau of Plant Industry, 1908-12, Chief, Bureau of Chemistry, 1912-21, United States Department of Agriculture.

PETER H. BRYCE, M. A., M. D.,

Consultant Nervous and Mental Diseases and Diseases of Nutrition; formerly Chief Medical Officer, Department of Immigration and Colonization, Ottawa, Canada; L. R. C. P., L. R. C. S., Edinburgh, 1880.

CHARLES V. CHAPIN, M. D., SC. D.,

Superintendent of Health, Providence, R. I., 1874-; Lecturer, School of Public Health, Harvard and Massachusetts Institute of Technology, 1913-; Professor of Physiology, Brown University, 1886-96.

HUGH S. CUMMING, M. D.,

Surgeon General, United States Public Health Service, Washington, D. C., 1920-; Director, International Sanitary Bureau; formerly Quarantine Officer, Hampton Roads, Va.; formerly in Bacteriological Department, United States Public Health Service.

LAVINIA L. DOCK, R. N.

Secretary, International Council of Nurses; on staff, Johns Hopkins Hospital, Baltimore, 1890-93, Cook County Hospital, Chicago, 1893-96.

FREDERICK P. GORHAM, M. A.,

Professor of Bacteriology, Brown University, 1913-; Bacteriologist, Providence Health Department, 1899-; Bacteriologist and Biologist, Rhode Island Shellfish Commission, 1913-.

RUDOLPH HERING, D. SC.,

Consulting Engineer, New York, 1888-; Assistant Engineer, Prospect Park, Brooklyn, and Fairmount Park, Philadelphia, 1868-71; Department of Public Works, Philadelphia, 1873-86; Chief Engineer, Drainage and Water Supply Commission, Chicago, 1886-88; President, American Public Health Association, 1912-13.

FREDERICK L. HOFFMAN, LL. D.,

> Third Vice President and Statistician, Prudential Insurance Company of America, 1894-; Ex-President, American Statistical Association; Vice President, National Society for the Study and Prevention of Tuberculosis; Director, Executive Committee, National Safety Council.

LELAND O. HOWARD, PH. D., M. D., LL. D.

> Chief, Bureau of Entomology, United States Department of Agriculture, 1894-; Honorary Curator, Department of Insects, United States National Museum, 1895-; Consulting Entomologist, United States Public Health Service, 1904-.

GEORGE MARTIN KOBER, M. D., LL. D.,

> Dean, 1901-, and Professor of Hygiene, 1890-, Medical School, Georgetown University; Acting Assistant Surgeon, U. S. A., 1874-86; Member, Consulting Staff, Children's Hospital, George Washington University Hospital, and Washington Asylum Hospital; President, Washington Sanitary Improvement and Housing Companies, 1916-.

CHARLES E. NORTH, M. D.

> Director, the North Public Health Bureau, and Secretary, National Commission on Milk Standards appointed by the New York Milk Committee.

GEORGE T. PALMER, M. S., D. P. H.,

> Epidemiologist, Department of Health, Detroit, Mich., 1919-; Chief, Investigating Staff, New York State Commission on Ventilation, 1913-17; Epidemiological Division, Surgeon General's Office, Washington, D. C., 1917-19.

EARL B. PHELPS, B. S.,

> Chemist and Bacteriologist, Sanitary Research Laboratory, 1903-13, Assistant Professor of Chemical Biology, 1908-13, Massachusetts Institute of Technology; Professor of Chemistry and Chief, Division of Chemistry, Hygienic Laboratory, United States Public Health Service, 1913-19.

SAMUEL C. PRESCOTT, S. B.,

> Professor of Industrial Microbiology, Massachusetts Institute of Technology, 1914-; Director, Boston Bio-Chemical Laboratory, 1904-; Director, Research Laboratory, United Fruit Company, Port Limon, Costa Rica; Chief, Division of Dehydration, Bureau of Chemistry, Washington, D. C., 1918-19.

MAZŸCK P. RAVENEL, M. D.,

> Professor of Preventive Medicine and Bacteriology, University of Missouri, 1914-; President, American Public Health Association, 1920-21; Chief of Laboratory, Henry Phipps Institute for Study, Treatment and Prevention of Tuberculosis, 1904-7; Professor of Bacteriology, University of Wisconsin, 1907-14, and Director, State Hygienic Laboratory of Wisconsin, 1908-14.

STEPHEN SMITH, M. A., M. D., LL. D.,

Founder and First President of the American Public Health Association; formerly Professor of Surgery and of Anatomy, Bellevue Hospital Medical College; Editor, 1853-60, *New York Journal of Medicine*; Editor, *American Medical Times*, 1860-4; Member, Council of Hygiene, New York City, 1864; organized Sanitary Investigation, which led to creation of Metropolitan Board of Health, 1866, of which he was a Commissioner.

PHILIP VAN INGEN, M. D.,

Clinical Professor, Diseases of Children, College of Physicians and Surgeons, Columbia University; Attending Physician, Children's Service, Bellevue Hospital; Chairman, Executive Committee, and President, 1919-20, of the American Child Hygiene Association.

LAWRENCE VEILLER, A. B.,

Secretary, National Housing Association, New York City; Director, Department of Housing Reform, Russell Sage Foundation.

GEORGE C. WHIPPLE, C. E.,

Professor of Sanitary Engineering, Harvard University, 1911-, Massachusetts Institute of Technology, 1914-; Secretary, School of Public Health, Harvard and Massachusetts Institute of Technology; Member firm of Hazen, Whipple & Fuller, Consulting Engineers, New York.

THE HISTORY OF PUBLIC HEALTH, 1871-1921

STEPHEN SMITH, M. A., M. D., LL. D.

First President of the American Public Health Association

O N the 17th day of last January, the commissioner of health of the city of New York, Dr. Royal S. Copeland, made the following remarkable entry in the official records of his department: "Generally speaking, where two persons died fifty years ago, out of every 1000 population, only one died last year (1920)"

He adds this comment on the statement: "It is interesting to note that this tremendous decrease in the death-rate is the direct result of preventive measures on the part of the sanitary officials."

In another entry the Commissioner states that every disease that the sanitary officials specifically attacked showed a markedly diminished death-rate.

The statement of the Commissioner authorizes the conclusion that during the decade 1861–1871 there was inaugurated a system for the conservation of the public health in the city of New York so radical and effective that it created an epoch.

Bass, the eminent medical historian, regards epochs as the essentials of history and urges their study by the passing generation. Eloquently he expresses this duty as follows:

Acquaintance with views and knowledge of epochs submerged in the shoreless ocean of time frees the mind from the fetters and currents of the day with its often oppressive restraints; widens the horizon for a glance into the past and an insight into the present of human activity; deepens a view for a comprehension of the ideas which guided the earlier and more recent physicians, and gives on the other hand to our daily professional labor a high consecration.

Deeply impressed with the historian's sentiments and their quite universal application to the medical profession, it has occurred to me that it will be appropriate to the present occasion, if I, now verging on my centenary, should devote my paper to some historical and personal reminiscences, long submerged in the "shoreless ocean of time," but essential to the introduction of the great epoch in sanitation which we now celebrate.

Anniversaries come and go, and in these late days, with apparently ever-increasing celerity. Too often we give these records of our successes and failures but a simple greeting and profit nothing by their recurrence. But the wise and prudent man regards the anniversaries which occur in his business as beacon lights which illumine his future pathway and enable him to avoid its pitfalls of failure and seize the fleeting moments of success. So let us on this most auspicious anniversary look backward and learn the lessons of experience which it teaches before we take a step into the uncharted future.

THE SECRET OF LONGEVITY

Prior to the years 1866–1871, which include the beginnings of the present century of preventive sanitation, the health and longevity of the people was regarded as due to the special physical endowments of each person. From time immemorial, "old people" have been asked the secret of their lives which has enabled them to live so long. The folly of this question is seen in the variety of answers given. Though in many instances very sensible replies were made, too frequently they are quite absurd.

It is stated that Franklin wrote that "an Angel visited Methuselah, then at the age of five hundred years, and informed him that he was to live five hundred years more and he should build him an house. Methuselah replied, 'If I am to live but five hundred years more, it is not worth while for me to build an house; I will live as I have done in the open air.'"

Moses, the great Jewish sanitarian, was believed to have revealed the divine law of life in these impressive words, "The days of our years are three score and ten; if by reason of strength they be four score years, yet is their strength labor and sorrow; . . . . ."
But Moses lived to see the futility of this law in his own person, for he safely passed four score years without "labor and sorrow." It

is written, "Moses was an hundred and twenty years when he died; his eye was not dim, nor his natural force abated."

Horace, the Latin poet, replied to the same question, "*Moderatus in Rebus,*" "Moderation in all things."

A recent American authority said, with characteristic emphasis, "I keep my stomach and brain busy."

THE SCIENCE OF LONGEVITY

The long period, unnumbered centuries, of ignorance and superstition as to the conditions affecting the public health, which promote or prevent longevity, came to an end with the development of the medical sciences effected by the scientists of the last and present centuries. Owen established the length of biological life by the development of the bones, fixing the normal life at five times the number of years required to perfect the bones. In man it requires twenty years to complete the process which makes normal or potential life one hundred years. This is the birthright of every child born fully developed.

Virchow's cell theory taught that the ultimate elements of all tissues of the body are living units of high vitality, made to perform a certain function, then to die and be cast out of the body as dead matter, their places being supplied immediately by new cells. Thus the tissues are being constantly renewed and within a given period the entire physical system is renewed. It is on the maintenance of this renewal that health and longevity depend. Finally, Pasteur unfolded the life-history of bacteria, the greatest health and life destroyers that man has to contend with.

On these fundamental principles, the science of preventive medicine, or civic sanitation, was established at the beginning of the century whose semicentennial we now celebrate. Incidentally or accidentally it became my duty to take the initiative and the responsibility in establishing in New York City scientific civic sanitation, by the enactment of the Metropolitan Health Law in 1866 and the organization of the American Public Health Association in 1871. These were the forces that gave the first impetus to the tremendous development which has its results in the death-rate of 1920. The events leading to the effective organization of these correlative institutions, the first legal, with power to make and enforce sanitary laws and ordinances, and the second, voluntary, for the purpose of increasing the number of scientific health authorities throughout the country, and coördinating their operations, are of such importance as to require notice in this historical sketch.

THE SANITARY CONDITION OF NEW YORK CITY IN 1860–1870

I came to New York from a small farm in the highlands of the state in 1850 for the purpose of completing my medical studies at the College of Physicians and Surgeons of Columbia University. I had selected medicine as my profession on the suggestion of my physicians as a preventive measure against the recurrence of a form of indigestion of which I had been a victim from childhood. To that advice I attribute my activities in middle life and the comparatively comfortable age to which I have attained.

Upon graduation, I joined the resident staff of Bellevue Hospital after a competitive examination, and after two years' residence in that great laboratory of disease of every kind and form, entered the field of private practice. During my term of service in Bellevue Hospital, a severe epidemic of typhus fever prevailed, due to an immense immigration of Irish people, among whom it first appeared following a famine. Ten of our staff of twelve suffered attacks, two of whom died. I was one of those who escaped. The pressure upon the accommodations of the hospital became so great that the commissioners established a fever hospital on Blackwell's Island, and I was appointed its visiting physician, being regarded as immune.

A FEVER NEST

Upon examination of the records of admission of patients, I discovered that from one tenement house upwards of one hundred cases had been received. On visiting the house, I found a veritable "fever nest." The doors and windows were broken, the cellar was filled with sewage, every room was occupied by families of Irish immigrants who had but little furniture and slept on straw scattered on the floor. I learned that the house was the first resort of immigrants, as there was no one in charge and hence no expense.

My first effort to vacate and close this fever nest was an application to the Police Department. During my interview with the president, the attorney of the board was called, and upon hearing the case informed us that the police had no authority to act in such cases, and he knew of no department of the city government that could legally take the steps which I proposed, namely, to abate a nuisance of such a kind.

I then determined to find the owner and endeavor to persuade him as a matter of public duty and humanity to put his house in proper sanitary condition. Visiting the tax office, I found that the taxes were paid by a wealthy gentleman living in Union Square. He received my request with a flat refusal to improve the house, alleging that it never paid anything and was a constant source of annoyance.

When I related the case, and my failures, to the secretary of the Citizens' Association, a powerful body of men, with Mr. Peter Cooper as president, organized to defeat the schemes of Tweed, then in full control of the city government, he was deeply interested and suggested that the reform of the Health Department was directly in line with the work of the Association. He suggested that I should join the organization and become a member of the "Council of Hygiene," a committee already in operation and named after a French commission. I followed his advice, was elected and assigned to the Council, and became its secretary.

A joint meeting of the Council and the "Committee on Law" was held, and I explained at length the great prevalence and fatality of typhus fever, and the discovery of a most prolific "fever nest," which there was no legal authority to abate as a public nuisance, in the opinion of the attorney and the Police Department. Intense interest was manifested and the subject was referred to the secretaries for a report. The secretary of the Law Committee was Dorman B. Eaton, Esq.

SANITARY INSPECTION OF THE CITY

On reviewing the situation, it was found that the opposition which had defeated previous efforts of sanitary societies that had introduced health bills into the Legislature was chiefly denials of the unsanitary condition of the city and the incompetence of the existing officials. To determine more definitely the kind of opposition which the committee would meet and be prepared to contest it successfully, the sub-commitee proposed that a health bill be introduced into the Legislature of 1864, for the purpose of enabling the joint committee to learn the strength of the opposition. This course was adopted and at the hearings on the bill given by the legislative committee every allegation of the advocates of the bill was denied by a score of "health wardens," as the inspectors of wards were called.

The result of this test induced the committee of the Council of Hygiene to recommend that the Association cause a sanitary survey to be made by medical inspectors of character and have their reports verified by a notary. The report was adopted and the work of supervision committed to me. I organized it at once and spent the summer in its supervision. My plan was the division of the city into thirty-one inspection districts and the appointment of a qualified inspector in each; the preparation of a schedule of objects to be inspected, which included streets, houses, as to families and their condition, out-buildings, vacant lots, and other points of possible danger to health. In fact it included every matter affecting the public health, with a final report summarizing the results of the inspection. These final reports made seventeen bound volumes, and have heen pronounced by high authority as the most complete work of the kind on record.

By direction of the Association, Dr. Elisha Harris, of the committee of the Council prepared a summary volume of the principal results of these reports. The entire expense of this inspection, as paid by the Citizens' Association, was upwards of $22,000.

The members of the Association were quite enthusiastic upon receiving the report of the inspection and directed the committee to prepare a new bill based on the results of this inspection. Naturally this duty was assigned to Mr. Eaton and myself, as it involved both medical and legal questions. We began our investigations by examining the existing health organization of the city with a view to incorporating in the new measure any available competent officials.

HEALTH ADMINISTRATION IN NEW YORK IN 1864

This inquiry revealed the fact that New York had no effective sanitary administration. There were numerous departments filled with active politicians, but not one had any expert supervision. There was a Board of Health when the aldermen were summoned to meet as such. The value of the Board was stated by Mayor Fernando Wood, an expert in city politics, to a medical delegation that requested the Mayor to call the aldermen as a board of health to take measures against an approaching cholera epidemic. The Mayor replied, "I will not call the Board, for I consider it more dangerous to the city than cholera." There was the Health Commission, with practically no well-defined duties. The "city physician" attended the neglected cases of sickness among the poor, a negligible number. The most conspicuous figure in the list of sanitary officials was the head of the Street-cleaning Department, who had an annual appropriation of nearly $1,000,000 dollars to expend upon his political followers. The sanitary inspection of the city was one of his duties and for this work he appointed scores of "Health Wardens," who were generally saloon-keepers. The qualification of these sanitary officials for their duties was tested by a legislative committee. One was asked to define the word "hygiene," and he replied, "the vapor which rises from stagnant water." Another was asked, "What do you do when you are called to a case of contagious disease?" He replied, "I go to the house and call the people to the street, where I give my orders, which are to burn sulphur; I never go into the house."

THE METROPOLITAN HEALTH BILL

As said above, the Citizen's Association directed the committee to prepare a new bill based upon the results of the inspection. This duty was assigned to Mr. Eaton and myself.

The first question to be determined was the creation of a sanitary district. The Police Department at that time had been changed from a municipal to a state organization, by creating a metropolitan district which included a large area adjacent to the city of New York. The original purpose of this change was due to the policy of the Citizens' Association to remove control of the police from Tweed, who ruled supreme in the city government. The Metropolitan Health District was accordingly created. At Mr. Eaton's request I drafted the new bill in the autumn of 1864. I was guided chiefly in its details by the English sanitary laws, then the most complete in operation. With some important changes and additions the bill was adopted by the Medical Committee of the Council and referred to the Law Committee. In the hands of Mr. Eaton, an expert in the construction of legislative documents, the bill was greatly modified both in literary form and subject matter. The feature of the bill which aroused most discussion was introduced by Mr. Eaton, and was written in language not understood by the medical members. He explained that in his experience health authorities were often obstructed by the courts, especially in the prompt abatement of nuisances. While he acknowledged that this provision of the bill was without precedent in legislation, he contended that when a health authority, whose duty was to protect and promote the public health, found any matter or thing "dangerous to life and detrimental to health," and had made an official record of the facts, and an order of abatement of the nuisance, there should be no authority having legal power to prevent the action.

Though the legal members doubted the propriety of endeavoring to secure legislation by such an effort to conceal the true intent and purpose of the law, it was admitted to be within the limits of legislative rules of procedure. The medical members of the committee supported Mr. Eaton's view, and the bill was reported favorably to the Citizens' Association, which adopted it after full discussion of the doubtful clause. The prevailing argument in the Association was that the courts were completely under the control of Tweed and injunctions would prevent the proposed Board of Health from abating nuisances.

The bill was introduced early in the session of the Legislature of 1865, by the appointment of Mr. Eaton and myself as a committee. The first hearing was before a joint committee of the two houses, with Senator Andrew D. White, the future president of Cornell University, as chairman. In opposition appeared a large delegation of city officials, chiefly health wardens. Mr. Eaton explained the bill and referred to me as prepared to demonstrate the unsanitary condition of the city, and the importance of the bill as the proper remedy for the relief from the evils of the high sickness and death-rate. I had provided myself with the written and certified reports of our inspection. The opposition was a blank denial of every specific statement I made. I was able to prove the correctness of our reports so effectively that the opposition ceased before the hearing adjourned. The only resource of the opposition was to ask for another hearing, which was granted. The hearing was favorable to the bill, for the opponents were compelled to admit the general accuracy of our charges. Favorable as the hearing had been, the bill was defeated in the Assembly.

The committee now commenced a campaign of education of the medical profession of the state preparatory to the Legislature of 1866. The profession was very sympathetic, and at the election in the fall of 1865, defeated the nomination of the opponents of the bill. The bill was introduced into the Legislature of 1866 and was strongly supported by the entire medical profession of the state. It had also in its favor the persuasive report that an epidemic of cholera had appeared in Europe and would in due time reach this country. Under the pressure of these forces, the bill was among the first passed, and in March the Metropolitan Health Board was organized. Coincident with this event, cholera appeared and was destined to prove the adequacy of scientific civic sanitation. In an incredibly short time after the first case of cholera was reported to the Board, the Disinfecting Department of the Board, equipped with ample material and trained attendants, was in charge of the premises. The patient recovered and no second case occurred. Many similar instances occurred, of which I was personally cognizant. The result of this new experience in the treatment of cholera was public confidence in the power of the Board to control and suppress the spread of contagious diseases. People who had fled from the city for safety returned; business was generally resumed, and for half a century cholera has excited little or no alarm here, even when it reaches Europe in its world-wide itinerary. During this half century, the Health Department of New York City, though under the administration of officials of widely different political faiths, has steadily increased in popularity. This is a remarkable history, when we consider its power of exhaustive inquiry into and control of the management of the business and domestic affairs of the people of every class. Its power has been contested in the courts, and its constitutionality was early decided by the Court of Appeals.

The great achievements of the Board were the under-drainage of the soil, which prevented stagnant water and relieved the city of malaria; the removal of the cellar population to homes in the open air and sunlight; the removal of offensive industries from residential districts to the rivers; and the enforcement of rigid sanitary regulations.

There is an old motto that reads "Public Health is Public Wealth." Its truth has recently been proved by the health authority of England. The report states that the total annual loss of time by the sickness and disablement of men is 8,916,000 weeks, and for women 5,149,941 weeks. "It may, therefore, be said that at least 14,066,000 weeks work are lost every year through sickness."

The American Public Health Association

As the result of a large correspondence with existing health authorities and persons interested in sanitation, largely in regard to the organization and operation of the Metropolitan Board of Health, I suggested that a national association with a membership of persons connected with existing health organizations, and citizens interested in sanitation, would greatly facilitate the enlightenment of the public and promote the appointment of more competent health authorities. The suggestion was so generally well received that I called a meeting of several of the more prominent sanitarians for an informal conference. The meeting was held in New York in the spring of

1872. The plan of organizing a national association was unanimously adopted, a meeting for that purpose was called, and a committee appointed to arrange details and report a plan. This meeting was held at Long Branch in the following September and was attended by delegates from all parts of the country. The plan of organization was adopted with some changes, I was elected president, and Dr. Elisha Harris, secretary. The first meeting of the organized Association was called to meet in Cincinnati in May, 1873. The attendance at that meeting was large, the proceedings attracted wide public attention, and the great work of the Association was begun.

AN INTERNATIONAL PUBLIC HEALTH LEAGUE

In 1894, I was appointed by President Cleveland a delegate to represent this government at the Ninth International Sanitary Conference called by the government of France. The object of this meeting was to formulate sanitary rules and regulations governing the pilgrims in their visits to Mecca. It was alleged by the French sanitary authorities that cholera was always introduced into Europe by infected pilgrims from the Ganges. At Mecca they communicated the infection to the pilgrims from Europe, who transported it to their countries. The Conference was in session three months and made a code of rules to be adopted by the governments which controlled the pilgrims, and appointed a commission to supervise their enforcement. This sanitary league of nations has effectually protected Europe from invasions of cholera.

The delegates from this country were so much impressed with the simplicity and probable results of this action that they applied to the president to call a similar conference in the interests of this country, to prevent the transportation of infected immigrants. He approved the suggestion but could not then take such action.

I beg to submit this proposition as one proper to be considered by this Association. If such a league could be established in good faith, many of the immigrant questions, now so disturbing, would be settled, greatly to the interest of both the immigrant and the countries involved, and there would be no more transmission of contagion.

May I be permitted reverently to suggest that our purpose has the same sentiment as was heard by the shepherds on the plains of Judea at the Nativity?   Then the "good will to men" was announced to be the salvation of the soul from sin by divine appointment; while we now learn that salvation from the sins of the body must be effected by man himself, who created them.

Let us apply ourselves to the task with renewed vigor, and thus enable those who will greet the centennial anniversary of this Association to hear from sanitary officials the good news that the death-rate of the year 1971 is limited to those afflicted with old age, or to disease or accidents unpreventable and incurable by any agencies known to science.

THE AMERICAN PUBLIC HEALTH ASSOCIATION
PAST, PRESENT, FUTURE

MAZŸCK P. RAVENEL, M. D., PRESIDENT

Professor of Preventive Medicine, University of Missouri

ADDRESS GIVEN AT THE FIFTIETH ANNIVERSARY
CELEBRATION MEETING

Of the altrustic instincts veneration is not the most highly developed at the present day; but I hold strongly with the statement that it is a sign of a dry age when the great men of the past are held in light esteem. (Osler).

IT seems most fitting that on this, the fiftieth anniversary meeting of the American Public Health Association, we should pause to pay homage to the lives and accomplishments of those who guided the course of our Association in its early years and won for it the proud place it now occupies as an instrument for public good. We may well review our work and take stock of our achievements in an earnest effort to determine how far we have justified our existence and attained our ideals.

The Association

had its origin in that natural desire which thinkers and workers in the same fields, whether of business or philanthropy, or the administration of civil trusts, have for mutual council, advice and coöperation. (Smith).

A preliminary meeting, attended by Doctors E. M. Snow, Providence, R. I., Chairman, J. H. Rauch, Chicago, Ill., J. Ordronaux, Roslyn, N. Y., Stephen Smith, N. Y., E. H. Jones, N. Y., C. C. Cox, Washington, D. C., and Carl Pfeiffer, N. Y., architect, was held April 18, 1872, at 301 Mott St., New York, at which an informal discussion on the formation of a national sanitary association took place. A larger and more formal gathering was decided upon, and on the evening of the same day, these gentlemen, with the exception of Dr. Snow, and the addition of Doctors Elisha Harris and Moreau Morris, New York, and Heber Smith of the Marine Hospital Service, met at the New York Hotel. At this meeting a Committee on Permanent Organization was appointed with Dr. Stephen Smith as chairman. This committee issued a call for the first regular meeting held at Long Branch, New Jersey, September 12, 1872, at which time a constitution was adopted, and Dr. Stephen Smith elected the first president.

Up to this time no public health organization existed on the American Continent, and public health practice, in so far as it existed at all, was empirical and lacked uniformity.

In his classic address before the International Medical Congress in 1876, Dr. Henry I. Bowditch states that National Sanitary Conventions, so called, were held in Philadelphia, 1857, Baltimore, 1858, New York, 1859, and in Baltimore, 1860, but ceased with the outbreak of the Civil War.

Only three states, Massachusetts, 1869, California and Virginia, 1871, and the District of Columbia, 1870, had established boards of health prior to 1872, and only twelve up to 1876, the date of Dr. Bowditch's survey. In only two states was registration of births, deaths, and marriages claimed to be made with any degree of accuracy, though twenty had passed some laws concerning registration. In 1873, 134 cities in the United States had some form of health board.

In England three epidemics of cholera, in 1831, 1849 and 1854, had brought the appointment of commissions of investigation. In 1848, following the report of a royal commission appointed to investigate outbreaks of disease in large towns, and to recommend measures for the improvement of the public health, comprehensive sanitary acts were adopted, a general board of health was established and medical officers of health were appointed.

In 1869 the famous Royal Sanitary Commission was appointed, and proposed for the first time a ministry of health, which failed to carry, but the Local Government Board was created in 1871. An epidemic of Asiatic cholera in 1832, resulted in a Provincial Act for the appointment of Local Boards of Health, and in 1849 this act was amended to provide for a central board of health, to continue during the pleasure of the legislature.

In America, though we had not advanced so far, the leaven was working, and in 1850 there was published the "Report on the Sanitary Condition of Massachusetts," written largely, if not wholly, by a layman, Lemuel Shattuck. It was a remarkable paper which suggested the appointment of a state board of health, and so well outlined the duties and functions of such a board that when the board was finally appointed in 1869, the secretary, Dr. Derby, found in the pages written twenty years before his inspiration and support. In 1870 Dr. Derby wrote the first paper ever published in this country under the direction of a permanent body appointed by state authority for the investigation of diseases and instruction of the public concerning them.

Such was the condition of things in the English-speaking countries when our Association was born.

In France, Pasteur was revolutionizing all former conceptions of disease by his discoveries, and the formulation of new theories.

In August and December, 1857, Pasteur published his first papers on lactic acid fermentation and alcoholic fermentation, showing that fermentation was caused by living organisms.

Discussions on spontaneous generation followed and persisted for several years. The proofs against it given by Pasteur settled the dispute for all time.

In 1865 he took up the study of silkworm disease, and soon brought it under control by methods based on his new discoveries, his experiments adding much to the knowledge already gained, and confirming the theories advanced.

In England, Lister, a surgeon, began in 1867 to put into practice the ideas he had gained as a student of Pasteur, and was able to report in 1869 that of forty patients who had suffered amputations, thirty-four had survived. Such good results were unheard of at that time, and were attributed by him entirely to antiseptic surgery, which was the practical application of Pasteur's theories to surgical practice.

In 1870–72 Pasteur pursued his studies on the fermentation of beer, and invented what is now called "Pasteurization," to correct unhealthy fermentations.

No more opportune time could have been chosen for the formation of our Association. The art of medicine was becoming the science of medicine, and modern preventive medicine was being born. The discoveries of Pasteur put an end to superstition and empiricism and substituted the bed-rock of science as a foundation on which has been erected the wonderful structure of medicine as it exists today.

Although begun and apparently designed largely as an association of administrative officers, it was inevitable that others should be attracted to the ranks. The science of bacteriology had come into existence as a result of Pasteur's work, and the laboratory soon became a prime factor in the study and prevention of disease. The germ of anthrax had been seen by Rayer and Davaine in 1850; Delafond, 1860, had shown its power of vegetation, and Davaine, 1863, its causative relation to the disease, while Koch, 1876, obtained pure cultures on artificial media and demonstrated the spores. Pasteur completed the demonstration, making anthrax the first disease in which the etiological relation of a germ to a disease was proved.

In 1877 the bacillus of malignant edema was discovered by Pasteur; in 1879 the germ of chicken cholera by Pasteur, and the gonococcus by Neisser. In 1880 the pneumococcus was discovered by Pasteur and by Sternberg independently, and the typhoid bacillus by Eberth.

Of even greater significance, perhaps, was the announcement in this year by Pasteur of a bacterial vaccine against chicken cholera, followed in 1881 by his epoch-making demonstration of vaccination against anthrax. This year brought also the discoveries of the pus-forming organisms, the staphylococcus and streptococcus, knowledge of which has revolutionized modern surgery and robbed maternity of its chief dangers. The year 1882 will always be notable for the discovery of the tubercle bacillus by Koch. Loeffler and Schutz isolated the germ of glanders in this year also. The year 1883 saw the discovery of the spirillum of Asiatic cholera by Koch, and the bacillus of diphtheria by Klebs, while 1884 was marked by two discoveries of great public health significance — the isolation of the diphtheria bacillus by Loeffler, and of the typhoid bacillus by Gaffky.

The influence of the new science on public health ideas and practice was paramount. In the pages of our *Transactions* one may find a veritable history of bacteriology, with its practical application to public health, and while the earlier discoveries came largely from abroad, our Association was not without representatives, notably in the person of Dr. George M. Sternberg, our president in 1886.

The Association from its inception has taken a broad view of its duties to the public, and has established an enviable record for public service. At the third Annual Meeting, held in Philadelphia, the following resolution was adopted:

That a committee consisting of a member of this Association from each state and territory of the Union . . . . be appointed to petition Congress, at its next session, to institute a bureau of health, to be located at Washington City, with a branch at the seat of each state and territorial government.

That this Association urge upon the governor and legislature of each and every state in the Union the importance of enacting laws creating state boards of health and providing adequately for sanitary administration.

Five years later, in 1879, under the impending danger of a yellow fever epidemic, Congress created a National Board of Health,* which functioned for the term of four years provided for in the act creating it, but was allowed to pass out of existence by the next Congress, in spite of petitions showing the need of such a body, the excellent results achieved during its short life, and the importance of its continuance.

We have been more successful with the states, and there is now no state in the Union without some form of a health department.

MEMBERSHIP

With the growth of the Association, it became increasingly evident that its objects could be best attained by consultation and coöperation with our neighbors, whose problems were much the same as our own; so at the St. Louis meeting, in 1884, Canada was invited to join with us, and became a constituent member — without question the most important measure taken since the formation of the Association.

---

*A review of the "Operations of the National Board of Health" is given in Volume VIII, page 71, of our *Transactions*, by Dr. J. L. Cabell, president.

At the Brooklyn meeting, in 1889, the secretary was instructed to communicate with the health authorities of Mexico, Central America, Cuba and Colombia, and invite these countries to coöperate in the work of the Association. Mexico alone responded, accepting the invitation, and at the Charleston meeting, in 1890, we had the honor of entertaining Dr. Domingo Orvañanos and Professor José L. Gomez as the official representatives of the Superior Board of Health of Mexico. In 1892, at the meeting in the City of Mexico, the amendment to the Constitution proposed in 1891 was adopted, and Mexico came into the Association fully. These two sister countries have added greatly to our strength, and have given many of our distinguished members and officers.

In 1902, at New Orleans, the newly formed Republic of Cuba was invited to associate with us, and for the first time practically the whole of North America was embraced in our membership, making us in fact, as in name, the American Public Health Association.

SECTIONS

The influence of bacteriology and the growing importance of laboratory work have been already referred to. Discoveries were announced in rapid succession. Laboratories rapidly became essential to health officers and boards of health for diagnostic purposes and the control of such utilities as water supplies.

Although the epidemic of cholera in London traced to the "Broad Street Pump" occurred as early as 1854, the typhoid outbreak at Lausen, Switzerland, in 1872, was the first to attract widespread attention to the danger of polluted water. Other outbreaks, such as those at Caterham and Red Hill, England, in 1879, at Plymouth, Pennsylvania, in 1885, and at Lowell and Lawrence, Massachusetts, in 1890–91, had turned attention to the study of water supplies. The notable experiments in water purification instituted by the State Board of Health at Lawrence, Massachusetts, were designed and carried out largely by members of our Association, under the administration of our former president, Dr. Walcott. Many papers and discussions became too technical for the general meetings.

At the Montreal meeting, in 1894, Dr. Wyatt Johnston called attention to the desirability of having more uniform methods for the conduct of laboratory work. The result was that a sub-committee of the Committee on Pollution of Water Supplies issued a call for a convention of American bacteriologists, which met in New York in June, 1895. A committee was appointed to draw up procedures for the uniform study of bacteria and the differentiation of species. This committee reported at Philadelphia, in 1897, and the report was published in 1898 — the first of the various "Standard Methods" now published by the Association.

A further result of this convention was the appointment of a Committee on Laboratory Work and Methods, at the Ottawa meeting in 1898, with Dr. Wyatt Johnston as chairman. In 1899, at the Minneapolis meeting, this committee reported and was discharged, its functions being taken over by the Section on Bacteriology and Chemistry organized at this time. Nearly one hundred enrolled in the new section at once, of whom approximately half were new members of the Association.

The Section has always devoted much attention to the standardization and improvement of laboratory methods, and its publications are regarded as official throughout the countries of North America.

The scope of public health was rapidly widening during these years, and the growth of the Association kept pace with it. New members with new points of view were constantly joining our ranks, and specialism was inevitable. In 1908 two new sections were organized, Vital Statistics and Public Health Administration. Three years later it became necessary to further specialize, and again, in 1911, two new sections were organized, Sociological and Sanitary Engineering. In 1914 the Section on Industrial Hygiene was formed, and that on Food and Drugs in 1917. If time and space permitted it would be most interesting to review the genesis of all the sections. They were preceded by special committees and reports, which gave evidence of the growth of the public health idea, as well as the sense of duty to the public which has always actuated our Association. All sections were formed in response to demands which could not be put aside.   At present there are requests before us for the formation of still other sections, most of which have a basis of valid claims on our attention, and with the further growth of the Association we must soon expect to see the number of sections increased.

PUBLICATIONS

Until 1895 the proceedings of the Association, together with the reports and papers presented at the meetings, were published as an annual volume under the title *Public Health, Reports and Papers of the American Public Health Association.*   From 1895 to 1898, inclusive, they were published as a quarterly, entitled, *Journal of the American Public Health Association,* the original title and serial number being retained for the annual volume.   In 1899 the annual volume was returned to, and continued until 1908, except that for three volumes, two in 1905, and one in 1906, the papers of the Laboratory Section were published by the *Journal of Infectious Diseases,* and bound as Part II of Volumes XXX, XXXI, and XXXII; and for one volume, 1907, these papers were printed by the *Americal Journal of Public Hygiene,* and bound as Part II of Volume XXXIII.   In 1908, beginning with Volume XXXIV, our papers were published by the *American Journal of Public Hygiene,* which became the official organ of the Association, and this was continued until the establishment, in 1911, of our own periodical, the *Journal of the American Public Health Association.*

There are 37 volumes of our transactions, reports and papers under the original title.   Of these, Volumes XXXIV and XXXV are reprinted from the *American Journal of Public Hygiene,* and XXXVI and XXXVII from the *Journal* of our Association, which continued the *American Journal of Public Hygiene.*   During the first twenty-five years of our existence we published twenty-two volumes, containing 695 papers and 9,117 pages of reading matter. From 1897 to 1911, when the *Journal* was begun, 13 volumes were issued, containing 827 papers and 6,826 pages.   The ten volumes of the *Journal* completed to date, 1911 to 1920, contain 1,106 articles,

136 reports, 229 editorials, and 11,379 pages, making a total of 2,993 articles and 27,322 pages of literature on health, in which every phase of the subject has been discussed by specialists and experts. These pages are not only a mine of information, but also a good history of the public health movement during the past fifty years. The reports of committees and papers read leave no matter of interest untouched. Our general meetings have been the forum before which many epoch-making discoveries have been presented or discussed. The volumes are in demand for libraries, and it is now very difficult to obtain full sets. A review of them would be most interesting and proper in this address, but the several fifty-year histories on public health topics which are to be presented at this meeting and published in our Jubilee Volume will doubtless cover much of the same ground, so that only a few points will be noted here.

As it were a beacon to guide the young Association, the first volume contains a paper by F. A. P. Bernard, LL. D., president of Columbia College, New York, on "The Germ Theory of Disease and Its Relation to Hygiene," giving an excellent presentation of the new discoveries and ideas concerning disease. Although written by a non-medical man, it was in advance of much of the medical opinion of the day, since it was followed by papers on "Sewer Gas as a Cause of Scarlet Fever and Typho-Malarial Diseases"; "Does Smallpox Become Epidemic, or Spread Only by Its Own Contagion?"; "Gases of Decay and the Harm They Cause in Dwellings," and others of the same type, especially concerning yellow fever.

In comparing the earlier volumes with those of today, one is struck by the fact that the most important topics discussed in the early years are scarcely ever mentioned now. The first volume, published in 1873, is given up largely to yellow fever and cholera. One finds it hard to believe that cholera was at that time widespread in the United States, and that it existed in more than two hundred towns and cities of the Mississippi Valley.

Year after year we find pages devoted to the discussion of yellow fever, with many diverse theories as to its origin and propagation, such, for instance, as that it originated *de novo* in the cities of America; that the cause was cumulative and due to uncleaned privy vaults; that it arose from bilge-water; that the body does not reproduce the poison of yellow fever; and that the poison may be developed by adding one or more of the excretions of the patient to decomposing organic matter under well-known conditions.

These discussions were set at rest for all time in a paper read at our Indianapolis meeting in 1900, by Dr. Walter Reed, entitled, "The Etiology of Yellow Fever: A Preliminary Note." We feel a justifiable pride in knowing that the discoveries therein detailed were the result of studies made by one of our former presidents, Dr. Carlos J. Finlay, and our honored fellow-member, Dr. Walter Reed, who, with Doctors Lazear, Carroll, and Agramonte, gave the final proofs. It is impossible to praise too highly the scientific acumen displayed, or the devotion to duty which led these men to place their lives in jeopardy by experimenting on themselves, one, Dr. Jesse W. Lazear, making the supreme sacrifice as a result.

Only those of Southern birth or Southern residence can fully appreciate what this discovery has meant. In his presidential address on our twenty-fifth anniversary, Dr. H. B. Horlbeck urged that the President of the United States be requested to send a commission of expert bacteriologists to Havana and Rio to study yellow fever. Three years later the method of transmission was proved, and the disease was rapidly brought under control. The causative germ for years eluded discovery, but apparently has recently been cultivated by Dr. Hideyo Noguchi. Yellow fever was first brought into the United States in 1693, and for more than two hundred years was the terror of the South. Our pages show what the disease has meant to our country, and an especially graphic portrayal may be found in a speech by Dr. Joseph Holt, president of the Louisiana Board of Health in 1886. We can at this time scarcely understand the justification of the "shot-gun quarantine" which yellow fever outbreaks brought into being. That human nature does not change very rapidly is shown by the action of the authorities of Aberdeen in 1585, who erected gibbets, —

One at the nearest cross, one other at the Brig of Dee, and the third at Haven Mouth, that in case any infectit person might arrive or repair by sea or land to this brough, or in case any indweller of this brough receive, house or harbor, or give meat or drink to the infectit person or persons, the man to be hangit, and the woman to be drownit.

The meeting at Buffalo, in 1896, was made notable by the paper of Dr. Wyatt Johnston of Montreal, "On the Application of the Serum Diagnosis of Typhoid Fever to the Requirements of Public Health Laboratories." He demonstrated there for the first time the feasibility of sending blood dried on paper long distances through the mails, and making correct diagnoses in cases of suspected typhoid fever, a practice now common in every public health laboratory.

I cannot but pause here a moment to pay tribute to Dr. Johnston in recognition of his services to the Association and to the cause of public health. His early death took from us one of our most useful and brilliant members, and cut short a scientific career already notable and full of promise.

LOMB PRIZE ESSAYS

In 1884, Mr. Henry Lomb, of Rochester, New York, set an example which we wish might have been followed by others, by offering $2,000 to be awarded as prizes for essays on subjects selected by himself.

The contest attracted wide attention, and more than fifty essays were sent in, coming from foreign countries as well as America.

The awards were made at the Washington meeting, in 1885, as follows:

1. Healthy Homes and Food for the Working Classes, by Victor C. Vaughan, Ann Arbor, Michigan.

2. The Sanitary Conditions and Necessities of School-Houses and School-Life, by D. F. Lincoln, Boston, Massachusetts.

3. Disinfection and Individual Prophylaxis against Infectious Diseases, by George M. Sternberg, Washington, D. C.

4. Preventable Causes of Disease, Injury and Death in American Manufactories and Work-Shops, and the Best Means and Appliances for Preventing and Avoiding Them. By George H. Ireland, Springfield, Mass.

These essays were published as a separate volume and went through three editions. The essay of Dr. Sternberg was revised and enlarged, and published in our *Transactions*, Volume XXV, 1889. For many years it was the leading work on disinfection in the English language.

In recognition of his services, Mr. Lomb was made a life member of the Association.

JOURNAL

For many years the need of a medium for frequent communication between workers in the field of public health had been felt. Neither the annual volume, the quarterly publication, nor the affiliation with the *American Journal of Public Hygiene* had satisfactorily filled this need, which was becoming increasingly urgent as the field of health work enlarged and the number of workers increased. At the Milwaukee meeting, in 1910, a resolution was adopted creating a Committee on Journal, authorizing and directing this committee to provide for the publication of a monthly journal. The first number was issued in January, 1911, under the title *Journal of the American Public Health Association*. In 1912 the name was changed to *American Journal of Public Health* which it still retains.* From the beginning it has taken a leading position among scientific journals, and the premier place among those devoted to health. Its value to the Association cannot be estimated, keeping our members in touch with the organization during the intervals between the annual meetings, and giving them during the year information of the new and important developments in public health. Since its foundation it has replaced the annual volume for the publication of reports and papers.

Since March, 1919, a monthly *News Letter* has been issued. To date 112,774 copies have been distributed.

---

*In 1891 a quarterly was established, entitled, *Journal of the Massachusetts Association of Boards of Health*, the first number of which appeared in January of that year, published by W. S. French, Newton, Massachusetts, who was probably also the editor. It was the official organ of the organization from which it took its name. Dr. Samuel H. Durgin, president of the A. P. H. A. in 1902, became editor in 1903. The next year Dr. H. W. Hill became managing editor, and under the direc-

STANDARD METHODS

The Association has from its inception striven for the adoption of uniform practices and standard methods. It has for many years had various committees at work, constantly trying out methods and selecting the best. As a result, we have published the following:

"Standard Methods for the Examination of Water and Sewage." The predecessor, and really the first edition of this publication, was the report of the committee appointed in 1895 to draw up procedures for the uniform study of bacteria, adopted at the Philadelphia meeting in 1897, and published in Volume XXIII, 1898, of our *Transactions*. In 1899 a committee was appointed with the view of extending the standard procedures to include not only determination of species of bacteria, but all other lines of investigation involved in the analysis of water. Progress reports were made in 1900, 1901, and 1902, two of which were published in our *Transactions* and one in *Science*. The final report was published in 1905, as Part II, Volume XXX, of our *Transactions*. Revision has been constant, and other editions have appeared in 1912, 1917, and 1920. The fourth edition was revised by committees of the American Public Health Association, American Chemical Society, and referees of the Association of Official Agricultural Chemists.

"Standard Methods for the Bacteriological Examination of Milk," first edition 1910; second, 1916; third, 1920. The third edition was revised in conjunction with committees from the American Dairy Science Association, International Association of Dairy and Milk Inspectors, and members of committees from the Society of American Bacteriologists and American Association of Medical Milk Commissions.

---

tion of Doctors Durgin and Hill the *Journal* grew and extended its usefulness. In 1904, Volume XIV, No. 4, it became the *American Journal of Public Hygiene*, still retaining its function as the official organ of the Massachusetts Association of Boards of Health. In 1907 it became the official organ of the Laboratory Section of the A. P. H. A., and in 1908 of the Association, including the new sections on Municipal Health Officers and Vital Statistics. In 1911 the new *Journal of the American Public Health Association* continued as the *American Journal of Public Health*.

I am indebted to Dr. Victor H. Bassett, of Savannah, Ga., for much of this record.

"Standard Methods for the Examination of Air," first report 1909; second, 1912; third, 1916.

"Pasteurization of Milk," 1920. Report of Committee on Milk Supply of the Sanitary Engineering Section.

"Model Health Code for Cities," 1921. Report of Committee on Model Health Legislation.

"Standardization of Public Health Training," 1921. Report of the Committee of Sixteen.

"An Index for Public Health Literature."

"Health Quotations."

THE PRESENT AND THE FUTURE

Our Association is at a critical stage of its existence. As a necessary part of our growth, we have assumed many obligations, while others have been thrust upon us. We have outgrown the period when one of our members could manage our affairs from his own home or office. We have taken our place along with other great national societies, with a whole-time secretary, who is also editor of our *Journal*, an associate editor, and an office staff. The demands upon us are constantly increasing, as a result of our growth and extending influence. It is a sign of health on which we must congratulate ourselves. Nevertheless, a greatly increased income is required to keep pace with our responsibilities.

The high cost of living has been keenly felt by us directly and indirectly. The cost of publication of our *Journal* and *News Letter* has doubled. Salaries have of necessity been increased, though still below what they should be.

In May of this year we moved our offices to New York, joining with some dozen other national organizations in leasing space in the Penn Terminal Building. Although the move increased our expenses considerably, we believe that the close association with other societies has advantages which will prove more than compensatory. New York is our great center of life and human interests, a city visited by many thousands throughout the year, and it is our hope that new interest will be aroused in our members by having our headquarters easily accessible to visitors from all parts of the country.

The urgent need of the Association is a greatly increased income. The most obvious method of obtaining this is by enlarging our membership, though it must be pointed out that for several years past the membership dues have added but little to our net income, since almost the entire amount is spent in service to the members. Drives for new members have in the past been successful, and our membership has increased in a most gratifying manner. The business depression of the past year has prevented us from making any extended effort to gain members, and has caused many resignations. Specialism in public health, which is much in evidence, is also a menace to our membership, since new societies are constantly being formed having for their object the consideration of some special branch of preventive medicine now represented by a section of our Association.

The platform of the Association is, in length, breadth, and thickness, sufficient to accommodate all who are interested in human conservation. (Rankin.)

Health is not the monopoly of any group or class. It is the common heritage, and should be the common property, of all, and one of the objects most dear to the heart of our Association is to give to everyone the store of knowledge we now possess. It is true today, as in the time of Hosea, that "people are destroyed for lack of knowledge." For some years we have been trying to finance a popular health journal, written in non-technical language, which would present to the public in attractive form and style those facts of life and good living which should be known to all. We have not yet succeeded, nor have we been able to interest any philanthropist in the plan. Perhaps the very broadness of our platform is an inherent weakness. It is generally easy to obtain money for the relief of suffering but hard to get it for the prevention of that same suffering. Some other societies which concentrate their efforts on the prevention of a single disease have been more fortunate in enlisting the interest of wealthy persons.

When Mr. Lomb gave the money for his "Prize Essays," he said: "I see what you want.   You have an abundance of light, but your light must be hidden under a bushel because you have no means to disseminate it.   I propose to assist you, if it is acceptable."   We continue to hope that some far-sighted philanthropist may be brought to appreciate the opportunities offered in this field, which has up to the present remained fallow.   Thus financed we are confident that the *Journal* would soon become not only self-supporting, but a handsome source of revenue, furnishing much-needed funds for the extension of our activities.

We were born at an opportune moment, and have lived in a period which for all time will be remarkable for its scientific achievement.   "For countless generations the prophets and kings of humanity have desired to see the things which men have seen, and to hear the things which men have heard, in the course of this wonderful nineteenth century. . . . . In the fullness of time, long expected, long delayed, at last science emptied upon him from the horn of Amalthea blessings which cannot be enumerated, blessings which have made the century forever memorable; and which have followed each other with a rapidity so bewildering that we know not what next to expect." (Osler).   It is good to have lived in such a period, but it is better to have taken an active part in the events which have made that period notable, and this we can with confidence claim, especially as regards the biological sciences, the unravelling of whose mysteries has meant so much to human welfare and happiness.

The Association has had a glorious past of service to the countries represented in its membership, and to mankind.   In 1890, with less than 550 members, it was rated as "the largest and most influential organization in the world in shaping public health opinions."   That we have maintained this position, I am confident.   The five thousand who now share the privilege of membership are the trustees of the future.   We owe a debt to those who have wrought and passed on, which can best be paid by maintaining the standards set by them and by following their example of unselfish devotion to the welfare of our beloved Association.

We cannot, if we would, stand still and point to our past achievements. *Noblesse oblige.* Our path leads forward, and the difficulties which confront us at this time must serve to stimulate our efforts to even greater accomplishment for the future.

The needs of the Association* were clearly and forcibly set forth by President Rankin last year. He showed the possibilities of a popular health magazine, and urged a change of attitude to the public.

"The time is at hand," he said, "when the public are no longer to be thought of as beneficiaries in the public health movement, but are to be trusted as participants."

I can do no better than endorse these words, and urge that the directors take active steps looking to the enlargement of our membership according to the general plan outlined, the chief features of which are a national parent organization, with state and county societies in close affiliation, all bound together by a common object — the conservation of human life — and kept in constant touch with each other through the medium of a great public health magazine. So may we prove ourselves worthy of our trusteeship, and erect to those who builded our Association and passed it into our hands a memorial worthy of their high aspirations.

In bringing this address to a close, it would be a grateful task to tell something of the history of those who have contributed conspicuously to the success of the Association. It has seemed possible, however, to do this only in the case of a number of our former presidents, and, with the single exception of Dr. Stephen Smith, our first president, the biographical sketches must be confined to those who are no longer with us.

If it should be felt by any that invidious distinctions have been made in speaking of some when all could not be included, I beg to remind such

. . . that in science, at least, great names are landmarks; and the owners of these names have traversed and gleaned in fields where many a devoted laborer has delved and sown, and pathetically sweated blood in his altruistic zeal. In science, at least, no man works in vain. Full many a one, worthy of an elegy, has given his whole life to establishing a fact or indeed only an item to a fact; his work unrealized, ridicule and even persecution oft times his only compensation, throughout perhaps in the meanest destitution, yet his life and his work have been absolutely essential to the building of a mighty fabric. (Huber).

American Journal of Public Health, April, 1920, p. 297.

The study of the lives of our past presidents has been an inspiration, but has brought home to me a keen sense of my unworthiness to succeed them and of my inability to fill the office once held by them. Dear to me as is the honor of presiding at this fiftieth anniversary meeting, I have many times wished that this tribute might have been written by a more facile pen, and one capable of paying adequate homage to their lives and accomplishments. Whatever may be lacking in expression I trust is made up for by the love and reverence which have prompted my hand.

It is rare for a society to be fortunate enough to have present at the celebration of its fiftieth birthday its first president. Such is our good fortune. We have at this meeting the man we delight to honor above all others, the man to whom, more than to any other, we owe our existence, our founder and first president, who charted our course and stood at the wheel during the early years of our voyage, who stands today an example of all that our Association holds most dear, a man preëminent both as a citizen and a sanitarian, Dr. Stephen Smith.

Stephen Smith (1823–   ) was the first president of the American Public Health Association, and to him fell the arduous task of organizing the newly formed Association and of guiding its early steps toward the goal of success. He was twice elected to succeed himself, and retired of his own volition.

Dr. Smith was born on a farm in Onondaga County, New York. Early in life he selected medicine as his profession, and began his studies while still a student in high school. In 1848 he attended lectures at Geneva Medical College. In 1849 and 1850 he was a resident medical student in the hospital of the Sisters of Charity, Buffalo, New York. He entered the College of Physicians and Surgeons in New York in 1850, and graduated in 1851. He won the appointment as interne in Bellevue Hospital, where he spent two years. In 1854 he became a surgical and clinical teacher at Bellevue, continuing this work until 1891. He was also professor of anatomy in Bellevue Hospital Medical College from 1863 to 1870.

In 1864 Dr. Smith was made a member of the "Council of

Hygiene" of New York City. The investigations of the Council were organized and supervised by him, and its report in 1865 so impressed and aroused the public by its revelations as to bring about the act of legislature, April 21, 1866, creating the Metropolitan Board of Health, endowed with almost autocratic powers. Dr. Smith was appointed a commissioner of the Board by Governor Fenton, and through successive reappointments remained a commissioner until 1875.

Dr. Smith drafted the bill for a national board of health, and on its passage in 1879, he was appointed a member by President Hayes, serving four years. He drafted the law establishing the New York State Board of Health, and was instrumental in securing its passage.

In 1881 Governor Cornell appointed Dr. Smith Commissioner of the State Board of Charities for the first judicial district. He served only a year, and resigned at the request of the Governor to be appointed State Commissioner in Lunacy, which post he held for six years. His work for the insane was characterized by enlightened humanity, and he brought about an entirely new method of treating those unfortunates, adding greatly to their welfare and happiness. On his recommendation the first training school for nurses in a state hospital was established in Buffalo in 1884. He was early an advocate of state care of the dependent insane, having drafted a bill in 1884 providing for the removal of the insane from county poorhouses and asylums to state institutions. He renewed his efforts in this direction in 1886, and in 1890 "The State Care Act" embodying his plans became a law.

In 1893 Dr. Smith again became a member of the State Board of Charities, by appointment of Governor Flower. Governors Black, Higgins and Sulzer reappointed him, and he served until his resignation in 1918, at the age of 95. From 1903 to 1913 he served as vice-president of the Board. Of the last hundred meetings of the Board, Dr. Smith attended ninety-six, though all of them were held after he was eighty years of age.

Dr. Smith began to write early in his career, and has been a fertile contributor to medical literature. From 1853 to 1860 he was editor of the *New York Journal of Medicine,* and from 1860 to

1864 editor of the *American Medical Times*. From 1878 to 1906 he was New York correspondent of the London *Lancet*. Early in the Civil War he published a *Handbook on Surgical Operations*, of which 15,000 copies were sold. In 1887 his *Principles and Practice of Operating Surgery* appeared, in 1908, his *Civil Obligations of the Surgeon*, and in 1916, *Who Is Insane?* was given to the public. His last book, *The City That Was*, a description of the shockingly insanitary conditions prevailing in New York before the creation of the Metropolitan Board of Health, was printed in 1911.

Few medical men have ever even approached Dr. Smith in the number of honors paid to him. Presidents, governors and mayors have repeatedly appointed him to important posts, or sent him on missions.

His friends and associates have frequently given public testimonials of their love and admiration. On his eighty-eighth birthday a banquet was given in his honor at Plaza Hotel, New York, by the medical profession and a large committee of citizens, headed by Governor Dix,

. . . in public recognition of his services as an educator and practitioner in the field of surgery, as a pioneer in securing the public health legislation which has given to this country its efficient system of sanitary administration, as a promoter of measures which have greatly improved the condition of the insane in the State of New York, and, finally, for his work in this Board (State Board of Charities) with two intermissions, since 1881, a period of thirty years.

On the occasion of his resignation from the State Board of Charities, at the age of 95, after seventy years of public service devoted to the improvement of health conditions in general, and to the bettering of conditions in the care and treatment of the unfortunates of his state and city, the Board adopted a minute which is a remarkable tribute to Dr. Smith as a man and citizen and makes a permanent record of his services to the state and to humanity. This minute was transmitted to the legislature with the fifty-second Annual Report of the Board.

In considering Dr. Smith's public services, one wonders at the extent of the work accomplished, especially when it is remembered that he was from early professional life a teacher and enjoyed an extensive surgical practice, but he never put the business side of his profession to the fore, and never allowed the glitter of gold to blind him to the needs of the lowly and the poor. In this lies the glory of his professional career and of his life.

To the members of the American Public Health Association, he is dear as our founder and first president. We are proud to honor him, and know that we honor ourselves in doing so. Our Association is under a debt to him which can never be forgotten. To him it owes its existence and the formulation of the principles which have guided it for fifty years and made it a great power for good to the people of the countries it embraces.

As individuals we owe a debt of gratitude to our first president for the example of a life singularly free from self-seeking, yet singularly fruitful in accomplishment — a life which must be an inspiration to all who study it. He has exemplified in his life a standard expressed by himself in these words:

Happy the man whose life, whether short or long, is filled with honest efforts to cultivate every art that benefits mankind, and has seized every occasion to apply it where and when it was most needful and useful in uplifting the race.

"There comes a time when all must feel the luring,
    Of life's mysterious, beckoning golden west,
Tho' friends be fond and dear our works immuring,
    We set our sails for one more glorious quest.

"Ask not when we shall sail — May or December —
    Our Pilot knows the one all-favoring hour;
When tides are still, when ashes coat the ember,
    We yield the tiller to a friendly Power.

"And if we go before or come behind him,
    To that fair land where golden sunsets lure,
Of our fond love we'll need not to remind him,
    But press again that hand, brave, true, and pure."

Joseph Meredith Toner (1825–1896) was our second president, succeeding Dr. Smith in 1875. He was born in Pittsburg, Pennsylvania, and received his medical education at the Vermont Academy of Medicine and Jefferson Medical College, graduating in 1853. In 1855 he settled in Washington, D. C. He was a student of medical history and a book-lover. To him was due the foundation of the library of the American Medical Association in 1868, the Smithsonian

Institution housing the volumes. He was a fertile writer himself, having written more than fifty papers on subjects of medical interest. He was particularly interested in medical biography, and had completed more than 4,000 sketches for his *Biographical Dictionary of Deceased American Physicians.*

His published papers cover a wide range of subjects including a number of public health interest. He wrote on vaccination and inoculation against smallpox and yellow fever; a paper on "Free Parks, Camping Grounds, or Sanitariums for the Sick Children of the Poor in Cities;" also statistical papers on physicians, medical associations and hospitals, and many biographical sketches. Notable among the latter is his history of the medical profession in the District of Columbia. He was a collector of books, and in 1882 gave to the Government his entire library, 28,000 books and 18,000 pamphlets. In recognition of his services Congress ordered both a bust and a portrait of Dr. Toner which are now in the Library of Congress.

He endowed the Toner Lectures in 1871, for the purpose of securing two lectures annually containing new facts valuable to medical science. They were published by the Smithsonian Institution. This was the first endowment of the kind in this country. He encouraged research by the donation of a medal to Jefferson Medical College to be awarded yearly to the student producing the best thesis based on original work. The faculty of Georgetown University received a medal also, to be given yearly to the student who should collect and name the greatest number of specimens in any branch of the natural sciences. Among other honors, he was made president of the American Medical Association. He died at Cresson Springs, Pennsylvania, in 1896, full of years and honors.

John Henry Rauch (1828–1894) was our fourth president, elected in 1877. He was born in Lebanon, Pennsylvania. His medical education was received at the University of Pennsylvania, from which he was graduated in 1849. His leaning toward botany manifested itself in his graduation thesis on *Convalaria Polygonatum.* In 1857 he became professor of materia medica in Rush Medical College, Chicago, and in 1859 professor of materia medica and medical botany in the

Chicago College of Pharmacy, of which institution he was a founder. He entered the United States Army during the Civil War and served with distinction. Upon his discharge in 1865 he returned to Chicago and took an active part in public health work, being one of the organizers of the Chicago Board of Health in 1867, and serving as a member until 1873. During this time he made valuable contributions to sanitary science, among which were "Drainage," "Chicago River and the Public Parks," and "Sanitary History of Chicago."

He became interested in improving the condition of the gold miners in Venezuela, and visited that country in 1870. While there he made valuable collections for the Chicago Academy of Natural Sciences. His versatility and broad training is shown not only by this work, but by the assistance given to Professor Agassiz in collecting material for his *Natural History of the United States*, and his collection, mostly piscatorial, made from the Upper Mississippi and Missouri Rivers. He served our Association as treasurer before becoming president. His social interests, like his scientific training, were broad. He was associated with the Relief and Aid Society of Chicago, and was a "pioneer in the fight against quackery" in this country.

He returned to the place of his birth when his health failed and died there in 1894.

Elisha Harris (1824–1884), our fifth president, was elected in 1877. He was born in Westminster, Vermont, and received his medical degree from the College of Physicians and Surgeons of New York in 1849. Six years later he was appointed superintendent and physician-in-chief to the Quarantine Hospital on Staten Island. He maintained throughout his entire life a keen interest in sanitation and hygiene, and was one of the first men in this country to realize the importance of vital statistics. He was a pioneer in this work. During the Civil War he was active in sanitation, and one of the organizers of the National Sanitary Commission. He invented a railway ambulance which was used during the Franco-Prussian War, and for which he received a bronze and a silver medal.

At the close of the Civil War he supervised a sanitary survey of New York City. His survey of the tenement houses was thorough, and did much to better the condition of the poor.

On the organization of the Metropolitan Board of Health in 1866 he was appointed register of records, serving until a change of administration caused his retirement. In 1873 he was made registrar of vital statistics, serving until a change in city politics caused his removal. In 1880, when the State Board of Health of New York was organized, he was made one of the three commissioners.

He was a prolific writer on matters pertaining to public health and sanitation, many of his papers showing a prophetic vision.

Our Association owes him a peculiar debt of gratitude. He was our first secretary, and served in that capacity until elected president. During the first years of its life, by his unselfish devotion to its interests, he did more to keep it alive and promote its welfare than any other man save only our first president, Dr. Stephen Smith.

He died in 1884 at Albany, N. Y.

James Lawrence Cabell (1813–1889) was our sixth president, elected in 1878. He was born in Virginia, and received his medical degree from the University of Maryland in 1833. He went to Paris for further study, and remained there until 1837 when he returned home to become professor of anatomy, physiology and surgery at the University of Virginia, holding this chair until 1856, when he took the newly established chair of anatomy and materia medica, though he continued to teach physiology and surgery, and for a time comparative anatomy. He retired from active work in 1889, having served more than fifty years. During the Civil War he had charge of the Confederate Military Hospital in Charlottesville, in which work he showed marked professional as well as executive ability. When Congress, in 1879, created the National Board of Health, Dr. Cabell was made president of it, filling the position with distinction.

He was not a voluminous writer, but contributed excellent papers to several medical journals, including some on public health topics. His portrait is in the library of the Surgeon General, Washington, D. C. He died in Albemarle County, Virginia, in 1889.

John Shaw Billings (1838–1913), our seventh president, was elected in 1879. He was born on a farm in Switzerland County, Indiana, and spent his early life there, attending the rural schools, and obtaining higher instruction in Latin, Greek and geometry from Mr. Bonham, a clergyman. At the age of fourteen he passed the entrance examination for Miami University, and graduated in 1857. He received his medical training at the Medical College of Ohio, at Cincinnati, graduating in 1861. He entered the United States Army, passing first of the candidates on examination. He served in the military hospitals in Washington for more than a year and for several months at the General Hospital in Philadelphia. He next served in the field with the Fifth Army Corps of the Potomac, and later for some months in hospitals at Fort Schuyler and on Bedloe's Island. In 1864 he was assigned to the office of the medical director of the Army of the Potomac, and in 1865 transferred to the office of the Surgeon General, where he remained for more than thirty years. He took great interest in statistics and has been called "the father of medical and vital statistics in this country."

His greatest accomplishments were the creation of the Surgeon General's library, which now ranks among the great medical libraries of the world, and the publication of the *Medical Index Catalogue*. Sir Thomas Barlow called him "the prince of medical bibliographers." It is due to him that the medical literature of the world is available to students.

Dr. Billings' talents were shown in many lines. He "achieved excellence and gained distinction in no less than six different fields." He studied hospital construction, and in 1876, his plan for the Johns Hopkins Hospital, marking a new departure in hospital design, was selected over all others submitted in competition. He designed also the Barnes Hospital at the Soldiers' Home, and the Army Medical Museum; the Laboratory of Hygiene and the William Pepper Laboratory at the University of Pennsylvania; and the Peter Bent Brigham Hospital in Boston.

He was director of the Laboratory of Hygiene and professor of Hygiene at the University of Pennsylvania, leaving in 1896 to become director of the New York Public Library, the consolidation of the Astor, Lenox and Tilden Foundations.

He made many contributions to medical literature in the form of papers and treatises published in various journals, and also wrote a number of books covering a wide range of subjects — historical, statistical, heating and ventilation, and a medical dictionary. It is given to few men to become eminent in so many fields of endeavor. He died in New York City after a brief illness in 1913.

Robert Clark Kedzie (1823–1902), the ninth president of our Association, was elected in 1881. He was born at Delhi, New York, and received his medical education at the University of Michigan, having been a member of the first medical class graduated from that institution, in 1851.

He became professor of chemistry at the Michigan Agricultural College and devoted much energy to the teaching of sanitation throughout the state. By sanitary conventions under the direction of the State Board of Health, he induced every community to study its own sanitary conditions. He fostered Farmers' Institutes, in which he taught the practical application of chemistry to the needs of small communities. One of his first studies concerned the supposed magnetic properties of water from flowing wells lined with iron tubing. Such waters were largely exploited for gain on account of their alleged medicinal value. His demonstration of the facts put an end to this superstition. He did much to save life and property by his studies on illuminating oil, and demonstration of proper methods for detecting the explosive grades. His interest in the public welfare is shown by thirty-two valuable papers on "Municipal Health," as well as by others on various topics relating to health and sanitary science. He died at his home, Lansing, Michigan, in 1902.

Ezra Mundy Hunt (1830–1894), our tenth president, was elected in 1882. He was born in Metuchen, New Jersey. He graduated in medicine from the College of Physicians and Surgeons, New York, in 1852. In 1854 he became lecturer on materia medica at the Vermont Medical College. He was elected president of the State Medical Society of New Jersey in 1864. He became secretary on the State Board of Health in 1877, and held that position many years, editing the *Annual Reports* and publishing a number of papers on matters of public health interest. He exercised a wide influence on the medical profession of the state, by whom he was held in high esteem.

He died at his home in Metuchen in 1894.

Albert Leary Gihon (1833–1901), our eleventh president, elected in 1883, was born in Philadelphia. He received his medical education at the Philadelphia College of Medicine and Surgery, graduating in 1852.

He entered the United States Navy in 1855. In 1861 he was promoted to the rank of medical inspector, and served during the Civil War largely in European waters. He was made commodore in 1895, and retired from active service the same year.

He was a pioneer in naval hygiene, and his book, *Practical Suggestions in Naval Hygiene,* published in 1871, was for some years a standard work. He published many articles on naval hygiene, public health, climatology and kindred subjects. He died in New York City in 1901.

George Miller Sternberg (1838–1915), our fourteenth president, was elected in 1885. He was born at Hartwick, New York, and graduated in medicine from the College of Physicians and Surgeons, New York, in 1860. He was appointed assistant surgeon in the United States Army at the beginning of the Civil War. He served with credit throughout the war, and at its close was in charge of the Government Hospital at Cleveland, Ohio, holding the rank of medical director. He remained in the army and saw service in many parts of the country, including a number of campaigns against the Indians. He went through the cholera epidemic at Fort Harker, Kansas, in 1867, and through yellow fever outbreaks at Fort Columbus, New York, and Barrancas, Florida, in 1873 and 1875. These experiences stimulated his interest in yellow fever and led to many investigations and publications on the subject. In 1879 he went to Cuba as a member and secretary of the Commission of the National Board of Health. He was a delegate to the International Sanitary Conference at Rome in 1885, and in 1887 was detailed by Congress to make investigations in Brazil, Mexico and Cuba relating to the cause and prevention of yellow fever. While his own investigations failed to throw light on the cause of the disease, he must be credited with the organization of the commission headed by Major Walter Reed, whose brilliant work proved the agency of the Stegomyia mosquito in the transmission of the disease.

Dr. Sternberg was a prolific writer of books and papers. His bibliography includes 143 titles, on bacteriology, disinfection, infectious diseases and matters of public health. His text-book on bacteriology was for many years the standard in America. He was one of the first in this country to make microphotographs, in which art he attained great skill, and on which he published one of the earliest books.

His principal books are *Manual of Bacteriology, Malaria and Malarial Diseases, Immunity, Protective Inoculations and Infectious Diseases and Serum Therapy*, and *Infection and Immunity, with Special Reference to the Prevention of Infectious Diseases*.

He will always be remembered as the founder of the Army Medical School in Washington, established while Surgeon General, which office he held from 1893 until his retirement in 1902.

In 1885 Dr. Sternberg won the "Lomb Prize" for his essay on disinfection, which was later revised and translated into several foreign languages. The experiments on which it was founded occupied his attention for several years.

The University of Michigan, in 1894, and Brown University, in 1897, conferred on him the degree of Doctor of Laws.

His later life was spent in Washington, where he died in 1915, aged seventy-seven years.

Emanuel Persillier Lachapelle (1845–1918) was the twenty-first president of our Association, elected in 1893.

He was a French Canadian, born in the parish of Sault-au-Recollet, at that time about six miles from the old city of Montreal, but now a part of the city.

He was educated in Montreal, and received his medical training at the École de Médecine et Chirurgie of that city, graduating in 1869. Later the honorary degree of Doctor of Laws was conferred on him by McGill University. He rapidly established an enviable reputation as a practitioner, but gave much time and attention to the advancement of the medical profession in his Province, and to the academic interests of Laval University, in the medical school of which he served as dean for some years.

In the Association he was best known as a sanitarian. The Provincial Board of Health of Quebec was organized in 1886, just after the memorable epidemic of smallpox in Montreal, and under his guidance as president has done scientific work of inestimable value to the Province. Among other positions of trust and honor held by him were the following: President of the College of Physicians and Surgeons of the Province of Quebec; superintendent and president of the Hospital Notre Dame; president of La Société d'Administration Générale; president of the Medical Council of Canada; president of St. Jean Baptiste Society; and Controller of the City of Montreal.

As the leading member of the French Canadian medical profession he was made by the French Government Chevalier de la Légion d'Honneur and Officier de l'Académie de France.

As a citizen he took part in many business affairs, serving as director of the Provincial Bank of Canada and of the Crédit Foncier Canadien-Français.

He was a fluent speaker and made many graceful addresses, but did not commit many of them to paper.

He was much beloved and respected, not only by his fellow-French-Canadians, but by citizens of all classes, to whom he had endeared himself by his personality, his patriotism and his benefactions. He died, after more than a year of illness at the Mayo Hospital, Rochester, Minnesota, in 1918.

Dr. William Bailey (1833-1911) was the twenty-second president of the Association, elected in 1894.

He was born in Franklin County, Kentucky, within a few miles of the State Capitol. His early years were passed on the farm. He received his education in the common schools, later attending the Kentucky Military Institute, teaching there for three years after his graduation. He then entered the Kentucky School of Medicine, graduating in 1857. He later resumed his medical studies at the University of Louisville, graduating in 1864. He came under the influence of a number of great men who have added lustre to American medicine, since Samuel D. Gross, Austin Flint, Daniel Drake, L. P. Yandell and other notable men were then professors in the two colleges from which he graduated.

After practicing medicine in Shelbyville for six years, he moved to Louisville, and became professor of materia medica and therapeutics, and later dean, in the Hospital College of Medicine. Ten years later he accepted the same chair in the University of Louisville, and after the death of Dr. Bell, became professor of the theory and practice of medicine in the same institution, a position he filled with credit for many years.

He was a strong medical society man, and a regular attendant of both local and state societies, became president of the State Medical Society in 1899. He was also a member of the American Medical Association and attended its sessions regularly.

Dr. Bailey was one of the pioneer sanitarians of Kentucky, and probably the first member of the American Public Health Association from that state. He took an active part in its councils, having been a member of the Executive Committee and its president. His interest never flagged to the day of his death.

When the State Board of Health was created in 1878, it was hoped that Dr. Bailey would be made a member in consideration of his prominence in this field, but his appointment failed through political conditions. In 1888, however, Governor Simon Bolivar Buckner took the Board out of politics and made Dr. Bailey a member. He retained his membership until his death, and for some time was president of the Board.

Dr. Bailey took an active interest in the civic affairs of his home city. For a number of years he was a member of the "Conversation Club" of Louisville, serving as its president, and frequently contributing papers and addresses. He was for ten years a director of the Louisville Trust Company. While not a voluminous writer he often contributed articles on public health topics to scientific journals.

He enjoyed a large medical practice, and was constantly in demand as a consultant.   He has been described as "one of the ablest, gentlest, kindest and most beloved physicians and teachers who ever practiced and taught medicine within the boundaries of his native state."

He died at his home July 15, 1911, following an injury.

Eduardo Licéaga (1839-1920) was the twenty-third president of our Association, elected 1895.   He was born in the city of Guanajuato, the son of Dr. Francisco Licéaga and Señora Trinidad Torres de Licéaga.

He was educated at the old College of San Gregorio, where he took the first prize in Latin, and later at the College of the State of Guanajuato, winning there prizes and honorable mention.   His medical education was received at the National School of Medicine in Mexico City, from which he graduated in 1866.   The Emperor Maximiliano bestowed on him the degree of Surgeon and a gold medal.

He soon won distinction both at home and abroad.   For many years he taught surgery in his alma mater, and became its director, serving from 1904 until 1910.   In 1913 he was made honorary director. For twenty-five years he was director of the Maternity and Infant Hospital.

He was a member of the following Mexican scientific societies: Lancasterian Company; Mexican Geographical and Statistical Society; the Medical Society of San Luis Potosi; the National Academy of Medicine; the Medical and Pharmaceutical Society of Puebla; the Medical-Surgical Association "Larrey"; Medical Society of Guanajuato; Medical Society of Jalisco; Medical and Pharmaceutical Society of Merida; and the Mexican Society of Surgery.

He represented Mexico at many international congresses, among which may be mentioned the Public Health Congress at Vienna, Austria; the Medical Congress at Moscow; the Tuberculosis Congress, and the Congress on Hygiene and Demography, both at Washington; the first and third Pan-American Congresses, at Washington and Havana, respectively, and international conventions at Washington, Mexico and Costa Rica.   From 1893 to 1913 he represented his country at the meetings of the American Public Health Association.

Many honors were bestowed upon him — Knight of the Order of Guadalupe in 1866; diploma as honorary member of the Mexican Geographical and Statistical Society; honorary member of the Physicians and Pharmacists of Merida; foreign member of the Academy of Medicine of Venezuela; honorary member of the Surgical and Medical Society of San Sebastian, Spain; degree of vice-president of the Mexican Society "Antonio Alzate."

He wrote numerous scientific papers on hygiene and public health, medicine and surgery. The National Academy of Medicine of Mexico made a special award to him for his work on "Dislocation of the Clavicle."

He was for many years president of the Board of Health of Mexico, during which time many active campaigns against disease were carried out and new measures inaugurated. He took an active part in writing the Sanitary Code of the City of Mexico, and was a member of the commission in charge of building the General Hospital of that city. During his administration antirabic vaccination was established, yellow fever along the Gulf Coast, and bubonic plague at Mazatlan were brought under control.

Most of the laws on sanitation which have been put into effect in Mexico for some years past were initiated by Dr. Licéaga. He had a long and honorable career, which was full of service to his country and mankind. The American Public Health Association joins with the people of Mexico in mourning his death.

He died in Mexico City January 13, 1920.

Henry Buckingham Horlbeck (1839–1901) was our twenty-fourth president, elected in 1896. He presided at our twenty-fifth anniversary meeting held in Philadelphia. He was born in Charleston, South Carolina. He took up the study of medicine under his father, Dr. Elias Horlbeck, and Dr. F. T. Miles. He attended three courses in the Medical College of the State of South Carolina, graduating in 1859. After serving as house physician in the Roper Hospital, he went to Europe, where he attended lectures under such men as Velpeau, Trousseau, Chassaignac, and Ricord. He entered the Confederate Army and was commissioned surgeon of the First Regiment, South

Carolina Volunteers, with which he saw service in some of the most severe campaigns of the Civil War. Dr. Horlbeck became secretary of the Board of Health of Charleston in 1880, and the next year health officer, a position he held up to the time of his death. He was particularly interested in yellow fever and quarantine.

He was a member of several learned societies, medical and literary. He wrote well but not voluminously, and was a finished speaker. His most notable publications were "Inaugural Dissertation and Prize Essay;" "Avulsion of the Arm and Scapula;" and "Maritime Sanitation at Ports of Arrival." He also prepared the *Annual Reports* of the Department of Health of Charleston.

He was a strong believer in cremation, and directed that his own body should be burned.

He died at his home in Charleston in August, 1901.

Benjamin Lee (1833–1913) was our twenty-ninth president elected in 1900. He was born at Norwich, Connecticut. He was educated at the University of Pennsylvania, taking the degree of A. B. in 1852, A. M. in 1855, and Ph. D. in 1876. He took courses under the Auxiliary Faculty of Medicine at the same University. He attended lectures at Jefferson Medical College in 1853–54 and at the New York Medical College, 1854–55–56, graduating from the last institution in 1856 and receiving a prize for his thesis on "The Mechanics of Medicine." He took postgraduate work in Paris and Vienna.

Dr. Lee was a pioneer in orthopedic surgery, and for some years devoted himself to the treatment of deformities and spinal diseases by mechanical means.

In 1885 he was appointed a member of the newly created Board of Health of Pennsylvania, was made secretary of the Board, and held that position until the Board was superseded by the Department of Health in 1905, when he became assistant to the commissioner.

From 1893 to 1905 he was secretary of the State Quarantine Board, and in 1898–99 health officer of the Port of Philadelphia.

He was a member of the Philadelphia County Medical Society, holding the offices of corresponding secretary and vice-president of the State Medical Society, of which he became treasurer, and of the

American Medical Association. He was at various times president of the American Academy of Medicine and the American Orthopedic Association.

He wrote a considerable number of articles on surgery and public health, and was editor of the *American Medical Monthly* for a time. His most important work as an author was, *The Correct Principles of Treatment for Angular Curvature of the Spine*, 1872.

He died at Point Pleasant, New Jersey, July 11, 1913.

Henry Dwight Holton (1838–1917), our thirtieth president, was elected in 1901.

Dr. Holton was born at Saxton's River, Vermont. He received his medical education in Boston and New York, having graduated from the University of New York in 1860. He began his career as a practitioner of medicine and surgery, in both of which he attained success and an enviable position. However, he early turned his attention to the prevention of disease and throughout his life was untiring in his efforts along this line.

As early as 1873 he began to work for the establishment of a state board of health in Vermont, having gone before the General Assembly of that year to urge the importance of such a step. Though his efforts failed of success, he showed no resentment nor discouragement, but year after year went before successive legislatures to present the cause he had so deeply at heart. Finally after fourteen years, in 1886, the Board was established. In 1896, Dr. Holton was appointed a member, and became secretary in 1900, serving until 1912, when he resigned that office, though he continued as a member until his death and manifested to the end the zeal and interest in the welfare of his fellows which was so marked a characteristic of his life. Only thirteen days before his death, the Board held a meeting in his sickroom, at which, in spite of illness, he showed all of his accustomed interest in the work.

To few of our members or officers does our Association owe as much as to Dr. Holton. He always took the keenest interest in its work and its success, and was ever ready to give, not only his time and counsel, but also to furnish material aid from his private resources.

During the trying time of reorganization and the founding of the *Journal*, Dr. Holton more than once made substantial donations, which tided the Association over trying periods. His gifts were always made without ostentation, and were unknown to the rank and file of the Association. At one time he gave 247 subscriptions to the *Journal* to local health officers in Vermont.

He served as treasurer from 1892 until his election to the presidency in 1901.

In recognition of his devotion and many services to the Association, he was unanimously elected to life membership at the Rochester meeting in 1915.

Dr. Holton was a member of many learned societies and was often honored by election to office in them, having been president of the Connecticut River Valley Medical Association, Vermont State Medical Society and Vermont Society, Sons of the American Revolution; president of the board of trustees, and chairman of the executive committee of the Pan-American Medical Congress, 1895, and member of the American Medical Association, American Academy of Medicine, American Medical Editors Association, American Academy Political and Social Sciences, British Medical Association and National Conference of Charities and Corrections. He was honored in his state by election to the State Senate in 1884, and the House of Representatives in 1888. He was professor of pathology and therapeutics in the University of Vermont from 1873 to 1886. The University conferred on him the honorary Master's degree. From 1872 to 1890 he served as trustee of the University.

He was a good citizen and served his community in many ways outside of his profession. He was president of the Vermont National Bank, and the Brattleboro Gas Light Company. For twenty-five years — fifteen years as chairman — he was a member of the school board of Brattleboro.

He was president of the Leland and Gray Seminary and president of the board of trustees of the Austine Institution for the education of the deaf and blind. This institution and the Brattleboro Home for the Aged and Disabled owed their existence chiefly to him, and were the objects of his especial care during the last years of his life.

The list of his activities, though incomplete, demonstrates the wide range of his interests, as well as the esteem in which he was everywhere held.

He was a prolific writer on medical and public health subjects, having been the author of *Posological Tables* (two editions), twenty-two monographs, and many articles in current medical journals.

He died of malignant disease of the pancreas at his home, February 12, 1917.   The Legislature, in session at the time, passed resolutions of respect and appreciation.

Walter Wyman (1848–1911), our thirty-first president, was elected in 1902.   He graduated in medicine from Washington University in 1873.   In 1876 he entered the Marine Hospital Service as Assistant Surgeon.   He was promoted to the rank of Surgeon in 1877, and became Surgeon General in 1891.

He was instrumental in founding the Sanatorium for consumptive sailors at Fort Stanton, New Mexico.   Under his administration the Service grew in size, efficiency and influence.   Perhaps his most important accomplishments were the development of the national system of quarantine already begun, and the fostering of scientific research on matters pertaining to public health.

He was a member of a number of learned societies, in several of which he held office, having been president of the Association of Military Surgeons and vice-president of the American Red Cross and the American Medical Association.   He was chairman of the International Sanitary Bureau of American Republics, and of the Committee on International Quarantine of the Pan-American Medical Congress, in 1904.   He was for some years a director of the National Tuberculosis Association, and during the International Congress on Tuberculosis, in 1908, was president of the Section on State and Municipal Control of Health Matters.

He was a fairly prolific writer of papers on the subjects in which he was particularly interested, writing for both scientific and popular publications.   He died at Providence Hospital, Washington, D. C., in 1911.

Carlos Juan Finlay (1835–1915) was our thirty-second president, elected at Washington, D. C., in 1903. He was born in Cuba, his father having been a Scotch physician and his mother a native of France. His early education was acquired largely in France, his medical education at Jefferson Medical College in Philadelphia, from which institution he received his diploma in 1855. Dr. S. Weir Mitchell, who had just returned from the laboratory of Claude Bernard in Paris, was his private preceptor. Dr. Finlay was much influenced also by Dr. John Kearsley Mitchell, then a member of the faculty, and the first man in this country to maintain systematically the germ theory of disease. Dr. Finlay practised for some time in Lima, Peru, later going to Paris for further study.

In 1881 he represented the Colonial Government of Cuba at the International Sanitary Conference held in Washington, where for the first time he made public his views on the transmission of yellow fever by an intermediary agent. At the outbreak of the Spanish-American War, he went to Washington to offer his services to the American Government. Though sixty-five years old, he took part in the campaign around Santiago, constantly urging the acceptance of his theories concerning the transmission of yellow fever. In 1898 he presented his views to the United States Army Medical Officers, and wrote a complete plan of campaign against this disease on the same lines which were followed after the final demonstration of the agency of the mosquito by Dr. Walter Reed.

Dr. Finlay began to study the cause of yellow fever certainly as early as 1872. In 1879 the American Commission of the National Board of Health visited Cuba. This commission held that the disease was infectious, that the germ was given off from the sick, and that it had to undergo some change outside the body before it could reproduce infection. These conclusions evidently influenced Dr. Finlay profoundly, for the next year he was working along new lines, and in 1881 advanced his new theory.

He gave to both the English and American Commissions his notes, records, and ideas, and furnished the eggs from which Dr. Reed and his associates reared their first experimental mosquitoes.

He had already fixed the species which was capable of transmitting yellow fever, having selected it on account of its town-dwelling habits.

But a still more beautiful piece of reasoning was the induction that it was the Stegomyia mosquito, out of the six or seven hundred species of mosquitoes, that conveyed yellow fever. (Gorgas).

Dr. H. E. Durham, of the English Commission, says:

It is incontestible that Dr. Charles Finlay, of Havana, was the first to undertake direct experiments to substantiate his ideas of the part played by the mosquito in the transmission of yellow fever. His method was to feed mosquitoes upon yellow fever patients (not later than the sixth day), and then after an interval of from forty-eight hours to four or five days, allow them to feed upon susceptible persons . . . .

Dr. Walter Reed of the American Commission says:

To Dr. Carlos Finlay, of Havana, must be given, however, full credit for the theory of the propagation of yellow fever by means of the mosquito, in a paper read before the Royal Academy in that city at its session on the 14th day of August, 1881.

We here desire to express our sincere thanks to Dr. Finlay who accorded to us a most courteous interview, and has gladly placed at our disposal his several publications relating to yellow fever during the past nineteen years, and also for ova of the species of mosquito with which he had made his several inoculations.

Many honors were paid to Dr. Finlay. His work was celebrated by a great banquet, given by the medical profession of Havana and the American Army Officers and presided over by General Leonard Wood, on which occasion a statue symbolic of genius was presented to him.

Jefferson Medical College conferred on him the degree of Doctor of Laws. He was made an honorary member of the College of Physicians of Philadelphia. In 1901 the Liverpool School of Tropical Medicine awarded to him the Mary Kingsley medal. The French Government made him an officer of the Legion of Honor. The Government of the Second Intervention, at the instigation of Col. Jefferson R. Keen, U. S. A., and in accordance with the recommendation of the First Medical Congress of Cuba, created for him the office of honorary president of the National Board of Sanitation and Charities, with a salary, both of which were to exist during his life and terminate with his death.

The name of Dr. Finlay must always be held in high honor not only as a man, but as an original investigator. His theories were based on carefully studied observations which show an acute mind. He held correctly that yellow fever was transmitted by the bite of a single species of mosquito, which he selected among hundreds, and he outlined a plan which has proved successful for the eradication of the disease.

Though it remained for Dr. Reed and his associates to give the final and conclusive proofs of Dr. Finlay's ideas, he was the first to show the correct methods of experimentation. He was the first to apply blood-sucking insects with the object of transmitting infection from the sick to the well.

Our Association has just cause for great pride in remembering not only his accomplishments, but that he was a member and our president. Dr. Finlay died in Havana August 20, 1915.

Frank F. Wesbrook (1868–1918) was the thirty-third president of the Association, elected in 1905.

He was born at Oakland, Brant County, Ontario. He was educated at the University of Manitoba, and obtained his medical education at the Medical College of the same institution, graduating in 1889. The next five years were spent in postgraduate study in England and Germany. For three years he was John Lucas Walker student at Cambridge University, the last year of his term having been spent in the laboratory of Prof. Carl Frankel at Marburg, Germany. In 1895 he was made professor of pathology and bacteriology at the University of Minnesota, and in 1906 became dean of the School of Medicine. This office he held until 1913, when he was made president of the University of British Columbia. He was for many years director of the State Board of Health Laboratory of Minnesota, and a member of the Advisory Board of the Hygienic Laboratory of the Public Health Service. He was a member of many scientific societies and Fellow of the Royal Society of Canada.

The honorary degree of LL. D. was conferred on him by the Universities of Manitoba, Toronto and California. Dr. Wesbrook was a frequent contributor to scientific journals, writing on bacteriological and public health topics, and later chiefly on medical education and education in general.

When the Great War broke out he entered the Officers' Training Corps, and was gazetted lieutenant, captain and later major.

He died in Vancouver, B. C., Canada, October 20, 1918.

Franklin C. Robinson (1852–1910) was the thirty-fourth president of our Association, elected in 1905.

He was born in East Orrington, Maine. His collegiate education was obtained at Bowdoin College, from which institution he graduated with honors in 1873, receiving an election to Phi Beta Kappa.

In 1874 he was appointed instructor of analytic chemistry and mineralogy in his alma mater. This was followed in 1881 by election to the Josiah Little professorship of natural science and the chair of chemistry and mineralogy. In 1855 he took also the chair of chemistry in the Medical School, holding these positions until his death in 1910.

Bowdoin College conferred on him the degrees of M. A. in 1876, and LL.D. in 1903.

Professor Robinson's work was largely as an expert chemist, and his work in public health was chiefly along chemical lines. He invented a formaldehyde disinfecting apparatus, said to have been the first practical one. He pointed out the danger of arsenical colors in wall paper, his demonstrations of which were so convincing as to bring about the passage of laws prohibiting the use of such colors.

He was an expert on water purification and was often called on for advice and testimony in this capacity. He was employed in the well known case between Jersey City and its water company. His experiments in this case established the use of bleaching powder as a germicidal agent for water purification.

An expert in toxicology and the determination of blood stains, his services were much in demand in criminal and other legal investigations.

He was a member of many scientific societies, among them being the American Chemical, the Society of Chemical Industry, the American Association for the Advancement of Science, the British Society of Chemical Industry, the New England Society of Chemical Teachers, and the American Public Health Association.

In the last he was chairman of the Committee on Disinfectants from 1897 to 1910, a member of the executive committee 1898–99, and president 1906.

Professor Robinson's interests were wide, and he devoted much time to the cause of education and the welfare of his community. He was a member of the State Board of Health from 1888 until his death, state assayer for several years, and chairman of the State Survey during the last two years of his life.

He was a founder and president of the Brunswick Public Library Association, took an active interest in the schools of Brunswick, and was largely responsible for the installation of a modern sewerage system in the city.

Domingo Orvañanos (1844–1919) was our thirty-fifth president, elected 1906. He was born in the City of Mexico, and educated at the College of San Gregorio and College of San Indefonso. He entered the National School of Medicine of Mexico in 1862, where he pursued his studies for five years, graduating in 1866. Later he took post-graduate work at the New York Polyclinic.

He was a member of the National Academy of Medicine; the "Pedro Escobedo" Medical Society; the Geographical and Statistical Society of Mexico; the French Society of Hygiene; the Supreme Board of Health of Mexico, and chief of the Medical-Climatological Department of the National Medical Institute. He was also professor of medical clinics in the National School of Medicine.

He at first devoted himself to diseases of the eye, but later took up internal medicine. He enjoyed a large practice among the wealthy, but with the wide philanthropy for which he was noted he gave much attention to the poor also.

He was the author of a number of papers published in the *Bulletin of the Superior Board of Health of Mexico:* "Notes for the Study of the Climate of Mexico," 1883; "Essays on the Medical Geography and Climatology of the Mexican Republic," etc.

Dr. Orvañanos represented the Mexican Republic at the Medical and Surgical Congresses held in Rome and Moscow. He was a member of the committee which prepared the Sanitary Code of the Mexican

Republic, and while a member of the Board of Health did excellent work for the advancement of public health, interesting himself especially in the improvement of dwellings.

He died in the City of Mexico April 1, 1919.

William Thompson Sedgwick (1855–1921), our forty-third president, was elected in 1914. He studied at the Sheffield Scientific School, Yale Medical School, and Johns Hopkins University, but did not graduate in medicine, preferring his beloved field of biology. At the age of twenty-eight he became assistant professor of biology at the Massachusetts Institute of Technology, finally becoming professor of biology and public health, and holding that position up to his death thirty-eight years later.

He was perhaps the first man in this country to apply biology intensively to public health problems. Bacteriological discoveries were constantly being announced, and the newly made professor naturally became enthusiastic over the future of this branch of biological science and its great importance in public health work.

The study of water supplies and sewage disposal early engaged his attention. He was made consulting biologist to the Massachusetts Board of Health (the first board to apply the new discoveries in bacteriology and chemistry to these problems) under the leadership of Dr. H. P. Wolcott, also a past president of our Association. At Lawrence, Massachusetts, an experiment station was constructed, and later a filter, the first municipal plant in this country to be scientifically designed and conducted. To the work at Lawrence we owe much of our present knowledge of the problems of water purification and sewage treatment, and many of our leading sanitary engineers may be called graduates of the Lawrence Station. In all of this work Professor Sedgwick played an active and important part. When in 1914, the State Board was replaced by the State Department of Health, he was appointed a member of the Council, and served on the Committee on Sanitary Engineering, and as chairman of the Committee on Food and Drugs.

In 1882 Professor Sedgwick was made a member of the Advisory Board of the Hygienic Laboratory of the Public Health Service. In

1918 he was commissioned Assistant Surgeon General (Reserve) in this Service. He was a member of the International Health Board of the Rockefeller Foundation. In 1920 he went to England as exchange professor at Cambridge and Leeds — as one paper put it, as "Ambassador of Health."

Professor Sedgwick will probably be longest remembered as a great teacher. He was far-sighted and enthusiastic, and had the great faculty of imparting his enthusiasm to his students. He was instrumental in establishing the School of Public Health of Harvard University and the Massachusetts Institute of Technology, serving as chairman of the administrative board from its foundation until his death.

He belonged to many societies, and served as president of the New England Water Works Association, Society of American Bacteriologists, American Association of Naturalists, and the American Public Health Association. His wide range of interests and sympathies is shown further by the positions he held, among which were the following: Curator of Lowell Institute, chairman of Pauper Institutions Trustees, trustee of Simmons College, president of the board of directors, Sharon Sanitarium, president, Boston Civil Service Reform Association, and member of the American Philosophical Society.

He was a prolific writer, his bibliography including more than two hundred titles. Among his more important works should be mentioned *The Principles of Sanitary Science and Public Health*, and *The Human Mechanism* (in conjunction with Professor Hough), both of which have for many years been standard text-books enjoying a wide popularity.

He died suddenly on the evening of January 25, 1921, after a busy day, at his home in Boston.

THE STORY OF PUBLIC HEALTH IN CANADA

PETER H. BRYCE, M. A., M. D.

Ottawa, Canada

WE are told by Sister Margaret Bourgeois, who came to Canada from France in 1653 to establish in Montreal *la Congrégation de Notre Dame*, for the education of girls, that Quebec had "five or six houses in Upper Town and in the Lower Town only the storehouses of the Jesuits and of the Montreal people. . . . . The poverty on all sides was pitiful." Yet within fifteen years, due to the energy of the great French minister Colbert, we find that the Intendant, Talon, had established law and order, that immigration had greatly increased, and that there were in 1670 about 6,000 French people in the country. A treaty of peace had been made with the Iroquois, and two years after Talon's arrival a Jesuit annalist writes: "It is beautiful to see nearly all the banks of our river St. Lawrence occupied by new settlements, stretching along more than 80 leagues."

Yet how, amidst the daily routine and common task, the minds of men are influenced in the sphere of the mysterious and supernatural is well illustrated by the accounts of the series of earthquakes during seven days in February, 1663, when, as the Indians described it, "the trees were drunk" and pious souls saw four demons tugging at the four corners of the sky, threatening universal ruin, had not a Higher Being come to the rescue. One favorite theory was that the devil was enraged that God was so well served in the colony, while the humbler view was that the earthquake was a solemn warning to the people to abandon their evil ways, which admonition was very much in order, for the struggle for the suppression of the liquor traffic in the colony was at its height between the Fur-Trading Company and good Bishop Laval and the church.

Indeed, it may be said that the first serious sanitary question in the colony was that of prohibiting the sale of spirits to the Indians, of

whom Madame Guyard, *Mère de l'Incarnation*, the founder of the
Ursuline convent, said in 1639: "When we arrived in the colony the
Indians were so numerous that it seemed as if they were going to grow
a vast people; but after they were baptized God called them to Himself
either by disease or by the hands of the Iroquois." Such has been too
often the self-exculpatory excuse of the white races in the treatment
of the native peoples in the world's history. But these beginnings
were the nucleus of what in the next hundred years became the various
settlements of Canada. This period saw a constant movement of
explorers and missionaries across the great inland seas, resulting in the
discovery of the Mississippi and the exploration of the continent to the
foothills of the Rockies.

Owing, however, to changing governors, due to court intrigues
under the *fainéant* king Louis XV, the colony, well organized under
Frontenac, with its state church and schools, its feudal laws with
seigneurs and *censitaires*, became the prey of corrupt Intendants and
oppressive officials. Exposed for fifty years to the vicissitudes of
European wars and the hostile *Bostonnais* to the south, the colony at
last, in spite of Montcalm's heroic defense, fell before the disciplined
armies of Great Britain. Following the fall of Quebec a constitution
was given to Canada in 1774, ensuring to the French people their laws,
religion and language. In 1791 the country was divided into Upper
and Lower Canada, and it was in 1795 that an act was passed in Lower
Canada "to oblige ships and vessels coming from places infected with
the plague or any pestilential fever or disease to perform quarantine
and prevent the communication thereof in the province." The act
further stated: "In case any ship shall come from any place visited by
the plague or any pestilential fever or disease, or has any person on
board already affected with disease, and should the commander or other
person having charge as aforesaid neglect to perform quarantine, he
shall be adjudged guilty of a felony and suffer death as in cases of felony
without the benefit of the clergy."

The story of Dr. Edward Jenner's discovery of vaccination in
1797 spread with amazing rapidity, and was not only of medical importance, but also, as the following sentence from "The Heart of Mid-
lothian" shows, had impressed even the literary world. Referring

to the meeting between Jeannie Deans and Queen Caroline, Sir Walter says: "The lady who seemed the principal person had remarkably good features, though somewhat injured by the smallpox, that venomous scourge, which each village Esculapius (thanks to Jenner) can now tame as easily as their tutelary deity subdued the python." An interesting account of the introduction of vaccination into Canada is given in the following letter supplied by a lady eighty-six years of age:

"Ottawa, July 29, 1921.

DEAR DR. BRYCE:

My son has asked me to give some leading facts which have come to my knowledge re the early introduction of vaccination into Canada, which I have much pleasure in doing.

My maternal grandfather, Dr. Jos. Norman Bond of Yarmouth, N. S., received from his brother in Bath, England, an intimate friend of Dr. Jenner, a small quantity of vaccine lymph in a letter in the early spring of 1802. I do not know exact date.

To test it my grandfather tried it on his own child, an infant of a few weeks old. It was apparently successful, but to further satisfy himself as to its efficacy, he inoculated the child with smallpox. Of course no smallpox made its appearance. He then introduced it into his general practice. This child grew to manhood and old age, and, being a doctor himself, was constantly exposed to smallpox of a virulent type.

We always considered it probable that this was the first case of vaccination in British North America, but in November, 1885, I came across, in the *Toronto Globe*, an extract from an old book entitled *Colonel Landman's Travels*. Colonel Landman was, I think, an army officer stationed at Quebec. He writes of receiving from England in the winter of 1801–02 vaccine lymph which he tried on the children of a friend named Blackwell. This may have been a few months previous to my uncle's case, or it may not; I have no precise dates.

In 1901 I read a very interesting article, copied into one of our papers from a medical journal of Philadelphia, written by Dr. Floyd Crandall, of 113 West 95th St., New York. It gave much information re the early introduction of vaccination into the U. S. A. Unfortunately I lost the clipping, but I distinctly recollect that it antedated by a short time its introduction into Canada.

My uncle, the child vaccinated in Yarmouth, was afterward Dr. Jos. Blackburn Bond, who died about forty years ago.

The above are the facts which I have gathered so far on this, to me, interesting subject.

Yours sincerely,

MARIA J. I. THORBURN"

The early years of the nineteenth century in Canada were clouded by the wars in Europe and finally resulted in wars at home. Yet it is noteworthy that in 1816 a board was formed to examine persons and license those fitted to practise medicine in Upper Canada.

Immigration was growing rapidly after the Napoleonic wars and many were reaching Canada by the St. Lawrence route. The year 1832 has always been for the writer an "*annus mirabilis.*" It saw the passing of the first Reform Bill in England, the completion of the first seventy miles of railway in Maryland, and the appearance of Asiatic cholera in America. Sir Edwin Chadwick, after an inquiry into the sweat-shops in the east end of London, was in that year appointed secretary of a commission to inquire into the English Poor Law. In February, 1832, was appointed in Quebec the first sanitary commission in Canada, consisting of Doctors Morrin, Parent, and Perrault. Later a Board of Health was appointed, which adopted quarantine and other regulations. Grosse Isle, thirty miles below Quebec, became a quarantine station, and a squad of soldiers with artillery was stationed there to compel ships to make pratique. The first cholera ship of the season, the *Constantia*, arrived in the St. Lawrence on the 28th of April from Limerick, and but 143 of the ship's 170 passengers were landed on the island — the other 27 had died during the voyage. By June cholera had reached Montreal, and rapidly spread up the St. Lawrence. Deaths were so many among the immigrants escaping from the famine in Ireland that no complete records could be kept; but there died in Quebec, of cholera alone, 2,208, and 1,843 in Montreal by September.

The immigrants ascended the river in open rowboats, tediously working their way up rapids and narrow canals. The accounts of sickness and death from the various landings have been handed down in many tragic stories. For instance, an official letter from Kingston of June 14, 1832, to Sir John Colborne, Lieutenant Governor, states that a public meeting had been held that day, and asks, in case of the existence of any public fund, that he would be good enough to place a sum at the disposal of the committee which had been appointed. Another letter of the same date was sent from Prescott, the landing at which passengers took the steamer for points on Lake Ontario, stating that boatmen and passengers had died at points below and that crews were deserting. This letter, also, asked for assistance. The Governor replied to these requests and placed £500 in the local banks. He asked magistrates and other respectable persons to form boards of health, the magistrates to assume all necessary authority. The *Journals* of the Legislature show that over $100,000 dollars was thus spent by order of the Governor. The year 1833 saw an act passed "To establish Boards of Health to guard against the introduction of malignant and contagious and infectious disease in this Province and the formation of Local Boards of Health." The *Courier of Upper Canada* has an item, dated April 17, 1833, stating that the Governor had constituted for Toronto and neighborhood a Board of Health of nine members, two of whom were physicians.

The provisions of the Act of 1833, of a wholly practical character, were somewhat enlarged in 1835, while in 1849, the year of the next outbreak of cholera, the act became "An Act to appoint a Central Board of Health." The act provided that at any time such a board could be formed by Order in Council; but the period was always fixed by the order. This temporary character was, however, in keeping with public belief at the time, which, in the absence of exact knowledge, ascribed epidemics to a special visitation of the Almighty, whether hortatory or punitive. Toronto papers of 1849 mark the arrival of the modern municipal politician, by reporting that a heated discussion of the act took place, it being considered unjust that the appointment of a board with attendant expense should be made compulsory. During the existence of the Central Board all local by-laws were suspended, and no act done under the Board could be set aside for lack of form or *certiorari*.

The next cholera year, 1854, saw the Central Board again appointed and its regulations precise and comprehensive. Pamphlets were issued covering the subjects of sanitation of houses, ventilation, clothing, diet and disinfection of clothes. The disease then appeared in immigrants at St. John, New Brunswick, and the old huts which had been used were kept on exhibition for many a year. In 1865 cholera again appeared in Europe and typhus was prevalent there in 1866. Again a Central Board was formed, the order being sent from the new capital of the

Confederation, Ottawa. It is worth noting that the medical officer of Toronto, then appointed, read a paper before the Canadian Institute in which he refers to cholera as the class of "zymotic diseases which multiply in the system."

The year 1867 saw the Canadian Confederation an accomplished fact; the formative period of Canada was largely over, and the developmental period had begun. Within ten years a series of provinces stretched from ocean to ocean, while a consciousness of nationhood began to possess a people of four millions holding half a continent in trust for posterity. It has already been said that 1832 was an *"annus mirabilis,"* but equally so was 1867. In this year we find Louis Pasteur, after testing with Claude Bernard the air of cholera wards in the Lariboisière Hospital for the germ of cholera, beginning his great study of pébrine, that disease of silkworms which was costing France millions annually, and we find the Board of Health of New York reformed and Dr. Stephen Smith made its first medical officer. In October, 1867, in the ancient capital of Quebec, the Canadian Medical Association was formed and a resolution adopted providing for the appointment of a strong committee on public health, to promote the establishment of a federal board of health. The birth of the Canadian Dominion was celebrated on July 1, 1867.

What during the fifty odd years since then has been accomplished in Canada can only be studied comparatively; but in no field, perhaps, more satisfactorily than in that of public health.

Already there had been the compulsory registration of marriages by the clergy in Upper Canada, and in Lower Canada registration of births and deaths in parish churches; but in 1869 Upper Canada, now the Province of Ontario, saw the passing of "An Act for the Registration of Births, Marriages and Deaths," whereby municipal clerks registered the same for a fee and made annual returns to the Provincial Secretary. Since 1870 there has been published an *Annual Report of Births, Marriages and Deaths*, this being the first important step toward systematic health work based on vital statistics.

The committee of the Canadian Medical Association, organized in Quebec City in October, 1867, brought in a report at the meeting in 1868 which contained the following:

Here and there in Canada the municipalites have taken steps to remedy existing affairs; but their efforts are too partial in their action and too limited in their scope to be productive of any important advantages. A necessity therefore exists for the introduction by the government of a comprehensive system of sanitary laws, not so complete, perhaps, as those of the Mosaic code nor so severe in the punishment of any violation of them.

But it soon became obvious that there had to be an evolution by progress from the simple to the complex in health matters as in Nature. Acute political changes in the seventies and the still-disputed question of the germ theory of disease made any evolution in public health slow. Although severe smallpox outbreaks and fatal scarlet fever took a heavy toll of lives everywhere, yet the vision of a public health service was never lost. A select committee of the Ontario Legislature met in 1878 to consider a report on the subject of "sanitary measures for maintaining and promoting the public health," and in 1881 an organized movement took place in Toronto among professors of hygiene and public spirited physicians, with the result that "An Act to Establish a Provincial Board of Health" was passed by the Ontario Government in 1882. Under the old existing law the municipal councils became committees of health. They might, however, delegate their duties to a committee who were to administer whatever municipal health laws existed, while the new Provincial Board had powers little more than advisory. During the two following years the board had succeeded in having only 50 local boards in 40 counties, and four salaried local medical officers. Hence, it was apparent that real progress was not possible without local boards being appointed compulsorily under statute, so that in 1884 "The Public Health Act of Ontario" was passed, adopting the English Consolidated Public Health Act of 1875 as its basis, while adapting existing Canadian health acts to the machinery of municipal government.

The autumn of 1884 saw a virulent smallpox outbreak which demanded the initiative and control of the Provincial Board. This body, moved by the terrible epidemic in Montreal in 1885, had by the end of the year been instrumental in the organization of 563 local boards in 600 municipalities, 283 medical officers, 160 sanitary inspectors, and many vaccination officers. The outcome of the organization was that although some 7,000 deaths due to smallpox occurred in the Province of Quebec in 1885, Ontario had only 18. This result in large degree depended upon the Act of 1884 being amended in 1885 to give the Provincial Board the right to investigate, and enforce, when necessary, local action in the case of an outbreak of contagious disease.

Evidently public health organization was making itself felt, and the next year saw the *Conseil de Santé* appointed in the Province of Quebec and a Public Health Act passed, modeled on the Ontario Act.

This addition to the fighting forces soon produced results, and 1887 saw a systematic quarantine inspection of every ship entering the St. Lawrence at Grosse Isle, before the ship could enter port. Almost every year afterwards saw progress in amendments to provincial acts dealing with phases of public health. Old-time legislation of a municipal character existed in the Maritime Provinces; but progress in public health there has been seen only during the last ten years. During this period Nova Scotia has appointed a full-time medical officer of health, and the Province has been divided into four health districts, each with a medical officer. Similar activity has been shown in New Brunswick, where a cabinet minister has been specially designated Minister of Health, a chief medical officer has been appointed, and a fully equipped laboratory established.

In the West, however, progress has marked every Province almost from its formation. Manitoba adopted the Ontario Health Act as its model about 1891, but owing to the large areas with sparse population, districts rather than townships became the units of health organization. The next to be formed was the Board of British Columbia. In British Columbia, owing to the mountainous character of the country, the scheme of utilizing the superintendents of the provincial hospitals as health officers in the rural districts was made use of, since such were already under part pay as provincial officials.

The public health work of the Territorial Government of the Northwest prairies during the early years of the Government was carried on chiefly under the Federal Director of Public Health, assisted by the Northwest mounted police and the authorities of towns; but on the formation of the Provinces of Saskatchewan and Alberta, in 1905, prompt action was taken in each to pass a public health act similar to that of Ontario. Nowhere have public health activities advanced more rapidly than in the three prairie provinces. Well equipped laboratories have been established and the work has been made effective by the appointment of a few all-time health officers and district nurses, working under the chief health officer. A number of district general hospitals were utilized as local centers, more or less closly supervised by the Provincial Health Department.

It is true that for many years the progress of public health in Canada seemed slow, but it maintained a pace at least equal to that in neighboring states. With her remarkable expansion from 1900 onward, when Canada in ten years increased 34 per cent in population, public health had many new demands laid upon it, while with increased provincial revenues various new duties were undertaken. One of the most notable grew out of the Ontario Sanatorium Act of 1900 providing for provincial aid and supervision of county sanatoria. Different provinces have erected provincial sanatoriums whose work was notably increased owing to the Militia Department subsidizing them for the care of tuberculous soldiers during the War. There can be no doubt that the remarkable results of modern preventive medicine in the various war areas, necessitating large expenditures for health purposes as a routine war measure, have served greatly to advance public health work as an ordinary function of government. Thus, in the Province of Ontario the first annual grant in 1882 was only $4,000 and provided for a part-time health officer. This has grown to an expenditure of $550,000 annually, and the staff numbers fifty officers. Those who had long been in the active work of public health in Canada had, as seen in a resolution adopted at Quebec in 1867, worked and waited patiently, hoping for the union of federal and provincial forces in the campaign against disease. Old theories regarding the limited jurisdiction of the Federal Government under the British North America Act, which for fifty years had been made to do service by the opportunist politician, were seen to be readily disproved when the essential need for united effort after the War was made apparent. Hence, during the session of Parliament of 1919 a bill for establishing a federal department of health was passed providing that a physician become the deputy minister of health. A number of existing services have been placed under the Department of Health and new branches dealing with various phases of public health are being developed. The Parliamentary grant for the fiscal year 1920-21 was $750,000.

This necessarily brief summary tells but little of the difficulties encountered in a new country having but few urban centers and a population, like that elsewhere, wholly uneducated as to the meaning and possiblities of public health work.

In the history of the American Public Health Association, prepared in 1915, and printed in the *Journal*, there has been told how even forty years ago much of the teaching was based upon views antedating the scientific era, and it was not till Pasteur's triumph in vaccinating against anthrax in 1881, Koch's discovery of the germ of tuberculosis in 1882, and Löffler's discovery of the germ of diphtheria in 1884, with Pasteur's crucial experiment with rabies in 1885, that public health took its place among the exact sciences.

The wars in South Africa and Cuba served to show how science, if not crystallized into effective methods for organized action has little meaning so far as the prevention of epidemics and deaths is concerned; but it remained for the Japanese, in 1904, to gather the first fruits from such methods. Ten years later the World War found the medical and sanitary services better organized in the armies of the combatants than any other branch. Thus the increase in the weapons of destruction was more than counterbalanced by the life-saving services of sanitation. The more elementary and relatively simple phases of public health work in cases of zymotic diseases have been elaborated and largely perfected during the last fifty years; but it remains yet for us to show that we have methods adequate to prevent those nervous and psychic diseases which seem to become greater and more prevalent with increasing urbanization of the people. The complexity of modern life and the greater demands made upon the emotional functions have tended to produce a neurotic population. If then, the devotees of Hygeia are to find adequate responses to their prayers, their approach to her shrine must be through the temple sacred to Minerva.

THE HISTORY OF BACTERIOLOGY AND ITS CONTRIBUTION TO PUBLIC HEALTH WORK

Frederic P. Gorham, M. A.

Professor of Bacteriology, Brown University; Bacteriologist, Providence Health Department

FIFTY years ago this very year, on March 29, 1871, Pasteur wrote to Duclaux:

> I have a head full of the most beautiful projects for work. The war has forced my brain to lie fallow. I am ready for new productions. Alas! Perhaps I am laboring under an illusion. In any case, I shall make the attempt. Oh! why am I not rich — a millionaire? I would say to you, to Raulin, to Gernez, to van Tiegham, etc., "Come! We will transform the world by our discoveries!"

The riches of Pasteur were not counted in francs and centimes, but in ideas and inspirations. It was not mercenary reward, but Pasteur's wealth of ideas, his fruitful inspiration, his stimulating example, that aroused his students and followers to answer his summons, and indeed, in the fifty short years following, the world has been transformed by their discoveries.

Knowledge of Microörganisms before the Time of Pasteur

We can hardly imagine how meagre was the information in regard to all microörganisms before the time of Pasteur. Probably the first record of the observation of bacteria is that of Athanasius Kircher (1602–1680) in his remarkably modern treatise, *De pestilentia in universum praesertim vero de Veneta et Patavina*, published in Venice in 1659. Kircher was the first to use the microscope in the investigation of disease, and he reports not only the presence of minute wormlike creatures in decaying meat, cheese, milk, vinegar, etc., but even attributes to them the production of disease, and formulates a theory of the animate nature of contagion.*

Science, 31, 1910, 264.

In 1683 Antony van Leeuwenhoek (1632–1723) described and figured organisms which we now know to have been bacteria.*

Whether or not Kircher and Leeuwenhoek really saw the bacteria with their 32-power lenses has been questioned, but one who reads Leeuwenhoek's vivid description can hardly doubt that he saw the same cocci, bacilli, and spirilla which we now find so easily in the material (tartar from the teeth) which he examined.

It was not until Ehrenberg (1795-1876) wrote in 1836 that the terms "bacterium" and "spirillum" were used in place of Leeuwenhoek's "animalcules," and not until 1849 that Joseph Leidy† placed these organisms among the plants rather than with the animals, as did also Perty in 1852, Robin in 1853, and Davaine in 1859.

CAUSES OF THE RAPID DEVELOPMENT OF BACTERIOLOGY

Following Leeuwenhoek's remarkable development of the simple lens and the resulting new observations of microscopic life, we find two lines of investigation stimulating and rapidly broadening the early development of our knowledge of the bacteria.

(a) *The theory of spontaneous generation.* The first was the idea of the spontaneous generation of life, which had been maintained in various forms through the writings of Anaximander of Miletus (610 B. C.), Empedocles of Agrigentum (450 B. C.), Aristotle (384 B. C.), Cardan (1542), and van Helmont (1577–1644), and which was first questioned by Francisco Redi in 1668, and still further doubted by Leeuwenhoek, but which was again opened by his discovery of the bacteria. It was around these organisms that the battle regarding spontaneous generation raged through the latter part of the eighteenth and the early part of the nineteenth centuries. The experiments of the contestants on either side led to the accumulation of much information regarding these organisms, and to the rapid development of methods of studying them. Needham, in 1748, and Spallanzani (1729-1799), with

---

*The Select Works of Antony van Leeuwenhoek, translated by Samuel Hoole, London, 1798, p. 118.
†Proc. Acad. of Nat. Sciences of Phila., Oct. 1849; Science, 40, 1914, 302.

their organic solutions in sealed flasks, Appert, in 1810, with his wonderful development of methods of canning and preserving foods,
Schultze, in 1836, and Schwann and Latour, in 1837, with their experiments on the effect of air upon decaying infusions, Schroeder and von
Dusch, in 1854, with their invention of the cotton plug, all contributed
materially to this development.

But the final settlement of the question of spontaneous generation
did not come until Hoffman, in 1860, and Chevreul and Pasteur, in
1861, experimented with their bent open tubes, and until Pasteur
further showed, in 1860, that a temperature higher than that of boiling
water was required to kill all organisms, and, in 1865, demonstrated
the fact of the presence of resistant bodies, now known as spores, which
were still further investigated by Cohn and Koch in 1876.*

(b) *The microbic theory of disease.* The second idea which stimulated the early development of our knowledge of the bacteria was their
supposed relation to disease production. Vague references to a
contagium vivum or *animatum* are as old as science itself. They are
found in Aristotle (384 B. C.), Varro (116-27 B. C.), Columella
(40 A. D.), Rhazes (860-932 A. D.), Fracastorio (1484-1553), who
published in 1546 his *De contagione et contagionis morbis et curatione,†*
Kircher, already referred to (1659), Plenciz of Vienna (1762), Farr of England (1839), Prof. J. K. Mitchell, father of Dr. Weir Mitchell, in
this country (1849), and Henle (1809-1885), an immediate predecessor
of Pasteur, who in 1840 published a theory of disease and who is usually
credited as the father of the germ theory of disease. But all of these
theories of disease were pure speculation. Not one of them was sub-
stantiated by experiment. Even for Henle, as Duclaux says,‡ "the
germ of the disease was not something superimposed upon the sick
person and independent of him; it was something belonging to him,
borrowing from him a sort of pathological vitality, and able to trans-
port it elsewhere". . . . "we find therein nothing of the new idea,
brought by Pasteur concerning the living virus, which can be cultivated
and modified outside of the organism."

---

*Cohn's Beitr. z. Morphol. d. Pflanzen, 1876-7, ii, 277-310.
†Science, 31, 1910, 500.
‡Pasteur–The History of a Mind, Duclaux. Trans. by Smith and Hedges, 1920, p. 229.

The true germ theory of disease had to wait until laboratory verification at the hands of Pasteur gave it a firm footing. The true story of the birth of the germ theory of disease begins when, in 1876, we find Pasteur taking up the study of the anthrax organism.

BIRTH OF THE GERM THEORY OF DISEASE — PASTEUR'S STUDY OF ANTHRAX

Even as early as 1850 Rayer, with the aid of Davaine, had seen the little rods in the blood of animals dead of anthrax, but without comprehending their importance. Again, in 1855, Pollender had repeated the observation and had even asked the questions, "Are they the infectious matter itself?" "Are they only the carriers of this matter?" or "Have they nothing to do with it?" Brauell, in 1856, with his observations of similar bacteria in putrefaction and his careless inoculation experiments, threw doubt upon the bacillus as the specific cause of anthrax. But Delafond, in 1860, came to the rescue with his careful experiments in cultivating the bacilli, and his demonstration that they were living organisms, and his attempt to show that they formed the spores or seeds, which were such a stumbling-block to investigators at this time. Davaine, in 1863, made the first inoculation experiment demonstrating that he could produce the disease by the transfer of the bacilli, and in 1876 Koch solved the problem of the spores. But it was left for Pasteur to demonstrate fully that the bacteria were the sole cause of the disease, and thus to lay the real foundation of the germ theory in his complete and thoroughly satisfying paper published on April 30, 1877, in the *Comptes Rendus de l'Academie des Sciences*.

While these studies on anthrax were progressing, other disease-producing organisms had been observed and described. Bassi, in 1837, had seen the corpuscles causing the pebrine disease of silkworms, later studied by Pasteur. Tulasne (1847-1854) and Kühn (1858) had demonstrated certain organisms in diseases of grain and potatoes. Klebs, in 1865, described the organisms present in purulent nephritis, von Recklinghausen and Waldeyer, in 1865, the organisms in metastatic abscesses, Rindfleisch, in 1866, the organisms in pyemia, and Obermeier, in 1873, the spirillum of relapsing fever.

But these were isolated observations unsubstantiated by convincing laboratory proof. Pasteur, in characteristic fashion, supported by his twenty years' experience in the study of the microbes of wine, beer, and silkworm diseases, soon outdistanced those who had already entered upon this field of work, and in his study of anthrax, not only thoroughly demonstrated the theory, but, in addition, contributed most fertile ideas of his own regarding the attenuation of viruses, the modification of the infecting organism, and the development of immunity.

EARLY BACTERIOLOGICAL TECHNIQUE

It is interesting to recall that before 1880 none of our modern methods of studying bacteria had been developed. All of Pasteur's work and the work of all his predecessors had been done by the unsatisfactory methods of dilution for securing pure cultures. Cohn used the method of dilution, Klebs used what he called the "fractional culture,"* and Solomonsen had devised a capillary pipette method.† Solid culture media for the isolation of pure cultures had not come into use. Vittadini, the mycologist, had used a gelatin medium for growing microörganisms in 1852, as had also Brefeld (1874) and other botanists. Klebs recommended its use for bacteria in 1873. But to Koch we owe the application of solid media to the isolation of pure cultures in 1875.

In April, 1876, Koch wrote to Cohn that he had worked out the life history and sporulation of the anthrax bacillus, and Cohn invited him to visit the laboratories of the University of Breslau. There he demonstrated the use of solidified gelatin for the isolation of pure cultures to Cohn, Weigert, Auerbach, Traube, Cohnheim and others, and in July 1876, Cohn published Koch's paper in his *Beiträge zur Morphologie der Pflanzen*, ii, 1876-7, 277-310.

*Arch. f. Exp. Path. 1, 1873.
†Bot. Zeit. 1879, No. 39, and 1880, No. 28

Koch in his invention of the solid medium method of isolation in 1875, first as a gelatin tube method and in 1883 as a plate method, laid the foundation on which all subsequent bacteriological investigation was erected. At about this time Hesse, one of Koch's collaborators, introduced the use of agar, and in 1887 Petri devised his well-known culture dishes. We owe to Koch also the application of the Abbé condenser and the oil-immersion lens to bacteriological investigation in 1878, while we cannot be too grateful to Weigert, who taught us to stain bacteria in 1871, and to use the basic anilin dyes for staining bacteria in 1875.

DISCOVERY OF ORGANISMS CAUSING SPECIFIC DISEASES

After these brilliant and fundamental contributions to bacteriological technique it is no wonder that the years immediately following saw the discovery, isolation, and cultivation of so many of the common disease-producing organisms.

1837   Bassi saw the protozoa of pebrine in silkworms.
1850   Rayer and Davaine saw the anthrax bacillus.
1847-1854   Tulasne described certain disease-producing organisms in plants.
1858   Kühn described certain disease-producing organisms in plants.
1863   Davaine produced anthrax by inoculation.
1865   Klebs described the organisms of purulent nephritis.
1865   Von Recklinghausen and Waldeyer described the organisms in metastatic abscesses.
1866   Rindfleisch described the organisms of pyemia.
1873   Obermeier discovered the spirillum of relapsing fever.
1877   Pasteur discovered the bacillus of malignant edema.
1877   Burrill, in this country, discovered the bacillus causing pear blight.
1878   Koch studied traumatic infection.
1879   Hansen and Neisser discovered the organism of leprosy.
1879   Neisser discovered the gonococcus.
1880   Pasteur and Sternberg simultaneously discovered the pneumococcus.
1880   Pasteur discovered the organism of fowl cholera and staphylococci in pus.
1880   Eberth and Koch independently discovered the typhoid bacillus.
1880   Laveran discovered the malarial plasmodium.
1881   Ogston discovered staphylococci in abscesses.
1882   Koch discovered the tubercle bacillus.
1882   Koch and Ogston discovered the streptococcus.
1882   Several observers reported the glanders bacillus, which was isolated in pure culture by Löffler and Schütz.
1883   Koch discovered the organisms of cholera and infectious conjunctivitis.

1883 Fehleisen obtained pure cultures cf streptococci in erysipelas.
1883 Klebs saw the diphtheria bacillus.
1884 Rosenbach demonstrated *Streptococcus pyogenes* in abscesses and oste-
   omyelitis.
1884 Gaffky obtained pure cultures of the typhoid bacillus.
1884 Nicolaier discovered the tetanus bacillus.
1884 Koch made his full report on tuberculosis.
1884 Löffler obtained pure cultures of the diphtheria bacillus.
1885 Emmerich isolated the colon bacillus.
1885 Bumm obtained pure cultures of the gonococcus.
1886 Escherich named the *Bacillus coli.*
1887 Weichselbaum described the meningococcus.
1888 Gärtner identified *Bacillus enieritidis* and *paratyphosus.*
1889 Kitasato obtained the tetanus bacillus in pure culture.
1892 Welch and Nuttall described the gas bacillus.
1894 Kitasato and Yersin simultaneously discovered the plague bacillus.
1897 Shiga discovered the dysentery bacillus.
1898 Theobald Smith differentiated bovine and human tubercle bacilli.
1905 Schaudinn and Hoffman described the *Treponema pallidum* of syphilis.
1906 Bordet and Gengou discovered *Bacillus pertussis* of whooping cough.
1919 Noguchi isolated the supposed cause of yellow fever, *Leptospira icteroides.*

EARLY AMERICAN BACTERIOLOGISTS

While these brilliant researches and discoveries were taking place abroad, workers in this country were not idle. Eagerly were the publications from the laboratories of Europe read on this side of the water, and many were the visitors from America to the laboratories of Europe. It did not take long for the results of this pioneer work to be accepted and extended in this country.

Bacteriology, the new science, hardly heard of in America before 1885, by 1890 had become well known. To Professor Thomas J. Burrill (1839-1916) belongs the credit of first introducing the study of the bacteria in his course in botany at the University of Illinois in the seventies. In 1877 he discovered the causative organism of the pear blight.* In 1878, Dr. William H. Welch, at Bellevue Hospital Medical College, and in 1879, Dr. T. Mitchell Prudden, at the College of Physicians and Surgeons, were studying and demonstrating the bacteria. In 1879, Dr. Daniel E. Salmon, of the United States Bureau of Animal Industry, was investigating the bacteriology of certain animal diseases.

*Trans. Ill. Hort. Soc. 114, 1877, and 80, 1878.

Dr. George M. Sternberg was the real pioneer American bacteriologist. No doubt stimulated by the discussions to which he listened while attending the annual meeting of the American Public Health Association at Richmond, Virginia on November 19, 1878, he began work that same year on a series of experiments to determine the value of certain commercial disinfectants. This involved much bacteriological techinque and a considerable knowledge of the bacteria which he learned in part from reading the publications of European laboratories but which he developed very largely for himself. This work, begun in 1878 at Walla Walla, Washington, continued in Washington D. C., and completed in the laboratory at Johns Hopkins, was the culmination of studies undertaken as chairman of a committee of the American Public Health Association which had made an appropriation for such investigations. The results were published in full in the *Transactions* for 1888, and were subsequently translated into several oreign languages. For t his work Sternberg received the Lomb prize, offered through the American Public Health Association and awarded at the Washington meeting in 1885. This was the beginning of the long and useful series of investigations in regard to disinfectants which have been made by members of this Association and which have led to our present method of scientific standardization.

In 1880 Sternberg was sent to New Orleans by the National Board of Health to investigate the microörganisms of the air in connection with his work on yellow fever, which he had begun as early as 1871. Although Sternberg's contributions to our knowledge of yellow fever were mostly negative, yet his name will be associated with that disease forever. It was necessary that some one hunt out and describe the large number of microörganisms associated with the disease in those days, and this Sternberg did, laying one after another of them aside, until he felt sure that a bacteriological origin for the disease could not be claimed.

It was Sternberg who suggested, appointed, and instructed the Yellow Fever Commission in 1900, which so brilliantly solved the problem of the spread of yellow fever by the Stegomya mosquito. It was not until 1919, however, that the search for the causal organism was completed when Noguchi isolated the *Leptospira icteroides*.

In 1880 Sternberg translated and published in this country Magnin's book on bacteriology, published in Paris in 1878, making extensive additions of his own.   This was the first American book on bacteriology.*   This was followed in 1892 by his *Manual of Bacteriology*, an exhaustive and authoritative work, prepared amid the exacting duties of an officer of the Medical Corps.   This book will ever stand as a monument to his energy and ability.

In 1881 Sternberg introduced to the American medical profession the bacillus of typhoid fever in a paper before the Association of American Physicians.   In 1882, at Fort Mason, California, for the first time in America, he demonstrated and photographed the bacillus of tuberculosis, discovered earlier the same year by Koch.   In 1881 he made his report refuting the claims for the Klebs-Tomassi-Crudeli bacillus as the cause of malaria, and in 1885, on his return as a delegate to the International Sanitary Conference at Rome, he demonstrated at Johns Hopkins University, for the first time in America, the living plasmodium of malaria discovered by Laveran in 1880.   In February, 1881, Sternberg discovered a pathogenic organism which he found constant in his own sputum and proved it to be identical with the organism described by Pasteur in January, 1881.   This organism was later proved to be the pneumococcus, the cause of croupous pneumonia. In 1881, before Metchnikoff's first paper was published (1884), Sternberg was the first to point out the fact that the white blood corpuscles devoured and removed from the body invading pathogenic bacteria.

Professor H. W. Conn became interested in bacteriology after hearing Professor W. G. Farlow lecture on the bacteria in Boston in 1880, studied under Councilman at Johns Hopkins in 1881, and began his studies on the organisms of milk in 1889, when Atwater founded the Storrs Agricultural Experiment Station.

In 1882-3 Professor William Trelease introduced some bacteriological work into his botany course at the University of Wisconsin using potato as a culture medium.   In 1882 Burrill published a pamphlet on bacteria giving the methods used by the French school of bacteriologists and the classification of Cohn.   Dr. Henry Formad

---

Bacteria: Magnin, Sternberg, 1880.

at the University of Pennsylvania in 1882 was teaching the diagnosis of the tubercle bacillus and the methods of cultivating bacteria after his return from Koch's laboratory, and in 1883 he with Dr. H. C. Wood, investigated an epidemic of diphtheria in Michigan but arrived at erroneous conclusions. In 1889 Dr. A. C. Abbott was Sternberg's assistant with Dr. Councilman at Johns Hopkins.

With the year 1885 courses in bacteriology began to appear in the medical schools and agricultural colleges. In this year, Dr. H. T. Detmers, who had been associated with Dr. Salmon in the Bureau of Animal Industry, went to Ohio and began bacteriological teaching giving his first course in 1886. In 1885, Welch became the head of the Pathological Institute of Johns Hopkins Medical School and took as his assistant Dr. Abbott, who had been Sternberg's assistant the previous year. Later Dr. George H. F. Nuttall became an assistant also, and in 1892 Welch and Nuttall announced the discovery of the gas bacillus, now know as *Bacillus welchii*. Dr. H. M. Biggs, in March, 1885, took charge of the Carnegie Laboratory, at that time attached to the Bellevue Hospital Medical College, and began instruction in bacteriology. Professor E. A. Birge, in 1885-86 gave courses in bacteriology at the University of Wisconsin and under him studied Professor H. L. Russell. Dr. T. M. Cheesman began instruction in bacteriology in Dr. Prudden's laboratory in 1885-86. Dr. J. E. Weeks spent 1884-5 in Berlin, and in 1885 Dr. H. Knapp brought bacteriological apparatus from Europe and asked Weeks to give a course in bacteriology, which he began in 1885 at the Ophthalmic and Aural Institute, then at 46 East 12th Street, New York. In 1885, Dr. H. C. Ernst gave a course of lectures on bacteriology at the Harvard Medical School. Prudden reviewed Koch's methods of studying bacteria in the *Report of the Connecticut State Board of Health for 1885* (pages 225-6). In 1866, Dr. Theobald Smith began lectures and laboratory work in bacteriology at the Medical Department of what is now George Washington University. Dr. B. Homes gave a course of lectures in bacteriology at the Chicago Medical School in 1888, and in 1889 became professor of bacteriology in the Postgraduate Medical School of Chicago. Professor L. H. Pammel gave lectures on the bacteria at the Veterinary School of the Iowa State College of Agriculture, and gave a general course in bacteriology in 1889. In 1889 Drs. V. C. Vaughan and F. G. Novy gave the first formal course in bacteriology at the University of Michigan. In 1888-9 Professor W. T. Sedgwick gave his first course at the Massachusetts Institute of Technology, Boston.

Relation of the Microbic Theory of Disease to Public Health Work

In spite of the brilliant discoveries of the causative organisms of most of the common diseases by European investigators, and the rapid dissemination of the knowledge of the bacteria and their behavior, these results for a long time had little effect upon the practices of public health officials either in this country or abroad.

Public health activities of various sorts began early in the history of civilization. Wherever people gathered together in communities the need of some sort of regulation for the protection of the public health was felt. In the colonies of America we find various sanitary activities recorded as early even as 1678, when Boston and Salem attempted to restrict the spread of smallpox. Later various sanitary regulations were put into force by cities and states mainly for quarantine against epidemics of smallpox, yellow fever, and the like. The public health movement on a large scale took definite form first in England with the Public Health Act and General Board of Health of 1848. In 1855 Louisana created a State Board of Health for the purpose of dealing with matters of quarantine. This was followed in 1869 by the creation of the Massachusetts State Board of Health, and in 1870 of the Virginia and California State Boards of Health.

The prevention of epidemics was the first and most important duty of these early sanitary authorities. Scavenging, sewers, and ventilation were the weapons depended upon to destroy the sources of contagion, then supposed to be filth, foul odors, and the decomposition and fermentation of animal and vegetable matter. This was the era of the filth theory of disease production, which continued for some thirty or forty years, and which is to-day just giving up its hold upon the health authorities of our cities and states. As Chapin says*:

Although there were some important truths in the generalizations of the early promoters of public health, and although their projects for civic betterment saved many lives and did much for human comfort and convenience, there were several errors which have had an unfortunate influence on preventive medicine and still have to-day. One of these is that disease breeds in filth instead of being merely carried in filth. Another is that all kinds of dirt are dangerous, not merely the secretions and excretions of the human body. A third unfortunate hypothesis is that infectious diseases are usually air-borne.

In the state of knowledge at the time, however, these mistakes were perfectly natural. The science of bacteriology had not arisen to throw its light upon these questions.

With the Public Health Act of England in 1875 we find the ideas of contagion becoming a little more scientific. That diseases are caused by germs that pass from person to person, and that their control requires notification and isolation were some of the new ideas beginning to take form. Immediately thereafter came the tremendous and sudden development of our knowledge of the organisms causing disease, the development of laboratory methods of discovering and diagnosing disease, and a knowledge of the means by which diseases are spread. Ultimately this led to correct ideas about the sources of contagion and the parts played by air, water, milk, and insects, in its dissemination. It is along these lines that we find the greatest contributions of bacteriology to public health.

(a) *Bacteriology of the Air.* The history of the bacteriology of the air must begin with that notable book in sanitary science, Tyndall's *Essays on the Floating Matter of the Air* (1881), and continue with Prudden's *Dust and its Dangers* (1890). Little by little the investigations of bacteriologists showed first that bacteria are not given off from moist surfaces (Nägeli, 1877), that they are not present in expired air (Tyndall, 1881), that they die quickly when dried (Germano, 1897). As a substitute for the theory of infection through the air there developed, first, the idea of droplet infection, announced by Flügge in 1897, and so admirably studied in this country by Winslow and Robinson in 1910; and, second, the idea that most of our communicable diseases depend upon

*Jour. Amer. Med. Assoc., Jan. 22, 1921, vol. 76, pp. 215-222.

rather close and immediate contact for their distribution. For emphasizing these ideas and showing their relation to public health practice we are indebted very largely to the teachings and writings of Dr. C. V. Chapin, which culminated in his book *Sources and Modes of Infection*, published in 1910.

Pasteur, in 1860, demonstrated the presence of living bacteria in the air. The first systematic attempts to study the microörganisms of the air were made by Maddox in 1870 and by Cunningham in 1873, who used an aëroscope which was a modification of one used by Pouchet (1858). Cohn, Pasteur, and Miquel (1883) used a method of aspirating air through a liquid, and still later came the plate method using Petri dishes. (1887) A notable contribution to the methods of studying the bacteria of the air was that made by Sedgwick and Tucker in a communication made to the Boston Society of Arts, January 12, 1888, suggesting the use of a soluble filter made of granulated sugar.

For the purpose of standardizing the methods of air analysis the American Public Health Association, in 1907, appointed a committee on Standard Methods for the Examination of the Air. This committee made its first report at the Richmond meeting in 1909, a second report of progress in 1912, and its final report in 1916. The researches carried on by the members of this committee, the investigations stimulated by it, and the standardization of methods developed, have all added to our knowledge of the chemistry and bacteriology of the air and their relation to problems of ventilation, hygiene and public health.

Another outgrowth of our knowledge of the bacteriology of the air has been the revolution which has taken place in our ideas of fumigation. Here again Chapin has taken the lead by bringing to the attention of sanitarians the facts worked out by the bacteriologists. If disease germs have but a short period of life outside the body, if they are not capable of living long in our surroundings, but are only carried about in the bodies of the sick and those exposed to the sick, why should the efforts of the health officer be devoted so largely to the disinfection of the rooms and houses after the termination of isolation? In March, 1905, Chapin abandoned terminal disinfection in Providence, except in special cases. It was not till 1915 that New York City followed this example, and later other cities gradually fell into line. Slowly the sanitary world has accepted the bacteriological facts championed by Chapin, and we find now that terminal disinfection is passing into general disuse, and more careful control of the sick patient and the contacts taking its place.

(b) *Bacteriology of Water.* Burdon Sanderson in 1871* had demonstrated the presence of bacteria in water. Miquel in 1880† devised the first exact methods for the enumeration of bacteria in water and even before this time had been using liquid media for the study of bacteria in water. Angus Smith of Manchester was the first in England to use Koch's solid media in water analysis. In 1885 Percy Frankland used Koch's methods of isolating bacteria in a study of London filtered water, and in 1887 Plagge and Proskauer studied in a similar manner the Berlin filters.

The filtration of drinking water was adopted as a sanitary measure long before the development of bacteriology. James Simpson, engineer of the Chelsea Water Company, constructed at London in 1829 the first filter for a public water supply. In 1856 an English company built filters for the Berlin supply. In 1866 James P. Kirkwood, C. E., went to Europe for the city of St. Louis to study clarification of river waters and made an elaborate report, *Filtration of River Waters* (New York, 1869). In 1871-2 the city of Poughkeepsie, New York, constructed the first filter in the United States, from designs by Mr. Kirkwood.‡ In 1874 Hudson, New York, and Columbus, Ohio, and in 1875 Toledo, Ohio, built similar filters. In claiming that Poughkeepsie built the first filter in the United States, Nichols says.§

I am not ignorant of the fact that a number of towns and water companies undertake to "filter" their water by passing it through broken stone, gravel, or gravel and charcoal, or even through sand and gravel. As far, however, as I have examined such arrangements, the most that can be said of them is that they act with greater or less efficiency as *strainers*, removing some of the coarser matters, the infrequency of the cleansing showing that the work done cannot be very great.

This may refer to such small filters as those at Greenwich

---

*Q. J. Micros. Sci. Oct. 1871.
†*Annuaire de l'Observ. de Montsouris* pour 1880, p. 492.
‡*Jour. N. E. Water Works Assoc.*, vol. 12, p. 209.
§*Mass. State Board of Health Report* for 1878, p. 152.

Connecticut, Ilion, New York, Nantucket, Massachusetts, and Mt. Vernon, New York, which Hazen says were very early in operation.

The first open filter of the slow sand type, scientifically designed was put in operation September 20, 1893, at Lawrence, Massachusetts. It was the joint work of Mills, Stearns, Drown, Sedgwick, Hazen, and Fuller, but most of all that of Mills.

Coagulation methods for the treatment of water were employed from very early times.   D'Arcet, 1831, in *Annales d'Hygiene Publique* gives an account of the purification of Nile water by adding alum and filtering through small household filters. Lime was used in Holland for filtering peaty waters through sand, and in England lime was used long ago for softening water by what was called Clark's process, and operated under patent. At the International Congress of Hygiene, before 1893, Anderson reported the use of a cylinder of iron through which the water passed, and by the rotation of the cylinder, which contained many small pieces of metallic iron, the water was purified. This seems to be the first form of a "mechanical filter."   In this country the first mechanical filters were operated in connection with paper and sugar mills. With the addition of coagulants it was soon found possible to remove bacteria by these filters. The first data of importance on this point were those secured by E. B. Weston in 1893-4 in Providence,[*] and in 1895-7 in much more elaborate studies at Louisville. In 1897, a mechanical filter was installed at Loraine, Ohio, and in 1898 at Elmira, New York.

The rapid adoption of filtration methods continued all over Europe and America. In 1903 it was estimated that 18 per cent of the water filters of the United States were of the slow sand type, 79 per cent of the mechanical type, and 3 per cent of special design. In 1900, 6.3. per cent of the urban population of the United States was using filtered water, in 1904, 9.7 per cent, and in 1911, 20 per cent. The last ten years have seen a much more general adoption of filtered water and a consequent decrease in the water-borne diseases.

The treatment of water by chlorination was first tried by de Morveau in France, and by Cruikshank in England, about the year 1800. The

[*]*R. I. State Board of Health Report*, 1894.

efficacy of chlorine as a disinfectant and deodorizer was well recognized during the early part of the last century, and in 1854 an English Royal Commission used it on the sewage of London. A committee of the American Public Health Association in 1885 reported it the best disinfectant available when cost and efficiency were considered. In 1889 Hermite introduced the use of an electrolized sea water under the name of Hermite fluid, and this was employed for domestic disinfection and for flushing sewers. Chlorine in various forms was employed in France and England for disinfecting sewage. In 1893 a plant for making chlorine from strong brine was set up at Brewster, New York, and the sewage from a small group of houses treated with it, before being discharged into a creek which flowed into Croton Lake, the water supply of New York City. This was the first time chlorine was used for the specific object of destroying bacteria.

After much work had been done in studying the action of chlorine on sewage at Hamburg (1898), Berlin (1907), by the State Board of Health of Ohio and the United States Department of Agriculture (1907), we find the most valuable contribution that of Phelps, who in 1906 at Boston, at Red Bank, New Jersey, and at Baltimore, in 1907, indubitably demonstrated the economic possibilities of sewage chlorination.

As far as can be definitely stated the first use of bleach solution in drinking water was that of Woodhead in 1897, who disinfected the distribution mains at Maidstone, England, after an epidemic of typhoid fever. The first systematic use of chlorine in water is due to Houston and McGowan in England, in 1904-5. Nesfield, of the Indian Army Service, recommended in 1903 the use of chlorine compounds to prevent the appalling loss of life from water-borne diseases such as occurred during the Boer War. His work is especially interesting because of his suggestion of the possibility of using compressed chlorine gas in steel cylinders as so commonly used at present.

In this country, about 1896, George W. Fuller experimented with chlorine in a Jewell Filter at the Louisville Experimental Station. The first commercial use of it was by George A. Johnson, in 1908, at the Union Stock Yards in Chicago. About the same time Johnson and Leal commenced its use at Jersey City, treating about forty million gallons of water per day.   During the next few years its use became very popular, and in 1911 over 800,000,000 gallons of water were being treated daily in some of the largest cities of North America, including Brooklyn, Albany, New York, Cincinnati, Columbus, Harrisburg, Philadelphia, Pittsburg, Erie, Hartford, Nashville, St. Louis, Kansas City, Montreal, Ottawa, Baltimore, and Minneapolis.   In 1918 it was estimated that over 3,000,000,000 gallons were being treated per day in North America.   The story of the use of chlorine in protecting the drinking water of the troops in the World War is a chapter by itself.

The development of the methods of filtering and disinfecting water has been possible only as the researches of the water bacteriologists have pointed the way.   The members of this Association have had a great deal to do with the improvement of the methods of water analysis.   Dr. Wyatt Johnston, of Montreal, was the first to call the attention of the American Public Health Association to the need of more uniform and efficient methods of bacteriological water analysis.   In 1894 the first step was taken at the Montreal meeting, when the Committee on the Pollution of Water Supplies closed its report with the suggestion of a coöperative investigation into the bacteriology of water. A committee for this purpose was immediately appointed, with a subcommittee to determine methods of laboratory procedure.   This subcommittee called a convention at the Academy of Medicine, New York City, June 21 and 22, 1895, for general discussion and formulation of laboratory methods, under the chairmanship of Dr. W. H. Welch.   Another committee was appointed by this convention to draw up a report. The committee met in New York City, February, 1896, to digest its material and outline its report, which was presented to the American Public Health Association at its meeting in Buffalo in 1896.   The report was subsequently withdrawn for further amendment and was finally submitted for publication at the meeting of the Association in Philadelphia in 1897.

At the Minneapolis meeting in 1899 another committee was appointed to extend the procedures to include all the lines of investigation involved in the analysis of water, bacteriological, chemical, and microscopic. Progress reports were made in 1900, 1901, and 1902. In 1901 the committee was instructed to revise the 1897 report. In 1905 the first edition of the report on *Standard Methods of Water Analysis* was published. A revised report, the second edition, was issued in 1912. The third edition was published in 1917. These committees worked in coöperation with similar committees of the American Chemical Society of American Bacteriologists. The fourth edition, with some changes in the bacteriological part, was published by the same committees in 1920. These reports are now the accepted standard methods of procedure in all laboratories doing water and sewage analysis, and represent one of the greatest contributions to the advancement of sanitary water analysis.

Bacteriology of Milk. The first work in this country on the bacteriology of milk was that of Conn in 1889. Bacteria had been observed in milk as long ago as 1659 by Kircher. Their relation to the sanitary quality of the milk was not recognized until long afterwards. Most of the early studies on the bacteriology of milk dealt with the question of fermentation, but in 1892 we find Sedgwick and Batchelder reporting on the numbers of bacteria found in Boston market milk. The American Public Health Association appointed a Committee on the Bacteriological Analysis of Milk in 1899. The first edition of the *Standard Methods for the Examination of Milk* was published in 1910, the second in 1916, and the third in 1921. The third edition was prepared in coöperation with committees from the American Dairy Science Association, International Association of Dairy and Milk Inspectors, Society of American Bacteriologists, and American Association of Medical Milk Commissions, and embodies the very latest methods of judging the sanitary quality of the milk from bacteriological analysis.

(d) *Insects and Disease.* Although as early as 1659 we find Kircher crediting to Mercurialis (1530-1606) the idea that flies may be agents in the transfer of disease,* and in 1879 Manson reporting the mosquito as a carrier of filaria, the first definite proof of an insect-borne disease was the demonstration in 1893 by Smith and Kilborne† of the

---

Science, 31, 1910, 264.
†*U. S. Dept. Agriculture Bureau of Animal Industry* Bul. 1, 1893.

part played by ticks in the transmission of Texas cattle fever. There had been many suggestions that malaria might be mosquito-borne earlier than this (Sanskrit Susruta, 5th century, A. D., Nott 1847-8, King 1883, Laveran 1891, Koch and others) but it was not until 1895 that Ross watched the development of a malarial parasite in mosquitoes. Laveran had already discovered the malarial plasmodium in the blood of malarial patients in 1880. W. G. MacCallum in 1897-8 demonstrated the sexual conjugation of the plasmodium at Johns Hopkins. In 1899 Grassi and Bignami proved that only the Anopheles mosquito carried malaria. In 1911, Bass and Johns of New Orleans announced that they had succeeded in cultivating the plasmodium in vitro.

The possible relation of mosquitoes to yellow fever seems to have been suggested first by Nott of Mobile in 1848. In 1854 Beauperthuy published in the *Official Gazette* of Cumana, Venezuela, an article stating very clearly the mosquito theory of the spread of yellow fever. To Finlay of Havana, however, we owe the first experimental work, a report of which was presented in 1882 to the Royal Academy of Medicine, Physical and Natural Sciences of Havana. In 1900 the American Yellow Fever Commission, consisting of Reed, Carroll, Agramonte and Lazear, appointed on the recommendation of Dr. Sternberg, commenced their investigations at Havana, and at once began to put Finlay's theory to the test. The proof of the theory and the phenomenal success attending its application to the eradication of yellow fever from Cuba, the Panama Canal Zone, and elsewhere is one of the most brilliant achievements of public health in the world.

In the past twenty-five years we have watched the battle against malaria and yellow fever fought and won by Ross in India, Grassi, Bignami and Bastianelli in Italy, Finlay and Gorgas in Cuba, and Gorgas in Panama, and now we find the International Health Board of the Rockefeller Foundation extending the field of operation into South and Central America and West Africa.

While the majority of insect-borne diseases are tropical and are but remotely interesting to us in the United States, we take particular pride in the investigations of Ricketts in 1907-8 on the transmission of Rocky Mountain fever by ticks.

The investigation of the relation of fleas to plague has also come to have more than an academic interest to us in the United States, for already in several instances plague has established itself on our shores. In 1897 Ogata found plague bacilli in fleas from rats dead of bubonic plague. This observation was confirmed by the German Plague Commission in the same year. Thompson and Tidswell in Australia, the English Plague Commission, Nuttall and others have little by little added to our information, until now the rat-flea-human method of spread of the disease is fully demonstrated.

The relation of flies to typhoid fever and other diseases was also suggested long ago. Raimbert (1869), Davaine (1870), and Ballinger demonstrated living anthrax germs on flies of various kinds that had been feeding on infected material. Nuttall (1897) showed that house flies could carry living plague bacilli for at least forty-eight hours after becoming infected. In 1886, Tizzoni and Cattani in Bologna, and, in 1892, Simmonds in Hamburg, demonstrated cholera spirilla on flies in a cholera hospital. Celli (1888) fed flies with pure cultures of typhoid bacilli and found virulent germs in the excreta. Sawtchenko in St. Petersburg (1892) found cholera germs in the feces of flies fed on a culture of the organism. Firth and Horrocks (1902) demonstrated typhoid bacilli on the legs and bodies of flies; Hamilton in Chicago (1903), Ficker in Hamburg (1903), and Klein (1908) recovered typhoid bacilli from flies in houses where there were cases of the disease. Sedgwick first called attention to the importance of flies in the control of the spread of typhoid fever in 1892.*

In 1895 Dr. George M. Kober pointed out the probable transference of typhoid germs from box privies to food supplies in his "Report on the Prevalence of Typhoid Fever in the District of Columbia." In the Spanish-American War General Sternberg issued orders to guard against flies. Veeder in his "Report on the Origin and Spread of Typhoid Fever in the United States Military Camps during the Spanish War" (1898) emphasized the importance of fly infection of food. Vaughan in 1900, as a member of the commission to investigate the cause of typhoid fever in the army camps, personally urged the import-

---

*Report Mass. State Board of Health, 1892, p. 736.

ance of the fly in the spread of the disease. The investigations of Packard (1874) and Howard (1896) in this country, and Nuttall (1899) and Newstead (1907) in England have added to our knowledge of the habits of the fly, while the studies of Sedgwick and Winslow in Boston (1902), Niven in Manchester (1903), Jackson in New York (1907), Sykes in Providence (1909), Ainsworth in India (1909), and Slack in Boston (1909) have all contributed materially to an understanding of the relation of the fly to the spread of disease.

(e)   *Carriers and Missed Cases.*   The germ theory of disease revolutionized medicine. The discovery that disease germs grow in the bodies of certain individuals without causing disease — that there are "carriers" of disease germs — revolutionized preventive medicine.

Pasteur and Sternberg as early as 1881 showed the presence of a virulent pathogenic organism in healthy mouths which later was proved to be the pneumococcus. Löffler, in his original paper on diphtheria (1884), reported the presence of the organism in a person who was not sick. In 1889 Roux and Yersin, and in 1890 Escherich called attention to the fact that diphtheria bacilli remain for considerable periods in the throats of convalescents. Park and Beebe of New York (1894), Müller (1896), Kober of Germany (1899), and the Department of Health of Baltimore (1899) reported diphtheria bacilli in the throats of well persons.

In 1900 Horton-Smith in England called attention to the chronic urinary typhoid carrier. The idea of the typhoid carrier as an epidemiological factor was directly evolved from the views set forth by Koch in his address of November, 1902. On his recommendation bacteriological stations were established in certain parts of Germany for the express purpose of testing in actual practice the thesis that the main source of typhoid fever in these typhoid-ridden districts was man himself, both during convalescence, and in the mild or missed cases of ambulant type. The discovery of the intestinal typhoid carrier was the natural outcome of the bacteriological study of convalescents. Frosch (1903) was the first to suggest the persistence of the bacilli in the intestinal tract and their relation to the infection of others. Drigalski (1903) and Dönitz (1904) established the hypothesis on bacteriological grounds, and it was Drigalski who first discovered a female chronic carrier who apparently had no history of an attack of typhoid fever.

Mild and atypical cases of nearly all the communicable diseases have now been recorded, carriers of many of them have been found, and there seems to be no reason why the carrier state may not exist in all of them. Any scheme of preventive medicine which fails to take the carrier and the mild or missed case into consideration is doomed to failure.

(f) *Immunity*. The fact that certain races of animals and men and certain individuals among these are more refractory to disease than others, and that the same individuals are at one time more resistant than at another, is the result of experience and observation from earliest times. Immunity, both natural and acquired, has long been known. The explanation of it and the methods of producing it or controlling it are some of the more recent developments of bacteriological science.

Although Jenner (1749-1823) had made the important discovery of cowpox vaccine as a preventive of smallpox in 1775, and had done the first human vaccination in 1796, it was Pasteur who, working for the first time with pure cultures of disease-producing organisms, could investigate the underlying causes of immunity. This he did in his study of chicken cholera immunity in 1879, and anthrax immunity in 1880.

In 1882 Metchnikoff began reporting his studies on the leucocytes but did not develop his theory of phagocytic immunity until 1884, while Sternberg already in 1881 had suggested the rôle of the leucocytes in removing pathogenic bacteria from the body, by devouring and destroying them after the manner of an ameba.*

Löffler had assumed the presence of diphtheria toxin in 1884. It had been partially isolated by Roux and Yersin in 1888, and in 1890-93 Behring and Kitasato developed the therapeutic inoculation of antitoxins and began their production on a large scale in 1894. Roux in 1892 was the first to use antitoxin from the horse in human cases.

Meanwhile the early serologists were investigating other proper-

---

*Proc. Am. Assn. Adv. Science, 1881. Salem, 1882, XXX, p. 83-94.

ties of the blood-serum in relation to immunity. Nuttall in 1886 first noted the bactericidal property of blood-serum. Buchner in 1889 showed that serum heated to 55°C. lost its bactericidal power. In 1894-5 Pfeiffer showed that specific protective substances are developed in the blood when cultures containing dead or living cholera spirilla or typhoid bacilli are injected into animals or man. Bordet in 1895 reported the method of activating serum which had lost its bactericidal properties by the addition of fresh serum from an untreated animal. In March, 1896, Pfeiffer and Kolle published their paper giving a method of differential diagnosis of typhoid fever by means of the serum of immunized animals. In 1898 Bordet, Gengou, and Durham extended the idea of bacteriolosis to include all cells in the process of cytolysis.

Following the introduction of diphtheria antitoxin by Behring in 1894 several important contributions to the control of diphtheria have been made by the bacteriologists. First came the suggestion by Theobald Smith in 1907 that a toxin-antitoxin mixture might be used in immunization, which was first put into practice by Behring in 1912, and which is now coming to be so generally used in the immunization of children. In 1910 Wesbrook, Wilson, and McDaniel published their valuable classification of the several different morphological types of the diphtheria bacillus. In 1913 Schick reported his cutaneous toxin reaction for determining the presence of immunity to diphtheria, which is now used in connection with the application of toxin-antitoxin immunization.

In 1901 Bordet and Gengou demonstrated the phenomenon of complement fixation which became the basis of Wassermann's complement fixation method for the diagnosis of syphilis (1906). Müller and Openheim (1906) applied the same method to the diagnosis of gonococcus infection, and others have extended it to glanders, meningitis, tuberculosis, and typhoid fever with greater or less success.

Agglutination of bacteria by immune sera was probably first noted by Charrin and Roger in 1889, but was first extensively studied by Gruber and Durham in 1896. Widal a few months later (June, 1896) reported its application to the diagnosis of typhoid fever, and in the same year Wyatt Johnston, of Montreal, suggested the dried blood method of sending specimens to the laboratory for diagnosis, and this method was adopted by the health department laboratories of Montreal and New York City in October, 1896, and is now used wherever typhoid diagnosis is undertaken.

In 1874 Dallera reported the peculiar eruptions following transfusions of blood, called serum sickness. In 1894 when diphtheria antitoxin came into use they were extensively noted. Heubner and von Bokay showed that they were due to the serum and not to the antitoxin. Magendi had already in 1839 observed a sensitiveness in experimental animals to successive inoculations of egg albumen. Richet (1902) extended the observation to other proteins and called the phenomenon anaphylaxis. Von Pirquet and Schick (1903) showed that serum sickness and anaphylaxis were the same sort of phenomena, Arthus (1903), Theobald Smith (before 1903), Rosenau and Anderson (1906), Otto (1906), Vaughan (1907), Besredka (1907), Gay (1908), Friedberger (1910), and others contributed to our further knowledge of the subject, which has recently developed into a more complete understanding of some of the peculiar diseases now called protein hypersensitiveness, such as certain forms of asthma, food idiosyncrasies, and hay fevers.

It was in 1905-6 that Jochmann made the first successful use of immune serum in cases of human cerebrospinal meningitis by the intraspinal method. The wonderfully successful results obtained in this disease by Flexner and his co-workers at the Rockefeller Institute (1913) are entitled to special mention in any history of the achievements of bacteriological science in America.

Vaccination against typhoid fever began in 1896, having been developed by Chantmesse and Widal in France in 1888, by Pfeiffer and Kolle in Germany in 1896, and independently by Wright in England in 1896. Wright introduced typhoid vaccination in the English Army in India in 1898 and during the Boer War in 1900, and Russell in the United States Army in 1909.

The true nature of the phenomenon of phagocytosis was pointed out by Wright and Douglass and to them we must credit the discovery of the opsonins in 1903, although similar substances were found independently by Neufeld and Rimpau, the same year, and called bacteriotropins. To Wright also we owe the method of determining the opsonic index of the blood (1900).

These are but few of the lines along which European and American bacteriologists and immunologists have been working during the last fifty years. Already the results of their studies are making an impression upon the public health work of to-day. Contagion is no longer feared as some intangible, unknown effluvium permeating the atmosphere against which we have no protection. Bacteriology has taught us that the communicable diseases are caused by specific microörganisms which live and grow in the bodies of men and animals and plants; that when these disease-producing microörganisms escape from their natural habitat they die more or less quickly; that the secretions and excretions coming rather directly from the bodies of the sick, and sometimes the well, are the real carriers of contagion. Bacteriology has taught us the parts played by the air, water, sewage, milk, and insects, in the spread of disease, and has developed for us special methods of protection. Not only this, but bacteriology has taught us accurate methods of diagnosing disease, methods of specific immunization against disease, and, last but not least, methods of curing disease and saving lives by the use of vaccines, sera, and antitoxins. Could we but number the cases of disease prevented, the lives saved, by the adoption of these ideas in public health work, we would know something of the debt which we owe to these indefatigable workers following in the footsteps of the illustrious Pasteur.

Glorious as has been this history, it is not complete without mention of the illustrious bead-roll of martyrs who sacrificed their lives in investigating the diseases with which their names are associated: Daniel A. Carrion, verruges; Jesse W. Lazear and Walter Meyers, yellow fever; Alexandre Yersin, and Hermann F. Müller, bubonic plague; Tito Carbone, Malta fever; Louis Ferdinand Thuillier, Asiatic cholera; Allan MacFadyen, typhoid and Malta fevers; J. Everett Dutton, African relapsing fever; Howard T. Ricketts, and and James Francis Coneffe, tabardillo; and Thomas B. McClintock, Rocky Mountain fever.

AMERICAN INSTITUTIONS, ASSOCIATIONS, and PUBLICATIONS

Pasteur's desire for millions to endow research has been fulfilled. Institutions and laboratories for investigation of disease have been established throughout the world. In 1872 Pettenkofer secured from the Bavarian government a grant of funds to establish his hygienic institute which was opened for study and research in 1878, the first of its kind in the world. The first research laboratory in this country was founded by Andrew Carnegie in connection with the Bellevue Hospital Medical College in 1884. The first hygienic laboratory in this country was the Laboratory of Hygiene of the University of Pennsylvania, Philadelphia, established in 1892. Among other institutions in this country we need only to mention the Carnegie Institution of Washington, the Harriman Research Laboratory of the Roosevelt Hospital of New York, the John McCormick Institute for Infectious Diseases of Chicago, the Community Health and Tuberculosis Demonstration Fund of the Metropolitan Life Insurance Company of New York, the Nelson Morris Memorial Institute for Medical Research of Chicago, the Rockefeller Foundation and the Rockefeller Institute for Medical Research of New York, to show how abundantly the millions desired by Pasteur have been supplied for the advancement of his beloved science.

The creation of public health laboratories by cities and states for the diagnosis of disease, for the preparation of curative antitoxins, sera, and vaccines, for the investigation of epidemics, for the control of water supplies and sewage disposal, and for research, has also progressed with remarkable rapidity. The first municipal laboratory in this country was established in Providence in 1888 by Dr. G. T. Swarts, who was then medical inspector under Dr. C. V. Chapin. At first this laboratory undertook only the study of water supplies and filters, and made an investigation of a typhoid epidemic caused by a polluted water supply, but later developed the general diagnosis work of a public health laboratory. Dr. Swarts was later elected secretary of the Rhode Island State Board of Health, and on September 1, 1894, he established the first state laboratory. Rhode Island was the first state to distribute free diphtheria antitoxin and preventive outfits

ophthalmia in babies.   In 1914 all of the states except New Mexico and Wyoming had established public health laboratories in connection with their boards of health.   The Hygienic Laboratory of the United States Public Health Service at Washington was authorized by Congress in 1901.

The universities and colleges of the country, especially those with medical schools, have contributed materially to the development of public health bacteriology.   Welch at Bellevue Hospital Medical College in 1878, and Prudden at the College of Physicians and Surgeons in 1879 were the first to establish laboratories for teaching and research. Now such laboratories are universally found in every institution worthy the name of college or university.

It was but natural that special societies should spring into existence to foster the acquaintanceship of the workers in bacteriology and public health, for the interchange of information, and for discussion of the subjects in which all were interested.   In 1899 the Laboratory Section of the American Public Health Association was organized, with Dr. Theobald Smith, chairman, and Dr. Wyatt Johnston, secretary. In 1899 also the Society of American Bacteriologists was founded, an offshoot of the American Society of Naturalists, with Professor W. T. Sedgwick, president, and Professor H. W. Conn, secretary.   In 1901 came the Association of American Pathologists and Bacteriologists, with Dr. W. T. Councilman, president, and Dr. H. C. Ernst, secretary. In 1914 the American Association of Immunologists was organized.

To mention only the American journals which have been founded for the distribution of information in the fields of public health and bacteriology we must include some of the best known in the world. The *Journal of Medical Research* was first started as the *Journal of the Boston Society of the Medical Sciences* in 1896, and in 1901 it became the official organ of the American Association of Pathologists and Bacteriologists.   The *American Journal of Public Health* was at first the *Journal of the Massachusetts Association of Boards of Health.*   In 1906 it became the *American Journal of Public Hygiene*, in 1911 the *Journal of the American Public Health Association*, and, finally, in 1921, the *American Journal of Public Health.*   The *Journal of Infectious Dis-*

eases was founded in 1904 by the John McCormick Institute for Infectious Diseases. The *Journal of Experimental Medicine* was begun in 1896, and in 1905 was published under the auspices of the Rockefeller Institute. The *Journal of Immunology* and the *Journal of Laboratory and Clinical Medicine* date from 1915. The *Journal of Bacteriology* was established by the Society of American Bacteriologists in 1916, and in 1917 the *Abstracts of Bacteriology* was begun by the same society. In 1919 came the *Journal of Industrial Hygiene*, and in 1921 the *American Journal of Hygiene*. In addition to these we have also the numerous publications of the United States Public Health Service, the United States Department of Agriculture, the state experiment stations, and the state and city boards of health.

Such is the record of the brilliant yet solid and substantial growth of bacteriology and its contributions to public health and human welfare. It is eminently proper that the names of those who have contributed to this growth, some of whom have sacrificed their lives in promoting it, be given places of highest honor in the records of the American Public Health Association.

AMERICAN MORTALITY PROGRESS DURING THE LAST HALF CENTURY

FREDERICK L. HOFFMAN

Third Vice-President and Statistician, Prudential Insurance Company of America

FOR want of time and opportunity I can not adequately discuss this important question. The literature of the subject is much more extensive than is generally known. The theoretical difficulties of the question are serious on account of the very complex nature of our population changes, both as to racial distribution and age composition during the intervening period. There are those who believe that the only true measure of mortality changes is the life table. Personally, I have never shared this conviction, which would set aside an enormous amount of much more conveniently available material. There are also those who believe that life insurance experience is a more accurate measure of mortality changes than the attainment of such changes by means of life tables based on the general population. This view is also opposed to my own, which rather leans towards the conviction that life insurance experience is primarily for life insurance purposes involving the calculation of pecuniary contingencies depending upon death or survivorship. It must be readily granted that all life tables for the general population suffer from the inherent uncertainty as regards the exposed to risk. It is of necessity assumed that the age, sex and race distribution of the population remains the same, or is modified according to known principles during the period intervening between two census enumerations. It is further assumed that the enumeration as to age, race and sex composition of the population has the same intrinsic accuracy as the mortality records derived from registration sources. But both of these assumptions may lead seriously astray. There is the further inherent uncertainty due to a mathematical compromise to give to life-table calculations an appearance of smoothness which may not represent the true facts in the case.

One of the most important observations on this aspect of the question is a brief and hardly-known essay entitled "Is There A Materially Greater Risk in the Assurance of a Select Life of from 40 to 45, than of a Select Life of from 20 to 25, for One Year?" by William Spens, contributed to the *Proceedings of the Institute of Actuaries*, Glasgow Scotland, November 25, 1850. Even more important is the question of the true mortality rate in late adolescence, which is possibly lower than in early adolescence, according to the calculations and investigations made by T. E. Young, the well-known actuary and author of a standard treatise on insurance. Although time and again attention has been called to the fact that the mortality between 18 and 21 may possibly be higher than, say, between 21 and 25, there has been very little critical discussion of a problem of the first importance in practical health administration. To permit of a graduated premium increasing with increasing age from 15 years upwards it is, of course, essential that a graduated increasing mortality curve should be used. The forced construction of such tables for life insurance purposes gives an appearance of increasing regularity in the death-rate during early adolescence which may be opposed to the exact truth of mortality experience. For public health purposes the precise death-rates by single years of life are absolutely essential, and the application of mathematical graduation processes is therefore not only uncalled for but possibly the means of giving wrongful impressions.

History of Mortality Table Construction

I need not on this occasion enlarge upon the sources and characteristics of the principal mortality tables, since this matter has been made one of admirable discussion by Henry Moir and his associates in behalf of the Actuarial Society of America (New York, 1919). I may recall that the first life table used for life insurance purposes was the so-called Northampton Table, constructed by Rev. Richard Price in 1771, who devised a more complete table in 1783. This was followed by the Carlisle Table, constructed in 1815 by Joshua Milne from materials contained in a tract published by Dr. John Heysham at Carlisle in 1797. Those who care to pursue this question further should consult *The Life of John Heysham, M. D.* and his correspondence with Mr. Joshua

Milne, edited by Henry Lonsdale, M. D., London, 1870. An exceedingly valuable primer on the construction of mortality and sickness tables has in recent years been written by Messrs. Elderton and Fippard, of the Institute of Actuaries, and published in London, 1914.

The earliest American life table was by Edward Wigglesworth, D. D., issued in the year 1789, under the title "A Table Shewing the Probability of the Duration, the Decrement, and the Expectation of Life, in the States of Massachusetts and New Hampshire, formed from Sixty-two Bills of Mortality on the Files of the American Academy of Arts and Sciences in the year 1789." Since this table is historically of the first order — though practically inaccessible to the average student — the entire text of the discussion is here included as a suggestion of the physical study of American mortality problems. Dr. Wigglesworth introduces the subject in the following observations:

On examination of the bills of mortality, on the files of the Academy, it appears that the Society are under obligation to a considerable number of gentlemen, in different parts of the commonwealth, for the attention which they have paid to this subject. Since their formula has been dispersed through the State, many gentlemen have communicated bills of their respective towns, or parishes, with a topographical description of the same, which will lead to an investigation of the natural causes which produce them, whenever it appears that particular diseases are endemial to any places.

Dr. Wigglesworth indicates a sound grasp of mortality discussion in that he emphasizes the danger of basing conclusions upon mere figures without a clear grasp of correlated facts affecting the numerical results He continues his remarks as follows:

Returns have been made from towns scattered along the seacoast, from Nantucket on the south, to Portland in Casco-bay on the north-east, and through the counties of Middlesex, Worcester and Hampshire, in a western direction. From Hingham, Ipswich, East Kingston, Dover, Portland, Edgartown, Waltham, Ashburnham, Brookfield, and Brimfield, they have been made for a long course of years. And though those which have been made from other places, are for a shorter term, yet, as they are from places very distant from one another, it is presumed that the result, from a combination of the bills, will give a very just representation of the increasing population of this state and New Hampshire, and the longevity of their inhabitants. At least, it will exhibit more authentick evidence on the last of these subjects than has, as yet, been laid before the publick. Should there be any error in the deductions there will be at least an approximation towards the truth; and the table will give the probability, decrement, and expectatation of life, among the inhabitants of this state and New Hampshire, with more accuracy, than has yet been done. Any errors in the deductions may be corrected, by taking the present result for the basis of a new combination with the bills that may hereafter be communicated.

Dr. Wigglesworth here shows a clear conception of the statistical law of large numbers and of the necessity that such calculations as were advanced should rest upon an adequate statistical basis, both as to number and area.

The number of deaths concerned was 4,893, of which 1,942, or 39.7 per cent, occurred during the first five years of life. The table in detail is given below:

WIGGLESWORTH LIFE TABLE (original data) 1789

Number of Deaths at Different Periods of Life out of a Total Mortality of 4,893

Under	5 years		1,942
Between	5	and 10	236
"	10	" 15	136
"	15	" 25	425
"	25	" 35	382
"	35	" 45	349
"	45	" 55	270
"	55	" 65	270
"	65	" 75	372
"	75	" 80	185
"	80	" 85	171
"	85	" 90	193
"	90	" 95	36
"	95	" 100	16

The foregoing data are commented upon as follows:

From these elements the table is formed, by taking the number of deaths as the radix of calculation. This would have given the proportional numbers of persons living, and dying at every age, from the birth to the latest extremity of life, had the annual number of deaths been equal to the births. But by the bills it appears that the births are annually double to the deaths. Therefore, the number of persons of each age, as given by the table, is less than is actually in life together, from an annual excess of 4,893 births. Consequently the expectation of life is less than just, especially in the early periods of life.

Few modern writers as candidly illustrate the inherent difficulties of life-table construction. The table itself, by five-year periods, shows the expectation of life as follows:

7

EXPECTATION OF LIFE ACCORDING TO WIGGLESWORTH
LIFE TABLE — 1789

Expectation at birth	28.15 years
at age 5	40.87 "
at age 10	39.23 "
at age 15	36.16 "
at age 20	34.21 "
at age 25	32.32 "
at age 30	30.24 "
at age 35	28.22 "
at age 40	26.04 "
at age 45	23.92 "
at age 50	21.16 "
at age 55	18.35 "
at age 60	15.43 "
at age 65	12.43 "
at age 70	10.06 "
at age 75	7.83 "
at age 80	5.85 "
at age 85	4.57 "
at age 90	3.73 "
at age 95	1.62 "

In concluding this historically most interesting and otherwise most instructive contribution to actuarial science, Dr. Wigglesworth observes:

The whole number of inhabitants, according to this table, is 140,182, of which 48,183 are persons under 16 years of age, and 91,999 above 16 years of age. By the enumeration of the inhabitants of Massachusetts, the whole number of free males under 16 was 95,453, and above sixteen, 87,189. Therefore, 35,851 persons under 16 must be added to those in the table under 16 to make the table accord with the enumeration, which will give 176,033 inhabitants, produced by an excess of 4,893 annual births. This addition will raise the expectation of a child just born from 28.15 to 35.47 years; of a child of 5 years of age from 40.87 to 48.46 years; of a person of 10 years from 39.23 to 43.23 years; of a person of 15 years from 36.16 to 36.50 years.

In other words, the probable factor of error diminishes with increasing age. Practically all life tables are seriously defective for the earlier years of life and most of the calculations are a matter of scientific conjecture. Beyond the age of 15 years the calculations are more trustworthy, and in adult life they are approximately acceptable as correct. In conclusion Dr. Wigglesworth remarks:

The annual excess of 4,893 births above the deaths, on a stock of 176,033 inhabitants determines the period of duplication to be 25 years and three-tenths of a year. At this rate, the inhabitants of the five New England states are probably increasing at this time by natural population without any consideration being had either to foreign or American accessions. Similar bills, kept in the other states with the same accuracy that they have been kept here, would determine their natural population with a degree of accuracy which would be of utility to the public, and would afford entertainment to persons of a philosophical disposition, both in Europe and America.

Did space permit I would be glad to deal critically with subsequent contributions to American mortality problems. Of interest in this connection are numerous efforts made to arrive at approximate mortality estimates on the basis of deaths alone, the latter over a wide field, for speculation and practical usefulness. Personally I have found mortality records without reference to the exposed to risk, when utilized with extreme care, of the greatest value in arriving at definite conclusions regarding the effect of the environment on the death-rate.

The only practical illustration of this method available for the present purpose is a table and chart for the island of Nantucket, Massachusetts, originally exhibited at the Panama-Pacific Exposition, San Francisco, in 1915. The table merely illustrates the results, but it is my intention, some time in the future, to present the details, inclusive of investigations made practically throughout the whole of the United States during a long period of years. The table and chart indicate a material increase in the average age at death, which, of course, is not the precise equivalent of a fall in the death-rate, but it is, nevertheless, an approximately trustworthy indication of sanitary progress.

THE REDUCTION OF MUNICIPAL DEATH-RATES

Vital statistics previous to the year 1850 must necessarily be accepted with extreme caution. Broadly speaking, there are no reasons for believing that in the main the data are not sufficiently accurate for the purpose of determining approximate mortality changes. For four cities mortality statistics are available for a practically unbroken hundred years, 1815-1914. These cities are New York, Philadelphia, Boston and New Orleans. Consolidating the statistics for these four

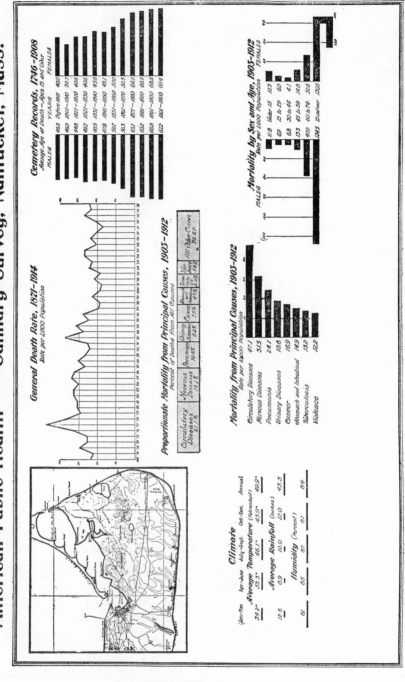

American Public Health ——— Sanitary Survey, Nantucket, Mass.

Statitican's Department, The Prudential Insurance Company of America

cities, the results are shown in the chart herewith reproduced, and which was also shown originally at the San Francisco Exposition. The chart indicates continuous health progress, reduced to 25-year averages, as follows:

The death-rate changed from 28.1 per 1,000 of population during the first quarter-century to 30.2 per 1,000 during the second quarter-century, 25.7 per 1,000 during the third quarter-century, and to 18.9 per 1,000 during the fourth quarter-century. For the last five years the crude death-rates per 1000 of population have been as follows:

1916	-	15.4
1917	-	15.6
1918	-	19.8
1919	-	14.0
1920	-	13.7

Considered individually, the quarter-century changes in the crude death-rate of the four cities vary necessarily from the collective averages. The most pronounced variation is in the case of the city of New Orleans, (1815-1914). The death-rate of this city during the first quarter-century was 52.9 per 1,000; during the second quarter-century 52.4 per 1,000; during the third quarter-century 32.3 per 1,000; and during the fourth quarter-century 23.9 per 1,000. During the last five years the death-rate has been 18.5 per 1,000 for 1916; 20.0 per 1,000 for 1917; 25.7 per 1,000 for 1918; 18.9 per 1,000 for 1919; and 17.6 per 1,000 for 1920. The data for New Orleans for the period 1820-1919 are also shown in graphic form in chart herewith reproduced.

Less suggestive, but not less impressive, are the statistics for New York, Philadelphia and Boston from 1815 to 1914. For New York, particularly, the rates have changed from 28.1 per 1,000 during the first quarter-century to 32.6 per 1,000 during the second quarter-century, to 27.5 per 1,000 during the third quarter-century, and to 18.4 per 1,000 during the fourth quarter-century. For Philadelphia the rates have changed from 23.7 per 1,000 during the first quarter-century to 21.9 per 1,000 during the second quarter-century, to 22.3 per 1,000 during the third quarter-century, and to 18.6 per 1,000 during the fourth quarter-century. For Boston the changes have been from a

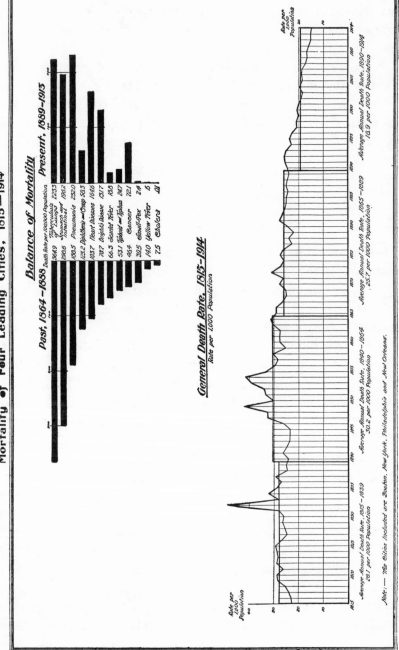

American Public Health —— Past and Present
Mortality of Four Leading Cities, 1815—1914

Balance of Mortality

Past, 1564 – 1888   Present, 1889–1913

General Death Rate, 1815–1914
Rate per 1000 Population

Note:— The cities included are Boston, New York, Philadelphia and New Orleans.

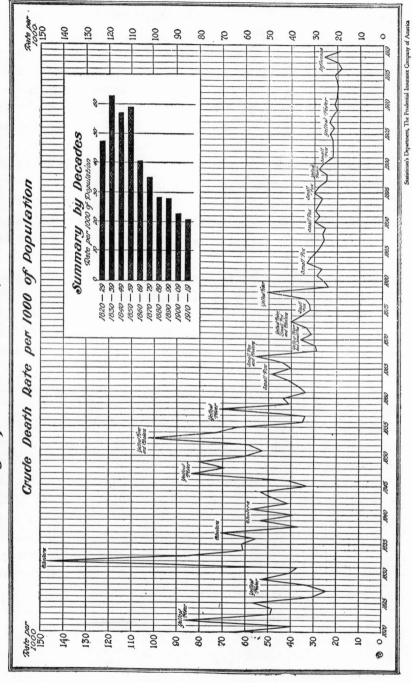

Mortality of New Orleans, La., 1820–1919

Crude Death Rate per 1000 of Population

Summary by Decades
Rate per 1000 of Population

Statistician's Department, The Prudential Insurance Company of America

rate of 21.3 per 1,000 during the first quarter-century to 25.0 per 1,000 during the second quarter-century, to 23.8 per 1,000 during the third quarter-century, and to 19.5 per 1,000 during the fourth quarter-century. The maximum death-rate attained in this country appears to have prevailed, as far as the records show, in the city of New Orleans during the year 1832, due to an epidemic occurrence of yellow fever and cholera that year. Perhaps nothing is more striking than the chart illustration of the earlier epidemic outbreaks compared or contrasted with the nation-wide pandemic of influenza in 1918. Regardless of the epidemic occurrence of this disease, the New Orleans death-rate during 1918 attained to only 25.7 per 1,000 but for Philadelphia, where the outbreak was particularly violent, a maximum rate of 23.9 per 1,000 was reached. The importance of this disease is best illustrated by the Philadelphia chart, which also gives the balance of mortality, a term first used, as far as I know, by the late Dr. Samuel W. Abbott in his analysis of the mortality of Massachusetts. The New Orleans death-rate of 1832 reached the almost incredible figure of 140.9 per 1,000, while during 1822 the attained rate was 88.2 per 1,000. During 1853 the rate, on account of yellow fever, was 118.4, never again reached during any of the subsequent epidemics.

The decade of 1851-60 was notable on account of high mortality rates, which practically marked the end of the era of almost universal sanitary apathy and neglect. The Massachusetts Sanitary Commission made its classical report in 1850 and this was followed in the subsequent decade (1865) by a notable contribution made by the Council of Hygiene and Public Health of the Citizens' Association of the City of New York. In 1857 the *Sixteenth Annual Report of the Massachusetts Registration Department* contained the first Massachusetts Life, Population and Annuity Table, prepared by E. B. Elliott, a noted acutary of his time. The table was introduced with some very interesting observations, from which I can only quote, for the present purpose, the following remarks:

The question here very forcibly arises, have the records of registration in Massachusetts, or in any considerable portion thereof ever been sufficiently complete to enable any one to determine with reliable accuracy, what law or laws do prevail over the mortality of the inhabitants of the state, or such portions of it? We consider this question, and its answer, taken in their broadest sense and application, as the most important practical consideration connected with our system of registration; and it affords extreme gratification to be able to give an affirmative answer to the question. Aside from its intrinsic value, it is creditable to the state of Massachusetts, because it is the *first* instance where such data have been thus furnished and thus used, in any considerable community on this continent. The great practical results in the variety of their applications, of such laborious deductions, will furnish, not only immediately but for years to come, the government and intelligent statesmen as well as others, with the means of determining many social and political questions of high practical value hitherto undeterminable.

The discussion includes some very useful references to early life tables, commencing with the one prepared by Halley, the astronomer and mathematician, in 1693, and the first English life table, constructed by William Farr, M. D., in 1843 from data contained in the *Report of the Registrar-General of England and Wales* and the Census of 1841.

It is a source of gratification to be able to make record of the fact that the first Massachusetts life table was constructed for the New England Mutual Life Insurance Company of Boston, and was originally published in the *Proceedings of the American Association for the Advancement of Science*, 1857. The table unquestionably represented a compromise on account of defects in the original data, but there are no reasons for questioning its intrinsic value as representing approximately the mortality experience of the period. The table was based upon a registered mortality of 16,086 deaths. Attention is called to the fact that the Massachusetts population had increased much more rapidly than the population of the principal countries of Europe, but there had unquestionably been a decline in the birth-rate since the earlier table of Dr. Wigglesworth was made public. The expectation of life for persons, with comparative data for Prussia, also compiled by Mr. Elliott, indicates higher values throughout for the Massachusetts commonwealth, excepting at ages 85 and over.

COMPARATIVE EXPECTATION OF LIFE
IN MASSACHUSETTS, 1855, AND IN PRUSSIA, 1839-41
E. B. ELLIOTT

Ages	Massachusetts	Prussia	Ages	Massachusetts	Prussia
0	39.8	36.7	60	15.0	11.2
15	43.0	41.2	75	6.8	6.0
30	34.0	30.6	90	2.9	3.0
45	24.6	20.4			

Among the interesting deductions from the tables presented, mention may be made of one conclusion:

The period of life in which the mortality of Massachusetts is greater than in European nations lies between about ages 16 and 37, which is perhaps the most important and valuable portion of human existence. These 21 years of early maturity and active adult life comprise that part which is characterized by the most energy and least experience in business transactions, and this fact is suggestive whether the peculiarities of the New Englander — his precocious business habits and the intensity with which he assumes and pursues responsible duties — render health and life more precarious at these ages than is apparent in older countries with different customs.

I cannot enlarge upon the interesting speculations advanced further than to say that the population of every new country, on attaining normal conditions of living, should naturally, as a matter of population selection, present a more favorable aspect than older countries, from which the more vigorous may have emigrated, while the evil consequences of population concentration assume a more serious form.

In connection with the census of 1880, the late Dr. John S. Billings communicated a number of interesting local life tables, which have never received the attention of which they are deserving as contributions to mortality knowledge. They were overshadowed by the importance attached to the American Experience Table, developed from the experience and records of thirty American life offices, under the direction of a committee of actuaries, by Levi W. Meech, actuary in charge. But life insurance experience can never serve as a substitute for general population data, and for practical purposes the tables constructed by Dr. Billings were of a higher degree of intrinsic value. The American experience represents the results contributed by thirty American insurance companies, an aggregate net number of policies or lives given as 1,027,529, of which number 46,543 had died. A revised edition of the American table was issued in 1886. As early as 1858 there had been issued a report exhibiting the experience of the Mutual Life Insurance Company of New York, representing the first fifteen years of the Company's experience. This is a really extraordinary document, unfortunately not as well known as it deserves to be, containing, in addition, much useful information on mortality contingencies. The author of this report was Sheppard Homans, an actuary of extraordinary ability, to whom the American actuarial profession, and life insurance generally, is under a lasting obligation. Other insurance companies contributed much useful information, readily ascertainable from the consolidation of tables by Henry Moir, in "Sources and Characteristics of the Principal Mortality Tables," published as Actuarial Study No. 1, by the American Actuarial Society, New York, 1919. In this work the American Experience Table, as originally constructed by Sheppard Homans, is stated to have been published in 1868, it being explained that the author had used the statistics deduced from the experience of the Mutual Life Insurance Company of New York, and, finding the figures inadequate at the older ages, arbitrarily adjusted the table, which, of course, limited its value. The American Experience Table, to which reference has previously been made was originally compiled by Levi W. Meech in 1881, giving it, therefore, a position of secondary importance.

The excessive mortality rate of American cities at this period no doubt suggested exhaustive inquiries on the part of life insurance companies, mention being made here only of the report on the "Vital Statistics of the United States," submitted to the Mutual Life Insurance Company of New York by James Wynne, M. D., New York, 1857. This exceptionally interesting publication includes observations on the influence of seasons and sources of moisture; on mortality; on influence of locality; on occupations, etc., typical of the thoroughness with which matters of this kind were dealt with at a period often assumed to have been far behind the present period. E. B. Elliott, who had constructed the original Massachusetts Life Table, was the author of a brief but important paper on "Deductions from Prussian Vital Statistics," contributed to *Hunt's Merchants' Magazine* of July, 1856. The full paper on Vital Statistics (Prussian Mortality) was presented at the annual meeting of the American Association for the Advancement of Science, Cleveland, 1856. Elliott also prepared the preliminary report on the "Mortality and Sickness of the Voluntary Forces of the United States Government during the Civil War," published as Memoir No. 46 of the Sanitary Commission, New York, 1862.

The fall in the death-rate during recent years to proportions considered absolutely unattainable a generation ago has naturally led to a diminution of public and scientific interest in mortality changes. During the early '90's it was an assumed basis of sanitary argument that a crude death-rate of 18 per 1,000 of population might safely be relied upon as an index of physical well-being approached by few communities. This view, among others, was held by the late Dr. Samuel W. Abbott, who, however, readily agreed that a further reduction was feasible without serious difficulty, although never anticipating an average death-rate for the registration area of less than 15 per 1,000. It is to the credit of Dr. Abbott, for many years secretary of the Massachusetts State Board of Health, that there was published in 1898 a Second Massachusetts Life Table, based upon the experience of the five-year period 1893-97. In introducing this table, Dr. Abbott points out that "The usefulness of life tables is not confined to the work of life insurance. A life table also serves as an index of the sanitary condition of the community out of whose data it is constructed." But, he points out, "The work of constructing a life table for any American state or city is necessarily less satisfactory in its results than the work of making similar tables for any of the civilized nations or communities of Europe, since most foreign populations are much more stationary than our own." This difficulty, of course, is inherent in the mortality calculations of all new countries, and particularly so in the case of a nation which has experienced so enormous an influx of foreign elements as was the case with the United States previous to 1915. The Massachusetts Life Table includes 240,215 deaths. It is evident, therefore, that a larger number must be recognized for the purpose of similar calculations. Dr. Abbott quotes a statement by Dr. Billings in the introductory remarks to Volume XII of the Reports of the Census of 1880:

The preparation for any given locality, race, or occupation *in this country,* of a life table which shall accurately represent the tendency to death or the probability of survival at each age, is practically impossible, because of the want of accuracy in the necessary data and because of the irregular migrations of the population. It should be clearly understood that all tables of vital statistics, including data derived from large numbers of people, even when these are obtained by the most accurate census possible, and by the most complete system of registration which can be enforced, give probabilities only, and that scientific accuracy is practically unattainable.

In explanation of the results of his investigation, Dr. Abbott remarks:

These figures present very decided differences as compared with those which were published in 1855 by Mr. E. B. Elliott. In those reports it was shown that the numbers dying before the close of the first year out of 100,000 born, were 15,510, or very nearly the same as those for the year 1895 for the same age. At the end of three years the survivors were only 74 per cent instead of 79 per cent as in 1895, and that one-half had died before the close of the 41st year instead of surviving to the 53d year, as in 1895.

In further explanation of the changes in the death-rate of Massachusetts, it is said that:

The death-rate of children under five, specially of those under one year of age, has not undergone very marked changes, but that of all ages from five to forty has very perceptibly diminished, while that of ages above forty has greatly increased. This result has been produced by the great reduction in the number of deaths from infectious diseases, including consumption, which occur in the early period of life from two years up to thirty. By this means a much larger ratio of the population than formerly survives to live throughout the useful and wage-earning period of life. This causes a material increase in the number of years lived at the later ages of life.

These persons being spared from the diseases incident to childhood, the relative mortality from the diseases of adult life and of old age is naturally increased.

This decided increase in the number of survivors throughout the useful ages of life has a marked effect upon the vitality of the population. It is undoubtedly due in no small degree to the increased attention which has everywhere been given in the past twenty-five years to public hygiene.

THE REDUCTION OF SPECIFIC MORTALITY RATES

The questions here involved require more extended consideration than I am able to give the subject at this time. Theoretically it is probably true that the diminution of the mortality from one prevailing cause increases the liability to death from another. Ultimately, of course, all must die, but it is precisely the point of view of preventive medicine that every disease can be reduced in relative frequency to the extent that the causative factors or conditional circumstances responsible for the occurrence are now understood and applied. It does not necessarily follow that because the mortality from tuberculosis has been diminished the mortality from cancer must increase. But in the case of Massachusetts and other New England states there are other and far more profound effects which require consideration. The composition of the population has undergone a profound change. The vast influx of French-Canadians with a high birth-rate, and of Portuguese with a possible degree of Negro intermixture, as well as the immense Italian, Syrian, Armenian, and Greek immigration, has unquestionably a decided effect upon the general death-rate, which can only be determined by painstaking and extended analysis. Still there can be no doubt that there has been a very substantial progress in the health of the state of Massachusetts during the past fifty years. There certainly has been a tremendous decline in infant mortality and a corresponding and equally pronounced diminution in the mortality from tuberculosis, while the reduction in the frequency of typhoid fever seems almost unbelievable, or, respectively, from a rate of 71.5 per 100,000 of population during the decade 1869-78 to 7.4 per 100,000 during the decade ending with 1918, and less than 5 per 100,000 during the last two years. Among diseases of children there is nothing more startling than the enormous diminution in the mortality from diphtheria which, during the middle 70's, reached a rate of nearly 65 per 10,000 for ages under 15 years, while the rate at the present time is less than 5 per 10,000. The tuberculosis death-rate of Massachusetts has declined from more than 40 per 10,000 of population during the early 70's to less than 15 per 10,000 during 1918.

These mortality reductions have been practically universal throughout the country. It would carry me entirely too far to consider in detail the decline in the death-rate of particular states and cities. Perhaps a suitable illustration for the present purpose is the gratifying mortality record of Chicago, showing the following results: Typhoid fever has been reduced from an average rate of 85.2 per 100,000 of population during 1851-60 to only 5.4 per 100,000 during 1911-20. This extraordinary improvement in mortality will be more fully realized when it is stated that a maximum typhoid fever rate of 175.1 was recorded for the year 1854. The mortality from all forms of tuberculosis also declined from a rate of 222.9 per 100,000 during the decade 1871-80 to 161.1 per 100,000 during the decade ending with 1920. During the year 1920 the rate was as low as 97.1 per 100,000, or the lowest on record

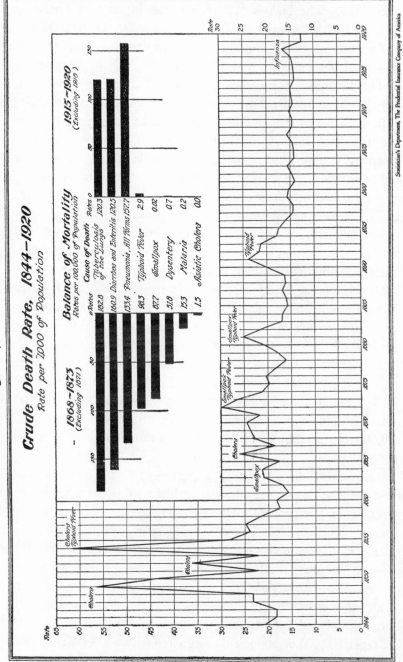

Mortality of Chicago, III.

Crude Death Rate, 1844–1920
Rate per 1000 of Population

Balance of Mortality
Rates per 100,000 of Population

1868–1873
(Excluding 1871)

Rates	Cause of Death	Rates
182.8	Tuberculosis of the Lungs	120.3
160.9	Diarrhea and Enteritis	120.5
133.4	Pneumonia, All Forms	152.7
98.3	Typhoid Fever	2.9
67.7	Smallpox	0.02
51.8	Dysentery	0.7
15.3	Malaria	0.2
1.5	Asiatic Cholera	0.0

1915–1920
(Excluding 1918)

Statistician's Department, The Prudential Insurance Company of America

since 1867. The highest tuberculosis death-rate was reached in the year 1872 with 296.9 per 100,000, or nearly 200 per 100,000 in excess of the rate for 1920. For pulmonary tuberculosis only, the rate has declined from 185.8 per 100,000 during 1861-70 to 130.6 per 100,000 during 1911-20. For smallpox the rate has been reduced to practically nothing against high death-rates from that cause during the years previous to 1894. The average rate has been reduced from 36.3 per 100,000 in 1861-70 to 0.1 during 1911-20. Cholera prevailed to an enormous extent during the early years of the record, or between 1851 and 1860, when the average rate was as high as 328.9 per 100,000. There have been no deaths from cholera since the last outbreak of the disease in 1873. Equally extraordinary has been the diminution in the acute infectious diseases of children. At ages under 10 the mortality from diphtheria and croup has diminished from a maximum rate of 579.5 per 100,000 of population under 10 during the decade 1881-90 to a rate of 172.8 per 100,000 during 1911-20, and a rate as low as 120.8 per 100,000 during the year 1920. The scarlet fever rate has been reduced from a maximum average of 629.2 per 100,000 during 1871-80 to a rate of 74.3 per 100,000 during 1911-20, and a rate of 34.7 per 100,000 during the year 1920. For measles the rate has been reduced from a maximum average of 128.4 per 100,000 during 1861-70 to a rate of 34.0 per 100,000 during 1911-20 and a rate of 16.8 during the year 1920. The mortality from whooping cough has declined from an average rate of 111.8 per 100,000 during 1861-70 and 1871-80 to a rate of only 28.5 per 100,000 during 1911-20.

Reviewing the mortality experience of the last half-century, most of the important diseases which are looked upon as preventable or postponable have been reduced. In other words, the diseases which are considered the efficiency test in health administration clearly emphasize that excellent and far-reaching results have followed initiative and energy in public health administration.

Equally satisfactory conclusions could be advanced with regard to all other important communities. In San Francisco, for illustration, the mortality from tuberculosis during the period 1884-88 was 323.6 per 100,000 of population compared with a mortality of 195.3 per

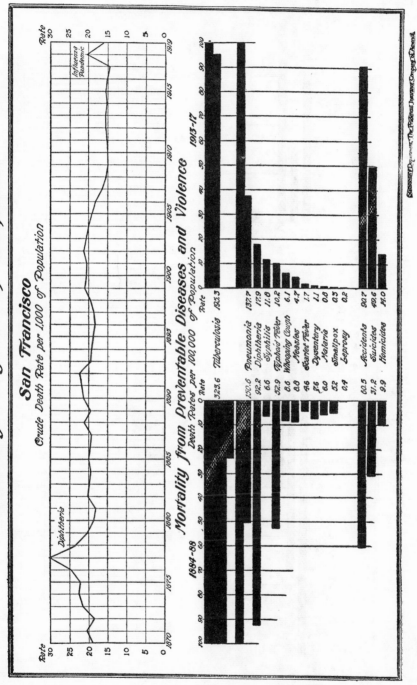

Sanitary Progress of California

San Francisco

Crude Death Rate per 1000 of Population

Mortality from Preventable Diseases and Violence

Death Rates per 100,000 of Population

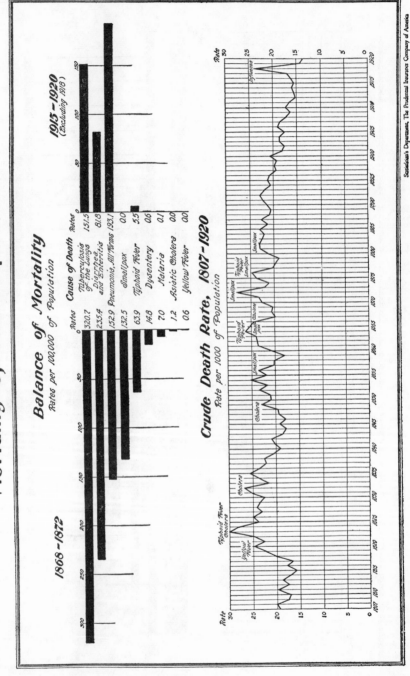

Mortality of Philadelphia, Pa.

Balance of Mortality
Rates per 100,000 of Population

1868-1872

1915-1920
(Excluding 1918)

Rates	Cause of Death	Rates
320.7	Tuberculosis of the Lungs	151.5
235.4	Diarrhea and Enteritis	81.8
152.9	Pneumonia, All Forms	193.1
132.5	Smallpox	0.0
63.9	Typhoid Fever	5.5
14.8	Dysentery	0.6
7.0	Malaria	0.1
1.2	Asiatic Cholera	0.0
0.6	Yellow Fever	0.0

Crude Death Rate, 1807-1920
Rate per 1000 of Population

Statistician's Department, The Prudential Insurance Company of America

100,000 during the period 1913-1917. Likewise there has been a reduction in the rate from pneumonia, diphtheria, typhoid fever, whooping-cough, measles, etc. The balance of mortality for New Orleans reveals similar results. Comparing the period 1864-88 with the period 1889-1913, the mortality from pulmonary tuberculosis has declined from 396.5 per 100,000 to 310.7 per 100,000; from diseases of the stomach,323.6 per 100,000 to 240.7 per 100,000; from smallpox, 136.9 per 100,000 to 11.6 per 100,000; from diphtheria and croup, 58.9 per 100,000 to 29.5 per 100,000; from typhoid fever, 53.6 per 100,000 to 48.9 per 100,000; from scarlet fever, 23.9 per 100,000 to 3.9 per 100,000.

I conclude these observations with the data for the city of Philadelphia, excluding, however, for the present purpose the influenza pandemic of 1918. Comparing the period 1868-72 with the period 1915-20 (exclusive of 1918) the mortality from pulmonary tuberclosis has declined from 320.7 per 100,000 to 151.5 per 100,000; for diarrhea and enteritis, from 235.4 per 100,000 to 81.8 per 100,000; for smallpox, from 132.5 per 100,000 to no deaths in the last period under observation; for typhoid fever, from 63.9 per 100,000 to 5.5 per 100,000; for dysentery, from 14.8 per 100,000 to 0.6 per 100,000; for malaria, from 7.0 per 100,000 to 0.1 per 100,000; for Asiatic cholera, from 1.2 per 100,000 to 0.0 per 100,000; and for yellow fever, from 0.6 per 100,000 to 0.0 per 100,000. These observations must be sufficient for the present purpose of emphasizing the mortality progress of the United States during the last half-century. No life tables for the nation as a whole are available for earlier periods to justify definite conclusions measurable in terms of greater exactness and precision. It is to the credit of Sam L. Rogers, director of the census from 1915 to 1921, and Prof. James W. Glover, University of Michigan, that a thoroughly trustworthy and comprehensive life table for the original registration states in the United States Registration Area and selected states was prepared for the census of 1910, based on the estimated population July 1, 1910 (24,131,759), and on the reported deaths in 1909 (353,576), in 1910 (377,015), and in 1911 (368,067). The original registration states include Maine, New Hampshire, Vermont, Massachusetts, Rhode Island, Connecticut, New York, New Jersey, Indiana and Michigan, and the District of Columbia.

It is observed in the introductory note by Mr. Rogers that "These tables, being based on the general unselected population, differ materially from tables derived from experience of life insurance companies, because the latter are based on risks selected through medical examination and otherwise." The tables constructed by Professor Glover have the advantage of being approved by an advisory committee appointed by the Actuarial Society of America, composed of John K. Gore, Chairman, Robert Henderson, Arthur Hunter, Emory McClintock, and Henry Moir. Special credit is also due to the former chief statistician of vital statistics, Dr. Cressy L. Wilbur. Since there are no comparative statistics for previous periods, it will be sufficient for the present purpose to give the expectation of life for the population of this registration area for both sexes for ages 15, 30, 45, 60, 75 and 90.

AGE	EXPECTATION OF LIFE
15	47.73 years
30	35.70 "
45	24.54 "
60	14.42 "
75	6.99 "
90	3.03 "

These results will bear favorable comparison with any other country in the world. Slight differences can not be considered as of material importance, in that the the mathematical methods employed in life-table construction may be sufficient to account for some differences, aside from the intrinsic trustworthy value of the data themselves. Those who may wish to pursue the study of this subject further should consult an important article entitled "Derivation of the United States Mortality Table by Osculatory Interpolation," by Prof. James W. Glover, contained in the *Quarterly Publications of the American Statistical Association* for June, 1910.

CONCLUSION

Much to my regret, want of time and opportunity precludes more extended critical consideration of a subject to which I have given attention for more than thirty years. In its final analysis, observational experience is as essential to sound judgment as statistical and mathematical calculations. The latter merely reduce to a measurable basis conclusions otherwise vague and indefinite, but nevertheless accurate, if used with restraint and caution, for practical purposes. No one who has observed the actual sanitary progress of American states and cities, even without the aid of statistical data, can fail to have arrived at the conclusion that profound changes for the better have taken place during the last fifteen years. But since it is not given to many to have passed through actual experience, the foregoing statistical data and charts may serve the useful purpose of substantiating the important statement that the United States, in all its essential parts, has made extraordinary health progress during the last decade, which would bear favorable comparison with any corresponding industrial nation of the world. Those who make much of European experience, and in season and out overemphasize what has been done in Germany, do so largely in ignorance of the conditions, which are a matter of common knowledge and recorded facts for this country. For this achievement, than which there is nothing more gratifying in our social and economic history, credit primarily belongs to a comparatively small body of energetic men, who at all times have left nothing undone to advance the cause of public health and preventive medicine, largely through measures and methods of community control. While more could have been done, the evidence is overwhelming that our own achievements are gratifying proof of an enlightened public consciousness in all that concerns the well-being of the citizen in the modern state.

THE UNITED STATES QUARANTINE SYSTEM DURING THE PAST FIFTY YEARS

HUGH S. CUMMING, M. D.

Surgeon General, United States Public Health Service

EARLIER PRACTICES

THE term "quarantine" is one that has been used to cover a variety of procedures. Originally it signified merely isolation — the segregation of those afflicted with maladies thought to be communicable. With the passage of time and the development of accurate knowledge of various diseases, quarantine procedure has undergone remarkable evolution. To the lay mind quarantine still conveys the meaning of detention only — restraint under isolation or with limited communication. To the sanitarian the term includes not only detention, but segregation and the application of disinfection or fumigation, and similar preventive measures based on definite epidemiologic information. Haphazard, arbitrary standards have given way to scientific, precise methods.

It is a matter of speculation as to what year or century restraint was first practised in order to prevent the spread of disease. It is known that isolation of lepers was practised in biblical time, but the measures taken were more or less imperfect. Whatever the efforts may have been in the earlier centuries to prevent the spread of disease, it seems probable that detention of ships and travelers was first practised by Venice in the early part of the fourteenth century, and the term quarantine had its origin in the Italian word "*quarante*," meaning forty, as forty days was the period of detention imposed upon infected vessels. As early as 1348 Venice had a system for the treatment of infected ships, travelers and merchandise. Venice established a quarantine station in 1403, and other ports on the Mediterranean followed this example, Genoa in 1467, and Marseilles in 1526.

At first, time was the main element depended upon for the elimination of contagion. The ship and its personnel and cargo were held isolated until the infection had run its course. Either because the time element alone did not prove effective (by reason, of the unknown rôle of the convalescent carrier), or because of the slowness of the practice, methods were adopted to expedite the elimination of the contagion. Fumigation by boiling aromatic substances came into vogue and sulphur fumes were employed rather generally during the eighteenth century.

During the Middle Ages all sorts of theories were advanced as to the dissemination of disease. The doctrine of "polluted air," in one form or another, was the one that had the greatest support, and preventive measures were directed toward the purification of the atmosphere. In 1710 England passed a rigorous quarantine act, and even as late as 1721 two ships from Cyprus, where plague was then prevailing, were burned in English waters by the sanitary authorities. In the early part of the nineteenth century, the English quarantine restrictions were greatly modified, and vessels were not subject to detention unless a communicable disease had occurred during the voyage or upon arrival. This procedure has been followed in England and continental Europe to this day.

The American quarantine practice is somewhat stricter, preventive measures being applied not only to ships actually infected, but also to vessels, cargo and personnel from infected ports or territory.

The earlier practice of quarantine seems to have been directed against leprosy, plague and syphilis, and it was not until the eighteenth century that European countries gave attention to cholera and yellow fever, the latter first making its appearance in Europe in 1723, at Lisbon.

In colonial days and during the nineteenth century, in fact up to 1878, quarantine function in the United States was entirely in the hands of the state and local authorities, and was carried out in accordance with the prevailing conception as to the communicability of disease.

It was but natural that prior to the discovery of the specific causation of the disease the methods employed were largely empirical. Following the discoveries of Pasteur, Koch, and their contemporaries, quarantine procedure was placed upon a more rational basis. In addition to the detention and isolation of the sick, those who had been in contact with them were detained for a period equal to the incubation stage of the disease, and measures were adopted to sterilize articles and places infected or thought to be infected. It was the era of promiscuous disinfection and fumigation, and "fomites" were thought to be of prime importance in the dissemination not only of smallpox, but also of yellow fever, plague, cholera and typhus. Ships were washed down with bichloride solution, even to the individual stones in in the ballast, and sulphur was burned in liberal quantities. It is rather interesting to read, in the *Annual Report* of the Marine Hospital Service for the year 1873, that the generous use of carbolic acid solution proved exceptionally effective in the treatment of yellow fever foci.

Although the purpose of fumigation had in view the destruction of bacteria and the disinfection of the environment in the measures applied against yellow fever, plague and typhus, we now know, in looking backward, that although the procedure was based upon a wholly erroneous conception of the etiology of these maladies, nevertheless the results were effective. The sulphur dioxide, futilely employed as a bactericide, was equally efficient in destroying stegomyia, the carrier of yellow fever, the louse, vector of typhus infection, and rats and fleas, transmitters of plague, as though the fumigant had been used for those specific purposes.

EVOLUTION OF MODERN PROCEDURE

Up until the early eighties of the last century quarantine measures were entirely administered by state and local authorities. The *Annual Report* of the Surgeon General of the Marine Hospital Service for the year 1872, however, refers to an order of the Secretary of the Treasury in which the attention of Marine Hospital Service officers, customs officials, and revenue officers was directed to the provisions of the Act of February 25, 1799, which enjoined federal officers to coöperate in the enforcement of quarantine laws and regulations.

On account of their duties in caring for sick seamen, officers of the Marine Hospital Service began to evince more and more interest in epidemics introduced through vessels from infected ports, and this was especially so with respect to yellow fever. The Surgeon General's report of 1873 devoted considerable space to studies of the epidemics in the South. As early as 1833 the Secretary of the Treasury was authorized by Act of Congress to employ additional revenue boats and officers to aid in the enforcement of quarantine laws and regulations, but the Act of April 29, 1878, may be considered as the first definite expression of Congress that the prevention of the introduction of infections diseases was a federal function. This Act provided that the Surgeon General of the Marine Hospital Service (Public Health Service) should draft rules and regulations governing the quarantine treatment of vessels from foreign ports; that consular officers should keep the Surgeon General informed as to the sanitary status of vessels departing for American ports, and should also furnish information each week as to sanitary conditions of the foreign ports at which they were stationed. Provisions were also made for the weekly publication by the Marine Hospital Service of the sanitary data furnished by consular officials, and also empowered officers of the Marine Hospital Service to enforce the national quarantine rules and regulations. This Act embraced all of the salient features of the recommendations submitted by Surgeon General Woodworth at the International Medical Congress in Philadelphia, 1876.

Appropriations were likewise made by Congress in 1878 for "investigating the origin and causes of epidemic diseases, especially yellow fever and cholera, and the best method of preventing their introduction and spread." In 1879 authority was given for the assignment of medical officers to consulates for the purpose of supervising the enforcement of sanitary measures applicable to ships leaving for ports of the United States. In 1882 an epidemic fund was created by Congress, to aid local authorities in suppressing epidemics, and from that time on a similar appropriation became an established custom.

In 1882, the Marine Hospital Service rendered material assistance in the maintenance of a sanitary cordon around Brownsville, Texas, where yellow fever was prevailing. This resulted, according to report of the Governor, in "allaying excitement along the border counties." He also stated that the "efforts made by the Marine Hospital Service were a perfect success in protecting the State from a general epidemic."

DEVELOPMENT OF NATIONAL CONTROL

Dating from 1882 the Marine Hospital Service gradually extended its public health and quarantine activities. Quarantine stations for detention and treatment of infected ships were established by the Service in 1883 at Ship Island (Gulf Quarantine) and at Sapelo Sound (South Atlantic Quarantine). These were the first national quarantine stations. In 1888 additional legislation was secured, providing penalties for violation of quarantine laws and regulations, and in 1893 there was enacted what may fittingly be styled the organic quarantine act. Previously, however, Congress had, in 1890, passed a quarantine law relating to the prevention of the interstate spread of certain infectious diseases, rules and regulations to be prepared by the Surgeon General. The Act of 1893 provided that no vessel from a foreign port should enter a port of the United States except in conformity with the provisions of the Act and rules and regulations made in conformity thereto, and that violations were punishable by a fine not exceeding $5,000. Masters of vessels were directed to secure from the consul or medical officer assigned to the consulate a bill of health, setting forth the sanitary history of the vessel, cargo, crew and passengers. The regulations provided that said bill of health should not be issued unless the vessel had observed all necessary sanitary requirements. The Secretary of the Treasury was directed to promulgate quarantine regulations governing the departure of vessels from foreign ports and their treatment at United States ports of arrival.

This Act also authorized the President to suspend travel from foreign countries to the United States if the sanitary conditions rendered such measure necessary. In the light of modern knowledge of the spread of disease, this radical measure is no longer deemed necessary, since the application of rational preventive measures provides adequate safeguards without material interference with commerce or travel. The Act of February 15, 1893, further authorized the Secretary of the Treasury to acquire the use of state quarantine property when tendered by proper authority, and to pay for the use of same. In June, 1906, Congress further empowered the Secretary of the Treasury to purchase quarantine stations operated by state or local governments when offered by the appropriate authorities, and to pay a reasonable compensation therefor.

The transition of a quarantine system, composed of units operated by the municipal or state authorities, to a compact federal organization has been gradual, but persistent. One after another cities and states have transferred their quarantine stations to the national Government, so that, with the passing of the New York Quarantine Station from state to national control on March 1, 1921, the Public Health Service now administers every station in the United States and in the Hawaiian Islands, the Philippines, Porto Rico, and the Virgin Islands. The desirability of a centralized control of quarantine stations appears so evident it seems strange that its accomplishment has been so long delayed. It is apparent that maritime quarantine should be administered uniformly so as not to prejudice or favor the commerce of a port. One of the objections to local control of quarantine is that there is frequent rotation in the position of quarantine officer, due to local political changes. In addition to its other advantages, national control of quarantine insures the availability of a large corps of trained quarantine officers, whose experience in quarantinable diseases and in quarantine technique has been increased by duty in foreign countries and insular possessions where such diseases mainly prevail. Federal control of quarantine further permits of greater coöperation with other branches of the Federal Government, such as the Immigration and the Customs Services. The Government is also better able to observe the obligations of international sanitary treaties, and to demand reciprocal action on the part of foreign signatories of such treaties.   Finally, as the object of quarantine is not only the protection of the local port, but the entire country, and since the benefits derived therefrom are not merely local in effect, the expense of the maintenance of quarantine stations should be borne by the country as a whole.

In no field of medicine is there a greater necessity for a highly specialized and trained personnel than in maritime quarantine, and the practice of appointment to the position according to a person's political affiliation, as was the common practice under local control of quarantine stations, created potentialities for serious mischief.

Above all other things the quarantine officer must be a capable diagnostician, and especially should he be familiar with those diseases for whose exclusion he stands responsible — plague, cholera, typhus, yellow fever and smallpox.   An accurate determination of any suspected illness on arriving vessels is not only most important for the purpose of safeguarding the port, but is likewise a serious matter to commerce, for errors in diagnosis, even though on the side of safety, may result in needless loss to the vessel's owner, every day a vessel is detained in quarantine meaning a loss of several hundred or several thousand dollars.   The cost of operating some of the larger transatlantic liners amounts to considerably more than $15,000 per day.

The quarantine officer must be a well trained bacteriologist, or else have one as an assistant, because the accurate diagnosis of plague, cholera and leprosy is essentially a laboratory procedure.   Likewise in yellow fever and typhus, while diagnosis is still largely dependent upon clinical evidence, laboratory tests are of great aid.   Also, the quarantine officer must thoroughly understand the manner of the spread of quarantinable diseases and be in a position to quickly familiarize himself with any special feature obtaining in an infected ship so as to speedily apply the essential preventive measures and not waste time in carrying out illogical or unnecessary measures.   He must be well versed in nautical matters and carry in his mind the sanitary condition of practically all the commercially important seaports of the world.   In addition to his professional equipment, the officer in charge of the larger quarantine stations must have administrative ability to operate the station proficiently and with reasonable economy. Above all, he should possess sound judgment, great tact, and at the same time show firmness and resourcefulness to meet the many emergencies that inevitably arise in quarantine administration. It must be clearly evident that the promiscuous selection for the position of quarantine officer of men untrained in the technical duties of the office, no matter how proficient in the general practice of medicine and surgery, is a very faulty custom.

The most striking feature of our existing quarantine system is the effective sanitary protection it affords, with comparatively small interference with maritime commerce or travel, the object aimed at being the maximum protection of the country with a minimum hindrance to commerce and the least inconvenience to the traveling public consistent with effective protective measures. The two objects are by no means inconsistent or conflicting. They are entirely practical in operation.

PRESENT DAY QUARANTINE REQUIREMENTS

According to the United States Quarantine Regulations, the strictly quarantinable diseases are confined to cholera, typhus, plague, smallpox, leprosy and anthrax (the latter applying only as to certain articles of cargo), for the reason, mainly, that these are considered as exotic pestilential diseases, easier to prevent of entrance than of eradication after their introduction. While this does not apply to smallpox, quarantine, nevertheless, tends to prevent the introduction of more virulent strains of the infection and protects against the greater prevalence of the disease.

With respect to infectious diseases of a minor nature, such as measles, whooping cough, scarlet fever, typhoid, venereal infections, etc., no special treatment of ship or contacts is provided for other than reporting to local authorities of the cases, so that they may be detained in local institutions until well.

Against the introduction of quarantinable diseases there are provided certain specific regulations, based upon a knowledge of the transmitting agency.

In cholera, chief attention is paid to the personnel, their food and water supply. The sick are isolated, with appropriate disposal of their excreta, so as to prevent any spread of the infection. Food and water are examined, and, if infected or deemed to have been exposed to infection, are either sterilized by cooking or boiling or otherwise are destroyed. The main reliance in the treatment of a cholera-infected ship, however, is placed on the bacteriological examination of the stools of passengers and crew. All persons who are found to be free of cholera vibrios are released. The sick and the convalescent and immune carriers are detained and isolated until bacteriological examinations become negative. This method is in marked contrast to the former practice, wherein all contacts were arbitrarily detained for a period of five days and then released if well — a practice that did not prevent the admission of carriers and at the same time imposed needless restraint.

In yellow fever the sick are isolated under screening and the contacts are released, if well, six days after last exposure, this to date from the assured destruction of mosquitoes (Stegomyia).

For the prevention of the spread of bubonic plague the destruction of rats and fleas is practised. The sick are detained at quarantine merely for treatment and to prevent public alarm, but comparatively little consideration is given in modern quarantine practice to the possibility of the spread of bubonic plague by passengers or crew.

In typhus, the sick and contacts are detained for the incubation period and treated for the destruction of lice found on their bodies or n their personal effects.

The former favorite practice of bathing with solution of bichloride of mercury and the disinfection of ships by chemical solutions have largely been abandoned and have given way to fumigation by sulphur dioxide, carbon monoxide, or hydrocyanic gas for the destruction of mosquitoes, rats, fleas, bedbugs and lice.

The Public Health Service has made notable progress within the past ten years in standardizing fumigation by cyanide gas and in improving the technique so as to render the procedure comparatively safe in the hands of trained personnel. Sulphur dioxide is a very safe agent, even in unskilled hands, but it is so lacking in power of penetration and of such slow toxicity as compared to cyanide gas or carbon monoxide that it necessitates prolonged exposure, and the compartment treated, whether the hold or superstructure of the vessel, must be clear of cargo or other articles. Studies made by the Service over an extended period clearly prove that sulphur dioxide, when used on vessels for the destruction of rats, is too ineffective to be utilized in the treatment of a plague-infected vessel.

Several thousand vessels have been fumigated at the various quarantine stations during recent years without accident, but an occasional casualty makes it evident that further safeguards must be devised to make the fumigant "fool-proof." When used in connection with a vacuum, cyanide gas is wonderfully effective in destroying, within a very brief exposure, lice, fleas, bedbugs, and other vermin.

During the past fifty years, therefore, our quarantine system has made great progress in the elimination of haphazard, untrustworthy practice and in the adoption of precise methods, and all this has been accomplished with a corresponding lessening of interference with public travel.

The American quarantine system is unique in the maintenance of a double line of sanitary defense. Through the application of preventive measures, at foreign ports of departure, to vessel, cargo, crew and passengers, under the supervision of a medical officer attached to the consulate, our ports are afforded a very substantial protection. The second line of defense by our domestic quarantine stations is and always will be our chief reliance. Naturally the system is by no means infallible — there is always the human element factor. The infection at a foreign port may be concealed or the quarantine officer may prove derelict, but the prevention of the introduction of yellow fever during the past sixteen years, despite its almost continued prevalence in Mexico, Central and South America, is a striking testimonial to the system and the personnel composing it. Not infrequently yellow fever ships have reached our home stations, but so far they have been apprehended and appropriately treated.

Achievements of the United States Quarantine System

On various occasions cholera has seriously threatened, but its advance has been stayed by measures enforced both abroad and at domestic quarantine stations. In 1911 the Public Health Service, working in conjunction with the state force at the port of New York, succeeded in preventing the entry of the infection, and this with but little interference to the traveling public. Thirty-five cases and twenty-seven carriers were detected through the inspection of arriving ships and the examination of the personnel. During the late summer and fall of 1911, 26,930 passengers and crew were subjected to a bacteriological examination, those that were free of the infection were immediately released, and those that were infected, whether actual cases or carriers, were held until free of the infecting agency, one convalescent carrier being held fifty-four days. Some of the carriers were detected on vessels on which, according to the history obtainable, no cases of cholera had occurred. Because of the measures carried out by this government at the port of New York, the Italian Government later on started examination for carriers and cases at the Italian ports of embarkation. As a result of this work, forty carriers were discovered at various ports and at various times among prospective emigrants. The latter were detained in segregated groups for a period of five days before embarkation, this procedure being in conformity with the requirements of the United States Quarantine Regulations. Similar measures have been carried out at Manila, the Hawaiian Islands, and on the Pacific Coast during those periods when cholera threatened from the East.

With our present-day knowledge of typhus and the realization that without vermin there can be no spread of the disease, it can reasonably be expected that in civilized countries the day of typhus epidemics is past. In the tenement quarters of many of our large cities, however, there exist conditions highly conducive to the spread of typhus. It is, therefore, important that every effort be made to prevent the introduction of the infection. From time to time the disease has threatened from a European source, but never more seriously than in the winter of 1920–21, when undue press publicity created widespread alarm in the public mind. On the cessation of hostilities in Europe it became evident that the developments of subsequent months would involve possibilities of sanitary significance to the United States. On account of military operations in Europe the sanitary conditions there had been more or less veiled, and while the areas occupied by the Allied forces were known to be fairly free of epidemic disease, it was a matter of speculation as to the condition in the areas occupied by the Central Powers and in the more easterly part of Europe.

During the war the public mind of the various nations party to the conflict and all the energies and resources of such nations were directed along military channels, and sanitation and public hygiene as a consequence were more or less neglected. On the resumption of commercial intercourse the expected happened. Typhus spread throughout continental Europe by means of returning soldiers, repatriated prisoners, and, to a less extent, by commercial travelers. Even before the armistice this condition of affairs was foreseen. Medical officers of the Public Health Service were sent to Europe to make preparation for the application of preventive measures at European ports of embarkation. All verminous persons coming from typhus-infected areas were required to undergo appropriate treatment, and detention when necessary, before embarkation. Notwithstanding this precaution, however, typhus appeared in some ten or twelve vessels bound for ports of the United States. In addition to the delousing measures applied at European ports of embarkation during the winter of 1920–21, there were similarly treated at American ports of arrival almost 100,000 persons. It is significant, however, that of the vessels on which typhus broke out there were only two vessels in which secondary cases occurred, and these two vessels were from a port where disinfecting procedure had not been carried out. Without a doubt had a similar situation obtained twenty or thirty years before there would have been almost an entire cessation of transatlantic travel. Yet, under modern quarantine procedure, the influx of thousands of travelers from typhus-infected areas of Europe (a greater immigration, in fact, than obtained for many a year past) occurred, with practically no danger of a sanitary nature to localities in the United States to which these people were destined.

Even more serious than the menace from Europe has been the typhus condition in Mexico during several years past. During 1917 and 1918 typhus created greater havoc in Mexico than its more recent appearance accomplished in Central Europe, but notwithstanding the proximity of the infected area lying to the south of us, and the thousands and thousands of travelers, the sanitary safeguards erected along the border were sufficient to prevent the introduction of the infection. For several years past the Public Health Service forces have disinfected (deloused) about 150,000 persons annually at the various ports of entry on the border. The quarantine forces along the southern border also serve to prevent the introduction of the highly virulent strain of smallpox that prevails in Mexico. For the past several years there have been vaccinated annually along the Mexican border between forty and fifty thousand persons.

The Public Health Service to-day operates in the mainland of the United States and its possessions approximately one hundred quarantine stations. At fully equipped quarantine stations there are provided facilities for the boarding and inspection of vessels and personnel; apparatus for mechanical cleansing of vessels; apparatus for disinfecting by steam, by sulphur, by formaldehyde, by cyanide gas, or by disinfecting solutions; also clinical laboratories, hospital for contagious and doubtful cases, steam laundries, detention barracks for suspects, bathing facilities, water supply, and a proper system for the disposal of sewage.

A brief reference to the operations of the national quarantine stations during the past year will afford one a cross-section view of the usual activities carried on by our quarantine system. At national quarantine stations there were inspected approximately 2,000,000 passengers and crew. Twenty thousand vessels were inspected, and 5,000 were fumigated or disinfected. Three thousand nine hundred eighty-six vessels arrived from infected ports, of which number approximately 47 had infection aboard. Somewhat less than 50,000 passengers and crew were detained and disinfected; 4,800 were either vaccinated or subjected to bacteriological examination. Along the Mexican border 55,000 people were vaccinated and 130,000 were disinfected (deloused). At the insular quarantine stations and at foreign ports over 10,000 vessels were inspected by officers of the Public Health Service, of which there were more than 1,500 fumigated, and more than a million and a half passengers and crew inspected.

Officers of the Public Health Service are stationed in the Philippines and in other parts of the Orient, including the coast of China, on the west and east coasts of South America, on the islands of the West Indies, and in all the chief ports of Europe, to enforce sanitary precautions against vessels, cargo, passengers and crew departing for ports of the United States. Whether it be the fumigation of a vessel at the plague-infected port of Hongkong in order to destroy rodent carriers of the disease; whether it be the fumigation of a vessel in the yellow-fever-infected port of Vera Cruz for the purpose of destroying mosquitoes on vessels sailing for ports of the United States; or the delousing of verminous passengers from the typhus-infected areas of Europe, this group of Public Health Service men, working in foreign countries, operates as a tremendous force in safeguarding the ports of the United States from the introduction of quarantinable diseases, and always with but the slightest interference to the traveling public or to the movement of traffic.

Of all civilized countries the United States appears at the present time to have a greater need of maritime quarantine protection than others. European countries are fortunate in having their ports comparatively, if not entirely, free of stegomyia, and hence the introduction of yellow fever is of no concern to those countries. Furthermore, the substantial stone construction on the water-front of the various European ports results in an automatic reduction of rodent population, thus serving as a barrier against the introduction of plague, while the protected water supplies at most of the European ports afford a rather satisfactory insurance against the spread of cholera. In contrast to this more fortunate condition of affairs, a large section of the United States is heavily infested with the yellow fever mosquito, and the intimate commercial intercourse with nearby countries where the disease is endemic necessitates constant surveillance at our southern ports of entry in order to prevent the introduction of the infection. The water-front construction at practically all American ports is of frame, and of such a type as to afford the greatest possible harborage to rats. The water-front along most of our ports is very heavily infested with rodents and affords the most favorable situation imaginable for the introduction of plague. Therefore, quarantine safeguards against the introduction of plague are not only necessary at the present time but will probably continue so for many years to come.

Typhus and cholera are the two epidemic diseases formerly greatly dreaded which today are regarded with much less concern. Nevertheless, there are many places where cholera would spread with the utmost facility if introduced, and the tenement districts of large American cities would probably afford as favorable a condition for the spread of typhus as any part of Europe.

The annual maintenance charge of the American quarantine system is comparatively small in contrast with the benefits and sanitary protection secured through its operation, and it seems improbable that it can be eliminated for many years to come, in fact, not until the internal sanitary condition of the United States is such that quarantinable diseases, even though introduced, can not spread.

HISTORY OF STATE AND MUNICIPAL CONTROL OF DISEASE

CHARLES V. CHAPIN, M. D., Sc. D.

Superintendent of Health, Providence, Rhode Island

PUBLIC HEALTH WORK IN THE SEVENTEENTH AND EIGHTEENTH CENTURIES

D URING the whole of this period, except, perhaps, during the very last years, public health work was occupied chiefly with attempts to control the spread of smallpox, with, perhaps, spasmodic efforts to quarantine against yellow fever. Little attempt was made to control other diseases. The methods employed were, in their main features, similar to those of the present time, namely, quarantine, isolation, immunization and disinfection.

Quarantine. The first sanitary legislation that I know of was the enactment in March, 1648, by the General Court of Massachusetts Bay, of a statute providing for maritime quarantine, because of the prevalence of disease in the West Indies. Owing to the cessation of the epidemic the act was repealed the next year. In 1699, another quarantine act was passed, but on account of its unusual character and stringent regulations was disallowed by the Privy Council. Soon after, quarantine acts were passed in several of the colonies and have remained on the statute books ever since. These laws were sometimes administered by the colonies and sometimes by the towns. Gradually maritime and interstate quarantine have been completely transferred to the Federal Government.

Inland quarantine in colonial times was usually adopted whenever smallpox appeared, but was rarely, if ever, effective, as indeed it is not now.

Isolation. The isolation of the sick was required by statute, or regulation, and interesting local provisions concerning smallpox were adopted in Boston and Salem as early as 1678. They forbade the selling of goods made by the infected family, or the exposure of any kind of infected material, and required contacts to stay at home. Notification by physicians was not required for a long time, though in 1721, in Rhode Island, keepers of houses of entertainment were compelled to report cases coming to their knowledge. The Massachusetts Act of 1701 provided for the "impressment" of houses to which patients might be removed and for furnishing nurses and attendants. We hear of pest-houses as early as 1743, and we hear of them now.

Immunization. In 1721 the Rev. Cotton Mather called the attention of the physicians of Boston to the favorable accounts from Europe of the artificial production of smallpox for the purpose of securing immunity. This was immediately put in practice by Dr. Zebdial Boylston, but at first the practice did not make much progress. In the latter part of the eighteenth century it became very popular and it is said that, in 1792, 8,000 persons were inoculated in Boston. With the introduction of vaccination, at the close of the century, inoculation fell into disuse.

Disinfection. Until very recently disinfection was held to be the sheet anchor of prevention and fumigation was supposed to disinfect. Naturally it was held in high esteem during the whole of this period. Disinfection was provided for in the Boston regulations of 1678, and in 1721 in Rhode Island the disinfection of infected goods was made compulsory. Strange to say, a very effectual method was prescribed, namely, exposure to the sun for at least six days. The popular method of disinfection during this period was, however, the method which has been used for two thousand years, or more, namely, fumigation by sulphur. During the eighteenth century smoke-houses were built at ferries and other places where travelers and their goods might be fumigated with sulphur, tar, or similar materials.

Prevention of Nuisances. The colonial legislatures very frequently enacted laws for the prevention and abatement of nuisances. There was such an act in Massachusetts as early as 1647, against pollution of Boston harbor. I have not, however, found an instance, before the very last years of the eighteenth century in which any suggestion is made in such a statute that the action was taken for the benefit of the public health.

OPINIONS WHICH GUIDED HEALTH WORK

As was stated above, during the seventeenth and eighteenth centuries, smallpox was the disease which was chiefly feared and this was plainly contagious, so that the chief purpose of preventive medicine was to prevent contagion.   At the close of the period entirely different views began to prevail.   There have always been leaders of medical thought who have insisted upon a close relation between dirt and disease, but they were not particularly prominent during the eighteenth century.   During the last decade, however, a series of epidemics greatly alarmed the public and attracted the attention of medical men. Influenza appeared in 1789, smallpox in 1792, scarlet fever prevailed shortly after and, still more terrifying, there were several epidemics of yellow fever in northern as well as in southern cities.   Benjamin Rush, the leading medical authority of the time and a man of the greatest influence, was led to the belief that yellow fever, and indeed most fevers, were due to the emanations from decaying animal and vegetable substances.   He held the most bizarre notions, as that a heap of decaying cabbages may cause an outbreak of malignant fever. He was largely influenced in his belief by the studies of Noah Webster on infectious disease.   The public health act of Massachusetts of 1797 gave the local boards of health authority to abate nuisances which in their opinion were considered dangerous to the public health. This seems to be the beginning of a period which was to last for three quarters of a century, during which it was generally believed that municipal cleanliness was about all that was necessary to preserve the public health.   The importance of contagion was forgotten, the entire attention of sanitarians was devoted to improving the environment, and only very slight attention was given to the individual or the means of protecting him from contagion.   These views were greatly fostered by the news which came from England in regard to the theory and work of English reformers. The writings of George E. Waring in the seventies of the last century did much to emphasize erroneous ideas in regard to the causation of disease by the gaseous products of decomposition, and particularly as regards the deadly nature of sewer gas. Writing in the *Atlantic Monthly*, he moulded the opinions of the more thoughtful laity, opinions which, in many instances, have persisted to the present day. Even as late as 1898 they so controlled the Federal Government that Waring himself was sent to Havana to stamp out yellow fever by cleansing the city. His untiring energy made Havana the cleanest city in the western world but yellow fever continued. Then the genius of Reed and Gorgas determined the true nature of yellow fever and eliminated the disease. The filth theory was dead and a new era opened for public health, an era in which shotgun methods of prevention are giving place to specific means of attacking each disease, based on a scientific study of causation.

THE NINETEENTH CENTURY AND LATER

As was shown above, the sanitarians of the nineteenth century, up to about 1870, were, except for maritime quarantine, occupied chiefly with the problems of municipal cleanliness. The severe outbreaks of smallpox in the early seventies once more called attention to the importance of contagion, and the attitude of English health officers, who now began to require the reporting of contagious diseases and to build hospitals for them, was early reflected in this country. Soon, too, the work of the bacteriologist began to give us definite knowledge as to the causation of the infectious diseases and to demonstrate that they are practically all contagious. Environment now received less and less attention and the individual more. The attempt to control contagion became the chief function of the health department for the next fifty years. It is gratifying to note that the early members of this Association, for the most part, were leaders in the new movement, and that the first few meetings were largely devoted to a discussion of specific measures directed against specific diseases, showing that the members very generally had gotten away from the notion then prevalent that the removal of filth is the one all-powerful method of combatting infection.

During the last twenty years or so, a new phase of public health work has been evident. Attention is being directed more and more, not only to persons, but to individual persons. Education has become one of the most important factors, and it is the education of the individual which is aimed at. Cure also must be personal and individual. The great health movements, like the movement against tuberculosis and that against venereal diseases, the hookworm campaign in the South, the prevention of infant mortality and the medical supervision of school children, all seek out the individual, teach right ways of living and offer treatment. The physician and the nurse are the chief agents in the new movement. They have taken the place of the sanitary inspector and the policeman.

THE DEVELOPMENT OF ORGANIZATION

During the seventeenth and eighteenth centuries there was probably no permanent organization designed to promote the public health and no officials who gave more than a small portion of their time to such matters. Whenever outbreaks of disease occurred, temporary committees or officers were appointed, or men voluntarily grouped themselves together to meet the emergency. It is said that a board of health was established in Petersburg, Virginia, in 1780. One was certainly established in Philadelphia in 1794, and in New York in 1796. The first comprehensive state enactment for the establishment of a local health department was that of June 22, 1797, in Massachusetts. Under it Boston established a board of health in 1799, with Paul Revere at its head. The growth of local health organizations was slow. A report, covering considerably over one hundred principal towns, made for this Association in 1873, gave only five as establishing a board between 1800 and 1830. There were thirty-two between 1870 and 1873. Chicago had no health department until 1867, and a considerable number of towns were without one as late as 1873. At the present time there is in every state some legal provision for local health organizations, though actually, in the great majority of small towns and rural districts, there is no board of health, or health officer, or else they are entirely inefficient.

State Health Departments. The conception of a state health department, which should investigate disease, guide and direct local health activities and remedy the sanitary defects of local government, is quite modern. It was first urged in Massachusetts in 1849 by a commission of which Lemuel Shattuck was the guiding spirit. It was not until 1869 that the State Board of Health was established in Massachusetts, the first permanent board of its kind in the United States. When this Association first met, only Virginia, California and Minnesota had followed the lead of Massachusetts. To-day every state in the Union has its health department.

COMPARISON OF IDEAS

Before proceeding to a brief consideration of the activities of municipal and state health departments, it will be instructive to compare present-day ideas with those of nearly half a century ago. In 1875 a committee of this Association prepared a very elaborate schedule for a survey of the sanitary condition of the principal American cities. The divisions of the schedule for this survey are given below. At the present time a committee of the Association is conducting a similar survey and a synopsis of its schedule is also given. A glance indicates how vast is the difference between what was thought of most importance as affecting the health of a city fifty years ago and to-day. The first nine items, as here given, are somewhat alike, though there are some noticeable differences. The last ten items are entirely different in the two schedules, and here again the differences are really far greater than at first they appear to be.

MUNICIPAL HEALTH SURVEYS

Schedule of 1875	*Schedule of 1921*
Water Supply	Water Supply
Drainage and Sewerage	Sewerage, Privies, Comfort Stations
Streets and Public Grounds	Street Cleaning

MUNICIPAL HEALTH SURVEYS — *Continued*

Schedule of 1875	*Schedule of 1921*
Habitations	Housing, Plumbing
Garbage and Excreta	Garbage
Slaughter-houses, Abattoirs, Manufactories and Trades	Nuisances
Public Health Laws	Organization, Finances
Vital Statistics	Vital Statistics
Location, Population, Climate	Contagious Diseases
Topography and Geology	Laboratory, Vaccination
Gas and Lighting	Infant Hygiene
Markets	School Inspecton, Working Papers
Public School Buildings	Industrial Hygiene
Hospitals and Public Charities	Health Centers
Police and Prisons	Public Health Nursing
Fire Establishments, Engines etc.	Food and Drugs
Cemeteries and Burial	Milk
Quarantine	Education, Publicity

In the following pages no attempt is made to narrate all that has been attempted by states and local communities to control disease, but the most important activities are touched upon and those which have been carried on for a long period of time, or are now prominently before the public. Less space is given to state activities, not because they are less important or less extensive. It is the local health officer who does the work which gives direct results. The states frequently feel constrained to do the same sort of work; that is, in one way or another, they do a large amount of local administrative work in which case, of course, it is exactly the same as that which the municipalities do. Again, a large part of state work consists in directing and stimulating local action and inducing the cities and towns to perform their proper functions.

HEALTH WORK OF CITIES

Nuisances. The ideas about dirt and disease which developed so rapidly during the last years of the eighteenth century became crystallized in the wording of the Massachusetts Health Act of 1797. The towns were to establish a health committee and health officer and their sole duty as prescribed was "to remove all filth of any kind whatever which shall be found in any of the streets, lanes, wharves, docks or in any other place whatever within the limits of the town to which such committee or health officer belongs, whenever such filth shall, in their judgment, endanger the lives or the health of the inhabitants thereof." The rules of the first board of health in Boston, adopted in 1799, carried out this idea, and referred to nothing except nuisances and the importation of bedding and feathers. The Massachusetts law served as the basis for sanitary legislation in many other states. There was no conception of the distinction between dangerous dirt and dirt not dangerous, and warfare was waged against everything decaying and everything which smelled bad, even if it was not the result of decay. Offensive trades were apparently considered the greatest menace. Pig-pens were a good second. The fight was against cess-pools rather than against privy vaults. Indeed, it was not until the closing years of the nineteenth century that we were taught by the new science of bacteriology that the improper disposal of human excrement is the one great and dangerous nuisance, far worse than all others. The health officials of New York City in 1849, in com-batting cholera, paid no more attention to privies than other nui-sances, and waged warfare on fat-rendering, slaughtering, manure piles and burying-grounds.

Gradually nuisance work received relatively less attention, but this was largely owing to the development of other lines. Neverthe-less, as late as 1900, I found that in a number of the principal cities in the country there were employed two hundred sanitary inspectors and only about sixty-five medical inspectors, the latter of whom were mostly part-time men. It is true, however, that the sanitary inspectors often placarded for contagious diseases, made inspection of the houses and fumigated.

Effective Nuisance Work. We have now learned that dangerous dirt is the dirt which carries human excretions. Work which preven-ted the passing of excretory effluvia from one human being to another was real health work, and of course the old-time health officers did much of it, though they wasted infinite time in removing dead cats and ash piles and in searching for sewer gas.

For years the public considered the abatement of nuisances the chief work of the health department, and many think so now, but where privy vaults have been abolished and good sewers installed there is no need for the health officer to waste his time on nuisance work.   Providence was the first city to recognize this and nominally turn over the prevention of nuisances to the police, though it must be admitted that the public still demands more or less attention from the health officer in such matters.   There are those who believe that nuisance prevention has been carried on so long and in the main so well by health officials that it is unwise to make a change, but it seems to me that the money and energy, both very considerable in amount, which are at present devoted to this, might be far better expended in other directions.

Plumbing Inspection.   The acme of the filth theory was the sewer gas bogy.   The sanitary engineers of the seventies of the nineteenth century believed that the tiniest whiff of this rather imaginary substance was deadly and must be kept out of our dwellings at any cost.   This idea gradually weakened with the development of bacteriology, until it was finally laid to rest forever by Winslow in 1909. We now know that sewer air is not dangerous at all.   Evil and error occasionally bring some good in their train, and it was the fear of sewer gas which led to the enactment of plumbing laws and the inspection of plumbing.   Poor and cheap plumbing is no economy and causes trouble and often nuisance even if it rarely causes death. Plumbing laws have compelled us to put good plumbing in our houses, though many millions of dollars have been wasted by unnecessary refinements, the outcome of the sewer gas theory.   Perhaps because of the articles on this subject in the *Atlantic Monthly,* Massachusetts was the first state to enact a law providing for the inspection of plumbing.   This was in 1877, and in 1881 Lawrence was the first city to adopt a complete plumbing code.   Of course most cities now have plumbing regulations.   In about half of the cities in which these regulations obtain, they are enforced by the health department. This is, however, no more a health function than the supervision of chimney construction, or the strength of walls, and should be a part of general building supervision, which it fortunately is in very many cities.

Water Supply and Sewerage.   The supply of pure water and the removal of human excreta through the sewers is one of the chief health functions of municipalities.   The early health officers devoted much attention to this, and during the middle of the nineteenth century most progressive urban communities, even some very small ones, established municipal water supplies and began the construction of a system of sewers.   Unfortunately, they did not understand what purity of water implies, and they did not appreciate that the chief value of sewers is lost if individuals are allowed to store up fecal matter in privy vaults.   Hence, it often happened that American cities made use of water from supplies grossly contaminated and suffered severely from typhoid fever and certain intestinal diseases, and would have suffered from cholera if it had gained a wider foothold in this country.   It is only during the last thirty years that, acting on newer knowledge, earnest efforts have been made to render our municipal water supplies really safe and quickly to get rid of all fecal matter through the sewers.

Contagious Disease Control.   During the first three quarters of the nineteenth century very little interest was taken in the direct control of the communicable diseases, though at the present time, probably most people, and certainly the present writer, believe that it is now the foremost duty of health officers.   As has been referred to, during the seventies there was a rapidly increasing interest in the prevention of contagion.

Quarantine.   Quarantine, particularly maritime quarantine, has been employed as a health measure since the settlement of the country. This subject will be discussed by another writer, but it seems worth while to say that, notwithstanding all its mistakes and shortcomings and unnecessary hardships at times, maritime quarantine has prevented devastating outbreaks of exotic disease and remains a powerful weapon for the protection of the public health.   At about the middle of the last century the term "external hygiene" was commonly applied to maritime quarantine, and "internal hygiene" to the prevention of the development of disease within the community. The conception of internal hygiene at that time was municipal cleanliness. Now we know that it is chiefly the prevention of contagion.

Notification. I think few people realize how recent are our methods for control of contagious diseases. It is true that notification, isolation, disinfection and immunization were employed against smallpox from the earliest colonial times. It is true, too, that some of the early colonial laws required the notification and control of smallpox or "other infectious or contagious distemper", but it is doubtful whether the law was ever applied except in smallpox, and certainly it was not in scarlet fever, diphtheria, typhoid fever, or measles. Notification of these diseases was first required in the seventies,— scarlet fever and typhoid fever in Brooklyn in 1873, and scarlet fever, typhoid fever, diphtheria and measles in New York in 1874. Typhoid fever was not made reportable in Boston until 1881, and in St. Louis not until 1889.

Diagnostic Laboratory. A bacteriological laboratory was set up in Providence by Dr. Swarts in 1888, which was utilized in the study of the typhoid outbreak of that year. The first diagnostic laboratory, however, was that of New York City, where Dr. Biggs offered to assist in the diagnosis of diphtheria in 1893. The example of New York was followed by a considerable number of cities in the following year, at which time, also, sputum examination was offered by the New York laboratory. Although laboratories grew apace, in 1900 there were nine of the forty largest cities of the country without laboratories and included among these was one of nearly half a million inhabitants. The laboratory is not only a prime necessity for the discovery of cases, but it has been of vast importance in stimulating the scientific spirit among public health officials.

Home Isolation. After notification, there gradually grew up in our cities a system of visiting the homes where disease existed, placarding, exclusion from school and places of employment and other restrictions of intercourse. It must be admitted that, at first, much of the visiting was done by sanitary inspectors who had no thought of tracing contagion, but merely reported on drains, cesspools and back yards.

Even to-day I know of a city of over a hundred thousand inhabitants in which the "epidemiological records" consist of absolutely nothing but a very brief statement of the sanitary condition of the house from which the case was reported.   Although the supervision of the ordinary contagious diseases has been extremely superficial and lax to a very large extent, there can be little doubt that it has really accomplished a great deal.   If this is so, it should give us encouragement to adopt more effective methods.

Real Control.   The former notion that the strict isolation of all cases of contagious disease notified by a physician would stamp out the disease has long since been shown to be wrong.   It is the carrier and mild case which do the harm.   Even as early as 1866, Stephen Smith recognized this and instituted house to house visitation in New York to discover the mild diarrheas, many of which were known to be real cholera.   More or less intensive search for cases has often been practiced in smallpox outbreaks, but Hill and Chesley, in Minnesota, were the first to show that, if success in the control of the more common infections is to be secured, it is necessary to go out and find the very great number of infected persons who are not seen by physicians or are not recognized by them as sources of danger.   They have shown that it is possible by such measures, carried out by skilled investigators, to accomplish much, at least, in the smaller communities and rural districts.   Their success warrants a much wider application of their methods.

Contagious Disease Nurses.   To nail a warning sign on the house does, I believe, in a large proportion of cases, accomplish a good deal and result in a fair degree of isolation.   To make it really effective, and in many other ways to get the best results, a fairly constant supervision is needed of the cases and also of all contacts and suspects. For this the visiting nurse is most useful, but it is only within a very few years that she has been employed at all for this purpose and in comparatively few places.   I know of no place in which a sufficiently large nursing force is continuously employed for the supervision of contagious diseases.

Hospitalization. Hospitals for the care of the common contagious diseases are an absolute necessity, although exaggerated ideas of their effectiveness have, at times, been held. It is now known that it is futile to attempt to stamp out scarlet fever and diphtheria by hospitalization alone. Though it is a needless expenditure of money to attempt to do this, yet for very many reasons, the hospitalization of a certain number of cases is of great importance and is dictated by humanity, as well as by the needs of public health.

As early as 1701 the Colony of Massachusetts required the towns to provide places for the isolation of smallpox, but it was two hundred years before such a requirement was made for other contagious diseases. Probably every considerable community has had its pest-house, but the building of modern contagious disease hospitals has progressed rather slowly in this country. As late as 1873 New York City, beside its smallpox hospital, had only two small wards on Blackwell's Island designed primarily for typhus fever. Even in 1900 there were probably not more than twenty-five or thirty such hospitals in the United States and these were mostly small.

Immunization. Inoculation against smallpox was practiced very commonly during the eighteenth century, and with the opening of the nineteenth vaccination took its place. This was usually offered by local authorities, but little attempt was made at compulsion. In fact, compulsory vaccination against smallpox has rarely been attempted in this country, except for school children, though it has very generally been required for the latter. Such laws are, however, greatly neglected in many communities. School vaccination does not insure a well protected community and it has some disadvantages, but it does protect the school children. During the last fifty years only one school child in Providence has had smallpox, and that was one of the exceedingly small number of children that, for one reason or another, escaped vaccination.

The value of antityphoid vaccination has been known for twenty years, but it was brought forcibly to public attention by its successful employment among our troops on the Mexican border. Since then it has been quite freely offered by state and municipal authorities, particularly in the South. Antirabic vaccination has been employed quite generally for about fifteen years. Vaccination against other diseases, as diphtheria, pneumonia and whooping cough is being tried out, but has not yet stood the test of long experience.

Disinfection. Fumigation has been practiced since the earliest colonial times. Until quite recently infected things were believed to be the chief factor in the spread of contagion and it never occurred to any one that infection might linger for a long time about persons while it disappeared rapidly from things. It is now known that little danger is to be apprehended from a house, or the things in it, after the people have become free from infection, and it is recognized that terminal disinfection alone is of little moment and that fumigation, as ordinarily practiced, is useless. Up to the present century, however, alleged terminal disinfection with sulphur, or formaldehyde, was considered to be one of the chief weapons against infectious disease. Moreover, disinfection was frequently applied not only to houses where there had been contagious disease, but supposed disinfectants were freely sprinkled in streets, yards and cellars to kill the disease-producing organisms of decomposition. This practice was in vogue in New York City up to the eighties of the last century. Providence, in 1905, was the first city to give up terminal fumigation, an example which has been quite generally followed, and most health officers have now come to believe that the procedure entails needless expense.

Instead of terminal disinfection, continuous disinfection all through the sickness is seen to be necessary to prevent the extension of the disease from the original case. Advice and directions are now generally given for this, but they will usually not be carried out without the advice and assistance of nurses given on frequent visits.

Venereal Disease Control. There is nothing in preventive medicine more important than this, but until very recently, little has been done. The modern movement against these diseases seems to have begun in California, where, under the leadership of Dr. Snow, these diseases were made notifiable January 1, 1911. By 1915 only a dozen states had made notification compulsory and little attempt was made at enforcing this provision. About twenty-five states were then offering free laboratory diagnosis for these diseases. It was the Great War which chiefly aroused the public to a realization of the tremendous harm which these diseases do and developed a backing sufficient for health officers to attempt what they long knew ought to to be done. The state health departments developed the greatest interest in the subject and with the aid of the Public Health Service every state is now carrying on an active campaign and stimulating local communities as far as possible. The chief features of the campaign are notification, the establishment of clinics, the education of the public and the enforcement of all police regulations which tend to make prostitution less easy. Results are already being obtained, but it is too early for any startling figures of wholesale reduction of these diseases.

The Anti-Tuberculosis Movement. The development of this movement has been one of the remarkable social phenomena of the times. It perhaps had its origin in the establishment of the Trudeau Sanatorium in 1885, and since that time the construction of sanatoriums and hospitals has proceeded with great rapidity. The first state sanatorium was built by Massachusetts in 1898. In 1908 there were 250 special sanatoriums and hospitals for this disease in the United States.

Sanatoriums are chiefly for cure, but prevention was early recognized as more important than cure. The discovery of the tubercle bacillus by Koch, in 1882, aroused the public to the dangers of contagion, and health officials devoted much attention to spreading information concerning the assumed modes of infection and to devising regulations to prevent it. As early as 1889, the New York Health Department distributed a very excellent circular and the next year began visiting cases.

The vision of Biggs, trained as he was in the scientific methods of the laboratory, led to more active methods based on his knowledge of the disease. He believed that the notification of cases, as in other contagious diseases, was a necessary first step, and this was required of institutions and requested of physicians, in 1894, in New York

City, although it was not made compulsory there until 1897. At the same time the examination of sputum was offered by the department, cases were visited and advice given, the proper care of sputum was insisted upon and hospitalization or removal to a sanitorium was secured whenever possible.

Although to Dr. Biggs, a member of a great municipal health department, belongs the credit of organizing official machinery for the control of this disease, and although a great number of local health officials are carrying out these measures, nevertheless it is also true that a vast amount of work is being done by voluntary organizations, many of them directed and managed by laymen, and that these also are furnishing the stimulus for much official work. The first state tuberculosis association was organized in Pennsylvania in 1892, but such organizations did not grow rapidly either in number or size for ten years or more, and the National Association was not organized until 1905.

As a large proportion of cases of tuberculosis are among the poor and as these are the ones that need most attention, it has come about that the dispensary is the most important feature of the anti-tuberculosis campaign and around it centers the work of the physicians and nurses engaged in the diagnosis, advice, care and control of the cases of this disease. The aim is to find every case of tuberculosis at the earliest possible moment and keep it under as favorable conditions for cure and prevention as the environment admits. Prevention of human infection and the raising of the resistance of the body are kept constantly in mind.

Besides the direct supervision of cases and contacts there is a large amount of valuable subsidiary work being done in connection with preventoriums, open-air schools, improved housing, social work, industrial hygiene, health centers, milk and food control, nutrition work and the like.

Milk Supervision. With the growth of cities, separation between the producer and consumer of milk became wider and skimming and watering more common. During the seventies of the last century there was a rather rapid development of municipal control to prevent this adulteration. Although such adulteration is largely an economic problem, it also has important health features and this was one of the factors leading to municipal action.

With the development of the science of bacteriology, it came to be seen that what makes good milk good is its freshness, cleanliness and freedom from bacteria. It was found that cleanly handling and prompt cooling mean few bacteria. As early as 1895, here and there, inspection of producers and dealers was begun by municipal authorities to try to improve the milk supply along these lines, and in 1895 a law providing for such inspection was enacted in Minnesota. As an aid in such inspection the score card devised by Woodward of Washington has become very popular. There has grown up a vast body of regulations and an elaborate system of inspection to secure clean milk. Among the most important measures are the fixing of a bacterial standard, the requirement of a low temperature, the establishment of a grading system and pasteurization. Most of this has been done during the last dozen years. Before that time the danger from bovine tuberculosis was very fully appreciated and many futile efforts were made to stamp out, or effectively control, tuberculosis in cattle. Now pasteurization has been substituted for this and a large number of cities require that all milk, except that from tuberculin-tested cows, shall be pasteurized. Efficient pasteurization and proper care of the milk afterwards not only disposes of the danger of the transmission of tuberculosis through milk, but of typhoid fever and other diseases as well. Chicago was the first city to require the pasteurization of all milk except from tuberculin-tested cows. The ordinance was passed in July, 1908, at the instigation of Dr. Evans.

Inspection of Provisions. From the very beginning of the modern sanitary era the inspection of markets and the articles there displayed for sale has been considered a very important sanitary function. It has been believed that fruits, vegetables, meats and all food materials subject to decomposition are, if not perfectly fresh, likely to be the source of serious disease. We now know that there is little evidence of this and much against it. Nevertheless, most of our cities maintain this sort of inspection. Market inspectors, even if they do not prevent much sickness and death, if they work wisely, can do much to promote cleanliness in the handling of food, which undoubtedly is of real sanitary significance. They also accomplish much in compelling care in the handling of such perishable material so that from an economic and aesthetic standpoint their services to the public are well worth what they cost.

Reduction of Infant Mortality. Fifty or sixty years ago, when from twenty to twenty-five per cent or more of all babies died during the first year of life, the seriousness of the problem was fully realized and the subject was freely discussed in the meetings of this Association, as well as in medical and other scientific meetings. The effort at official control has been of slow growth. Perhaps the first attempt was the appointment by the New York Health Department, in 1876, of a summer corps of physicians to search the tenement houses for infant sickness, the purpose being curative rather than preventive. The effort was not particularly successful. Owing to the rather exaggerated importance attached at that period to the rôle of milk in the causation of infant mortality, it was but natural that the first steps toward improving matters should have been directed to milk. The rapid development of a knowledge of infant diseases, of infant feeding and of infant care by pediatricians was perhaps the underlying cause of the movement. Even in the eighties of the last century many cities issued useful circulars on the care of infants and, it is said, that as early as 1892 most of the mothers in New York had learned the desirability of heating milk before feeding. Because of the belief that good milk was the most important factor in the preservation of infant life, stations began to be established where it would be possible for mothers, especially among the poor, to obtain milk of the best quality. It is said that the first milk stations were established in 1872 by the New York Diet Kitchen Association, and Koplik had one in connection with a dispensary in 1889. The greatest interest was given to the movement by Nathan Straus who began, in 1893, to establish his extensive system of stations in New York. The municipality itself did not provide stations until 1911, but meanwhile the first municipal station was established in Rochester in 1897. Probably milk stations are still chiefly maintained by private effort, though the municipalities are doing more and more. In 1910, 43 agencies were maintaining such stations, and in 1916, 110.

It was soon seen that the milk furnished at the station would do comparatively little good unless its proper use was directed and the mother well instructed in every phase of infant care. Hence, the physician and nurse became the most essential feature of these stations. Now the consultation for well babies, at which milk is not sold, has largely taken the place of the milk station as first established. In 1916 there were in 142 cities 95 organizations maintaining such consultations as compared with 110 maintaining milk stations. Home visiting by nurses has also been a natural and rapid development. At the same time there has been a great development of and improvement in clinics for sick babies.

The reduction of infant mortality has been phenomenal. In New York City it fell from 273 per 1,000 live births in 1885 to 94 in 1915. In recent years it has been noted that little reduction has taken place in deaths occuring during the first month of life, and it is realized that improvement can be made in this regard only by better care of the mother before and during childbirth; hence, the development of prenatal clinics, the supervision of midwives and other efforts to secure better obstetrical care, especially for the poor. The popular interest in all these phases of child hygiene has grown immensely during the last few years. A bureau of child hygiene has been established in many a municipal health department, the first of which was in New York in 1908. Similar bureaus have been established in many states, and the work has also been taken up by the Federal Government.

Medical Supervision of School Children. Medical inspection of schools, so called, began in the United States in 1894, though it was practiced to a considerable extent in Europe before that time. Doubtless there had previously been some spóradic work in the United States. Thus the Board of Education in New York, in 1871, had a physician to look after the health of the teachers and certain other health matters. In 1894, as a result of much contagious disease in the preceding year, Dr. Durgin, of Boston, began a system of medical inspection of school children in that city. The primary purpose was to seek out unrecognized cases of contagious disease. For the first decade school inspection made slow progress, but since then it has been extremely rapid. In 1910 it had been introduced into four hundred cities. In 1899 an act was passed in Connecticut providing for testing the vision of all pupils, and in 1906 an act was passed in Massachusetts making general school inspection compulsory.

It soon became apparent that although school inspection discovered a certain amount of unrecognized contagious disease, it had far greater possibility for good in other directions. The idea rapidly gained ground that it is the duty of the community to look after the general health of its school children, particularly those in the public schools. This sort of school supervision now takes cognizance of such matters as vision and hearing, the presence of enlarged tonsils and adenoids, the general nutrition of the child, its mental condition, the state of its teeth, the state of the heart — in fact, everything connected with the child's physical well-being. In many cities a more or less thorough physical examination of the child is made at certain intervals.

At first physicians only were employed in this work, but as soon as the outlook broadened and the general health of the child, rather than the prevention of contagion, became the chief function, it was seen that nurses would be of great value, not only in helping to find cases to be referred to the physician, but particularly in transmitting to the family advice given by the physician and in following up the case to encourage the family to do as advised. Nurses do not seem to have been employed in this country until 1902, when they were first made use of in New York City.

There is naturally great difficulty in persuading parents to secure proper medical attention for their children and many cities have found it necessary to establish special clinics for school children. Cure, as contrasted with prevention, has thus been forced upon health officials. The work of school inspection has met with a good deal of opposition from many practicing physicians who claim that it is taking the bread out of their mouths.   Thus far, this certainly has not been so, for very little practice has been diverted from private physicians which they would have had without inspection, and on the other hand a great deal has been given to them by inspection.

The benefits of school inspection are difficult to show by means of statistics, but teachers and health officers alike feel sure that they are very great.   According to Gulick, of 234,349 abnormalities discovered in New York in 1911, 37 per cent were remedied.   In Providence last year, of 2,237 eye defects, 33 per cent were remedied, and of 7,346 other defects, many of which, however, were quite minor, over 50 per cent were remedied.   In the aggregate, throughout the country, an immense amount of good is done every year by the improvement of the physical condition of school children through medical supervision.

Distribution and Administration of Serum.   Probably the chief cause of the phenomenal decline in the death rate from diphtheria has not been due to control of the spread of the disease, but to the use of antitoxin.   That this valuable remedy has been so easily accessible has been due to the action of city and state officials.   In December, 1894, the New York *Herald* antitoxin fund was turned over to the New York City Health Department and during the next year the department began to make, distribute and administer the remedy. Many cities followed this example, and although few cities have found it necessary or wise to make antitoxin, a good many have distributed curative serums of various kinds.   Recently, however, this health function has more generally been performed by state health departments.   The experience of some cities has shown that it is not enough to distribute these serums freely, but that many more lives can be saved if the health department stands ready to administer them. Even now, in most of our cities, many deaths from diphtheria take place because too many practicing physicians are negligent in the use of antitoxin.

Cure of Sickness.   One of the most important of the growing health activities of municipalities is the care of the sick.   A number of cities maintain general hospitals and dispensaries and otherwise care for the sick poor, though this duty is for the most part not placed upon the health department. Most of our curative work is done by voluntary organizations. For a long time it was believed by everybody that preventive medicine should keep its hands off curative medicine, and many health officers, most of the general public and nearly every practicing physician still think so. On the other hand, there are many experienced and sagacious health officials and publicists who believe that cure and prevention ought to be combined to a considerable extent in the same administrative unit. It is a fact that, for one reason or another, health officials, perhaps generally reluctantly, have been led to establish clinics for tuberculosis, for venereal diseases, for the treatment of the defects of school children and for various other purposes. These undertakings, rapidly extending, have served to bring the health department in close touch with the people and to gain their confidence, and also to render instruction, as well as all preventive work, easier and more effective. This is now frankly admitted by very many and the idea is embodied in what is popularly called the "health center," the establishment of which is now strongly urged as a legitimate health measure.

Other Activities. There are many other activities besides those which have been discussed which are occasionally carried on by health departments, oftentimes for a short period only and perhaps only in a few cities. Some of these have little to do with public health. Others give promise of being of great importance, but owing to comparatively short experience with them it is not possible to form very definite conclusions as to the methods employed and the results obtained. Still others are of local significance only. Among such functions may be mentioned the control of drug addicts; war against nostrums; campaigns against mosquitoes, flies and rats; supervision of eating places, as regards both the food handlers and the eating utensils; the prevention of noises; the prevention of accidents; the campaign against cancer; efforts to lessen the evils of heart disease; the supervision of baths and laundries and the regulation of baby boarding-houses. Scarcely a year passes when new lines of work are not undertaken by health officers with vision and enthusiasm.

It is well indeed that our health activities are not too thoroughly "standardized" and that such experiments can be freely made under varying conditions.

HEALTH WORK OF STATES

Organization. The first permanent State Board of Health was established in Massachusetts in 1869 just twenty years after it had been so strongly urged by Lemuel Shattuck. Now every state has a health department in its government. State health departments do not for the most part come into such intimate contact with the people as do municipal health officers. In the beginning it certainly was not intended that they should.

Investigation and Advice. The first conception of a state board of health was that its chief business should be the investigation of the causes of disease and the giving of advice to the people, and especially to the legislature and the municipal governments. Following the example of Massachusetts, many state health departments adhered to this conception and held aloof from executive action for a long time. For many years the Massachusetts department carried on a great variety of investigations, some of which were connected with matters of the greatest importance, such as the effect of alcohol upon health, ventilation, the bad effects of housing and the mode of spread of smallpox, typhoid fever and other diseases, and the reduction of infant mortality. Most important of all were the studies on the purification of water and sewage, and for a long time these served as a standard throughout the world. Although the board had not the authority to compel action by cities and towns, as many state health departments now have, its influence was so great that Massachusetts and the neighboring states forged ahead of the rest of the country in the protection of public water supplies and the disposal of sewage. On the whole, investigation of the sources of disease has not attained very brilliant results in the hands of most state health departments, as their energies have been largely forced into other channels whether they wished it or not.

Public Health Education. The giving of advice, meaning thereby the general education of the public in matters relating to public health and personal hygiene, has developed rapidly during the last twenty years. The need of such popular education was very early appreciated both by educators and sanitarians. As early as 1843 Horace Mann strongly urged teaching knowledge of the body and the means to maintain health to every pupil in the public schools. Municipal as well as state health officials have been interested in such educational work, but the latter have gone into it more systematically and have accomplished more. Lecturers, press notices, bulletins, almanacs, health trains, automobile clinics and a hundred different ways of attracting the attention of the public and bringing home to them the principles of preventive medicine have reached an enormous development during the last few years. Much good has been accomplished though, some of us fear, not a little evil. The health propagandist too easily falls from the ways of the scientific teacher into those of the commercial advertiser. Nevertheless, the well directed propaganda of many health departments has surely accomplished a great deal of good and has paved the way for more effective community action in the future.

Much of this educational work has taken the form of special campaigns for definite objects. Campaigns of great importance, like the reduction of infant mortality, the prevention of tuberculosis, the fight against venereal diseases and for the eradication of hookworm disease have been organized on a large scale in many states, during the last ten or twelve years, and have stimulated local activity in many cities, towns, and counties in the state where the campaign was being carried on.

Safe Disposal of Excreta. One of the most extensive and revolutionary of these campaigns has been that carried on in the Southern states for the sanitary disposal of human excreta. The teaching of Stiles as to the importance and prevalence of hookworm infection and the demonstration by Ashford of wholesale methods of cure stimulated the South to action, initiated in the states of Florida and Mississippi. The work was too stupendous for official health agencies then existing and would probably have languished, but for the splendid aid given by the Rockefeller Sanitary Commission. At about the same time the work of state and federal officials in Virginia and elsewhere showed that the same fundamental causes which led to the presence of hookworm infection led also to the prevalence of typhoid fever and the diarrheal diseases. It is through state health channels that the necessity for the proper disposal of excreta is being brought home to each individual citizen with the result, during the last few years, that typhoid fever and other fecal-borne diseases have been rapidly disappearing.

Engineering. Although the state control of water supplies and sewage disposal is of the most importance in those states where there is a large urban population, there is no state where it is not to some extent necessary. This subject, as its importance demands, is being discussed in a separate article by Professor Whipple. It is sufficient to say here that under the lead of Massachusetts the lethargy of the people in regard to the dangers of drinking impure water has been dissipated and that thousands of towns and cities have in one way or another, usually under the advice and perhaps under the direct compulsion of the state health department, freed their water supplies from infection and have thus done their part to banish typhoid fever and remove the menace of cholera forever.

Development of Local Health Activities. Although much remains to be done to promote the health of even our best ordered cities, in general, the sanitary development of urban communities has been far and away ahead of that of rural sections. Over one half of our population live in small communities where efficient health work is difficult. Probably the most important duty of state health authorities, at the present time, is to secure as good sanitary work in the country as in the large cities. This was very early realized, and papers read before this Association in 1873 emphasized the problem. During the last few years state health officers have been earnestly engaged in attempts to solve it. In a few instances the state has boldly taken over all health work, thus eliminating the local governments altogether. In other cases the state attempts to have a share in appointing local officials, fixing salaries and determining expenditures, perhaps forming artificial districts for this purpose. The state may coöperate with the local communities by bearing a part of the expense, or by doing the work for the local government. It is well that all these experiments should be tried, for thus only can we learn what is best. Already much has been accomplished, although it is but a fraction of what must be done if the best part of our country is to have the advantages for the maintenance of health which are often afforded even the slum-dwellers of our great cities.

Aid for Communities and Individuals. There are many things necessary for the proper working of health machinery which it is extremely difficult for small communities to provide for themselves, and the state has accomplished much in rendering assistance in such cases. A most important example of such assistance is the laboratory. Every city of 50,000 inhabitants should have its own diagnostic laboratory, but for smaller communities the state stands ready to assist with its own laboratory, sometimes increasing its value by having branch laboratories. The state's chemical laboratory, too, is ready to assist even the smallest place in solving its water, sewage, food and milk problems. The use of antitoxin and other serums and of vaccines, like typhoid vaccine and rabies vaccine, would have been extremely slow in many places if it had not been for their distribution by state health officials. Many thousands of lives are to the credit of our state boards of health because the prompt administration of diphtheria, tetanus or meningitis antitoxin has been by them rendered possible. Hundreds of cases of blindness have been prevented by the free distribution of drops to be put in the babies' eyes. These are a few examples of how the state aids small communities that would find it difficult to help themselves.

Vital Statistics. The proper registration of births, marriages and deaths may not seem to the public to have any very close connection with stamping out smallpox, or the prevention of typhoid fever, yet it is the first and most important health work that any community can do. Sanitary science will never progress, and even the knowledge we have cannot be intelligently applied, without a fairly accurate system of vital statistics. It is the bookkeeping without which every business venture great or small would soon be wrecked. Massachusetts was the first state to establish an efficient system of vital records, and the maintenance of such a system must always depend upon state control and supervision. At present more than three quarters of the population are living within the registration area for deaths, and the birth registration area is rapidly increasing.

Other Activities. Many other activities are engaged in by state departments of health which it is impossible to discuss in this limited space. Some of these have accomplished much. Some promise much. Some are local or sectional. Among these may be mentioned the control of plague, efforts to prevent pellagra, the elimination of trachoma, the supervision of public institutions, of hotels, camps and common carriers, attempts to reduce the nostrum evil, to teach sex hygiene, to develop industrial hygiene, and to maintain the purity of milk and other food.

RESULTS

Thus have cities and states sought to control disease. The yellow fever nightmare will terrify no more. There has been practically no cholera since 1873. Smallpox, which in former epidemics sometimes attacked half the population, is a negligible cause of death. Typhus fever is a very rare disease. Plague has not been able to gain a foothold.

The death-rate in New York city in 1869 was 28. In 1919 it was 12.93. This means the saving of 28,000 lives a year. There are no national statistics extending back fifty years, but in the last twenty years there has been a fall in the death rate of the rapidly expanding registration area of 4.7 per 100,000 living. This is equivalent to the saving of nearly 400,000 lives a year. Typhoid fever is a vanishing disease. The diarrheal diseases caused four times as many deaths fifty years ago as now. Scarlet fever mortality has fallen ninety per cent. Diphtheria has decreased nearly as much, and the mortality from pulmonary tuberculosis has been cut in two. Infant mortality in our better cities has dropped fifty per cent. Not all this, it is true, is due to conscious community effort, but is in part, dependent upon economic and other unknown causes. Nevertheless, if only one half of this life-saving is to be credited to health work the dividend on the money and energy employed indicates good business.

Figures do not measure the terror of epidemics, nor the tears of the mother at her baby's grave, nor the sorrow of the widow whose helpmate has been snatched away in the prime of life. To have prevented these not once, but a million times, justifies our half century of public health work.

FIFTY YEARS OF WATER PURIFICATION

GEORGE C. WHIPPLE, C. E.

Professor of Sanitary Engineering, Harvard Engineering School

THE history of water purification in the United States is intimately connected with the general movement to improve sanitation and public health as well as with the rise of modern science. No excuse is therefore necessary for referring to these subjects by way of introduction.

The great sanitary awakening occurred in England about the middle of the last century. Following the social uplift, sometimes called the New Humanity, which occurred in the twenties and thirties, came the sanitary surveys of Sir Robert Rawlinson, the public health activities of Sir John Simon, the statistical studies of Edwin Chadwick, and the medical investigations of Dr. Southward Smith in the forties. The English public health system dates from 1848. The new public health inspiration crossed the Atlantic and in the late forties occurred the investigations of Lemuel Shattuck, which culminated in that remarkable document, the *Report of the Massachusetts Sanitary Commission** of 1850. But the movement in the United States became side-tracked for a time because more important issues were before the public.

During and after the Civil War the problems of sanitation were attacked anew. A Citizens' Association made an investigation of the sanitary condition of New York City in 1865. The Massachusetts State Board of Health was established in 1869. The American Public Health Association was founded in 1872. Meantime a new demand for public health measures had arisen. The Civil War had left an aftermath of

---

*Long unavailable, but now reprinted in *State Sanitation*, Harvard University Press.

disease.   In particular typhoid fever, which had been so prevalent in the armies, was scattered throughout the country.   Many a returned soldier had become unwittingly a typhoid carrier.   The typhoid fever death-rates throughout the country were very high.   In Boston the typhoid-fever rates from 1855-60 were between 40 and 50 per 100,000; during the sixties they were above 60 for a third of the time;   in 1872 the rate was 86 per 100,000 — high figures these for a city like Boston. The rates in other cities were equally high, sometimes much higher.

It should be remembered also that it was during the last half of the century that modern science began its remarkable development. Several events marked the new era, the most important, perhaps, being the publication of Darwin's *Origin of Species* in 1859.   With it came the wide application of the inductive system of reasoning, of the experimental method.   All sciences darted forward as a result of the impetus given by the new ideas.   In the late sixties and early seventies Pasteur made his great discoveries.   These were followed by the work of Koch and others in the eighties, and the science of bacteriology soon arose. The experimental method was at once applied to the field of sanitation, including water purification.   Although filtration had been used for a part of the London supply as early as 1829, the benefits of the process were not appreciated nor its action fully understood for many years after that date.   Following a cholera epidemic in 1839 filtration was extended rapidly and in 1855 was made compulsory for the London metropolitan district.   It was the rise of the science of bacteriology and all that went with it which caused the modern development of this greatest of the sanitary arts,—the art of water purification.

Fifty years ago the quality of the existing water supplies in the United States was low, judged by modern standards.   Clearness and freedom from color, taste and odor were the ruling standards, and even these were often not complied with.   In some regions a good deal of attention was being given to lead poisoning and to hardness.   Water analysis was confined to the mineral constituents.   The germ theory of the transmission of disease through the agency of sewage-polluted water had not arisen.   In this country water purification was practically an unknown art.

BEGINNING OF FILTRATION IN THE UNITED STATES

But the dawn was already breaking. In 1866 James B. Kirkwood, a civil engineer, was sent to Europe by the city of St. Louis to study the new methods which had been coming into use in England and Germany, for besides the London filters there were at this time filters in many of the English and in most of the large German cities. Kirkwood's report, the first important document on filtration published in this country, may be said to mark the beginning of the history of water purification in America. His plan for filtering the muddy water of the Mississippi River, which was based on his European observations, was not adopted by St. Louis. It was fortunate that the plant was not built, for later studies of the filtration of such waters have shown that it certainly would have failed. Several other filters, however, were built as a result of his report, notably the Poughkeepsie filter which was constructed in 1872 to clarify the water of the Hudson River. This filter was the most successful of several which were built about that time.

In 1878 Professor William Ripley Nichols went to Europe to study water purification for the Massachusetts State Board of Health and his report was printed in the *Annual Report* of that year. Five years later his notable book on *Water Supply* was published. In this he discussed not only the problem of filtration, but that of tastes and odors as related to the algæ. In many ways the book was a pioneer in its field. For a considerable time the center of interest in matters connected with water purification was in Massachusetts. In 1887 the State Board of Health established an experiment station at Lawrence and the purification of water as well as the treatment of sewage was studied from all possible angles,—engineers, chemists and biologists contributing to the investigations. The experiments were made upon the relatively clear but polluted water of the Merrimac River. Some of those prominent in connection with this work were Hiram F. Mills, Frederick P. Stearns, Allen Hazen, George W. Fuller, H. W. Clark, Edwin O. Jordan, Mrs. Ellen H. Richards, Professor Thomas M. Drown, and Professor William T. Sedgwick, the last two acting in an advisory capacity. This was the first important scientific study of the subject of water purification in America and its results did much to develop the art.

While these experiments were under way, a notable epidemic of typhoid fever swept down the Merrimac valley and included the city of Lawrence which took its water supply from the river. It soon became evident that a filter was needed and in 1893 a sand filter designed by Mr. Mills was put into operation. This filter was built as a single bed without roof and involved certain complicated arrangements of coarse and fine sand, ideas which have not been followed in other plants; in fact, the filter has been largely rebuilt in recent years. This filter proved to be a great object lesson to the country, as it showed conclusively that polluted water could be made safe for drinking. It was a practical demonstration of the ideas which had been developed at the Lawrence Experiment Station.

Hazen, after his Lawrence experience and after conducting experiments at the World's Fair in Chicago, spent a year in Europe studying foreign practice, and out of this came his book on *Filtration*, which for a generation was the leading authority on the subject. Unfortunately, it is now out of print.

Meanwhile filtration had been developing in another direction in regions of the country where the water supplies were muddy. In 1883 Charles Hermany conducted some experiments in the filtration of the water supply at Louisville, Ky. In 1884 Alpheus Hyatt obtained a patent on the use of sulphate of alumina as a coagulant and in the same year a mechanical filter using such a coagulant was built at Somerville, New Jersey. Although mechanical filters had previously been used for clarifying water for industrial purposes, this was the first application of the method to a public water supply. The name of Professor Albert R. Leeds should be remembered in connection with the early development of this process, as he was its real inventor. A mechanical filter was built for the water supply of New Orleans, but failed to meet the requirements and was removed at great loss to the promoting company. Several other installations were made in different parts of the country. Some of these early mechanical filters gave fairly good results; others failed. It became evident that the process was not only useful but necessary for the purification of muddy waters, and also that engineers had not learned how to employ it successfully. Then science came to the rescue. In 1893 Edmund B. Weston made some tests of mechanical filters for the city of Providence, which should be remembered as the first carefully conducted tests with this type of filtraton. In 1895 to 1897 Charles Hermany of Louisville again studied the problem of filtration, this time with the assistance of George W. Fuller and a corps of engineers, chemists and bacteriologists acting for the Louisville Water Company and several companies interested in the construction of mechanical filters. These experiments, conducted on the water of the Ohio River, resulted in a notable report published by Mr. Fuller. The Louisville experiments were devoted to a study of the theory of the filtration of clay-bearing waters and the use of coagulation and sedimentation in connection with mechanical filtration. The principles thus established have served as the basis of the mechanical filters which have since been constructed in the United States. Various devices employed in mechanical filtration were also tested at Louisville and their weaknesses pointed out.

The experiments at Lawrence and Louisville demonstrated the fact that different kinds of waters require different methods of purification; that while slow sand filtration can be successfully used with a relatively clear water like that of the Merrimac River at Lawrence, coagulation must accompany filtration in the case of muddy waters such as those of the Ohio and Mississippi Rivers. With this thought in mind there followed a series of tests in different parts of the country. At Pittsburgh Hazen conducted experiments to compare the relative advantages of sand and mechanical filtration for the water of the Allegheny River. His report was published in 1899. Fuller made further experiments in mechanical filtration in Cincinnati in 1898. Experiments were also made at Washington, D. C., at Superior, Wisconsin, at New Orleans, at Philadelphia, at Reading, at Boston, and elsewhere. It was a time of experiment, and much of this experimental work was done by men who had received their early training in Massachusetts.

PROGRESS OF FILTRATION

The first large slow sand filter to be constructed after that at Lawrence was designed by Allen Hazen for the city of Albany, New York, to treat the water of the Hudson River. This filter was put in service in 1899. It differed in several respects from that at Lawrence, but especially by having a masonry cover, experience having already shown that the cold weather of winter interfered with the operation of open filters like those at Poughkeepsie and Lawrence. The Albany filter has in many ways served as a model for the sand filters which have since been constructed in the United States, such as those at Washington, Philadelphia, Providence, and many other cities.

The first important mechanical filter to be constructed along modern lines was that of the East Jersey Water Company at Little Falls, New Jersey, which was put in service in 1902 to purify the water of the Passaic River. As long as the basic Hyatt patent was in force the construction of mechanical filters had been confined chiefly to those built by private companies, but after the expiration of this patent in 1910 the art of mechanical filtration advanced rapidly. A large mechanical filter was built for the Hackensack Water Company in New Jersey in 1904 and many others followed.

It will be seen, therefore, that it was just about the beginning of the twentieth century when water purification in the United States really began to advance as a practical measure. The last decade of the nineteenth century had been one of experimentation. The work done by the chemists and bacteriologists was to be taken up by the engineers and pushed rapidly. Since 1900 there has been a great increase in the use of filtration. In 1870 practically no filtered water was in use in this country. In 1880, 30,000 people in cities having populations above 2,500 were using filtered water. In 1890 its number increased to 310,000; in 1900, to 1,860,000; in 1910, to 10,805,000; and in 1920, to at least 20,000,000. At the present time more than one third of the people living in cities that contain 2,500 or more inhabitants are using water which has been filtered. The number of filters in the country is probably not far from 800. At first, filtration developed in those cities which were supplied with relatively clear water and naturally the method of sand filtration was used, but since then the increase in the use of mechanical filters has been more rapid, largely for the reason that there are more places in the country where water supplies are of such a character that coagulation is necessary or desirable.

Efforts have sometimes been made to show that the two methods — namely, slow sand filtration, sometimes called the English system, and mechanical filtration, sometimes called the American system — were rival processes, each with its advocates, this idea being spread chiefly by the private companies interested in the sale of mechanical filtration devices. In the minds of the best sanitary engineers, however, these two processes have never been regarded as rivals, but rather as alternate processes, each of which has its own appropriate field of application. The ideas demonstrated by the early experiments that sand filtration is in general the most appropriate method for the purification of relatively clear waters and that mechanical filtration with coagulation is best adapted to the treatment of muddy or colored waters are as true to-day as they were twenty-five years ago. As a matter of fact, local conditions of many sorts have to be considered in deciding upon the type and design of a filtration plant. In addition to the character of the water to be treated, consideration has to be given to the availability of sites, the cost of land, and various financial considerations involving the initial cost of the operation, and the like. Continued study of the subject and experience gained at the various works which have been constructed have given to sanitary engineers data which enable them to determine the best combination of processes for any particular situation. Our country is so large and the water supplies in the different sections vary so greatly in their original quality that many supplementary processes such as aeration, sedimentation, coagulation, disinfection, and various chemical processes have been developed. No history of filtration would be complete without reference to some of these processes, but space does not permit them to be discussed in detail.

PROCESSES SUPPLEMENTARY TO FILTRATION

Aeration— that is, the exposure of water to the air in drops or in thin films — was practised long before the days of filtration. At one time it was thought that actual purification of the water took place. It is now known that aeration has little effect on the bacterial content of water but that its chief benefits are in supplying oxygen to water which is deficient in this gas, the removal of dissolved carbonic acid, and the removal of the odors due to microscopic organisms. Sometimes natural aeration is utilized, but in a number of instances, notably in the Catskill supply of New York City, very extensive aeration plants have been constructed. Prior to the design of these plants experiments were made by the writer to determine the underlying scientific facts of aeration and by the engineering staff of the New York Board of Water Supply to determine the best type of design. It seems probable that this feature of water purification will receive greater attention in the future than it has in the past.

Sedimentation is also an old process of water purification which was used long before the days of modern filtration. Although many sedimentation plants have been built in this country in connection with slow sand filters and mechanical filters, no scientific basis of design has yet been worked out. The most notable contribution to the subject was a paper by Allen Hazen on "Sedimentation," published in the *Transactions of the American Society of Civil Engineers* in 1904. Although this paper stimulated some experimental work, much remains to be learned in regard to the rate of subsidence of small particles in water, the nature of currents through basins as affected by length, depth, area, rate of flow, temperature and other factors. The whole subject of baffling also needs further scientific investigation.

Coagulation with alum is an old process, dating back to ancient times. Modern practice has included the use of other substances than alum— notably lime and sulphate of iron, a combination found to be specially useful with the muddy waters of the Middle West. Lime and soda have been used in connection with alum, sometimes to supply alkalinity to very soft waters and sometimes in connection with water softening processes. Inasmuch as the cost of chemicals is an important item in the cost of operation of filters, much attention has been given to the subject of coagulation. At the present time the problem is being attacked anew with the aid of some of the latest ideas of physical chemistry. For many years coagulants were added to the water to be filtered in soluble form, and it was a decided improvement when about fifteen years ago Hazen, Weston and others began to study and use the dry feed method of controlling the application of chemicals to the water. Another advance in the art was that of making the coagulant at the filter instead of purchasing it in dry form. C. P. Hoover, at Columbus, Ohio, was the pioneer in this field. Coagulation is generally employed with mechanical filters but sometimes with slow sand filters and sometimes in connection with sedimentation only.

Akin to the problem of clarification by coagulation and filtration is that of color removal. This problem has long been studied, but is not yet fully solved. In 1890 experiments on filtration made at the Chestnut Hill Reservoir of the Boston Water Works under the direction of Desmond FitzGerald included studies of decolorization. Much attention has been given in Massachusetts to the natural processes of bleaching as it occurs during storage in reservoirs. Natural processes are important, but they have their limitations. Up to the present time no better chemical method of decolorization than by the use of alum has been found, although this has not been altogether satisfactory, especially when the water to be treated is soft as well as colored. This whole problem of decolorization is now under review. Experiments have shown the colloidal character of the coloring, and the problem is now being attacked along the lines of colloidal chemistry. The problem of decolorization is especially important in New England, and in the western regions north of the glacial drift, where the waters of the streams are relatively clear, but soft and colored.

When alum first came into use as a coagulant there was a strong prejudice against it in the medical profession. The public had already passed through a lively agitation in regard to alum in baking powders, and the subject was one upon which even laymen had strong convictions. The suggestion of using alum in the St. Louis water brought out the newspaper headline, "We don't want puckered water." In Washington and Philadelphia the protest of the doctors led to the choice of sand filtration instead of mechanical filtration. This popular prejudice long ago subsided, as experience has shown that no evil effects have followed the use of alum; but curiously enough, however, a contrary change of opinion has recently occurred in regard to the alum reaction, this time from chemists and sanitary engineers themselves. Sir Alexander Houston, director of the laboratories of the Metropolitan Water Board of London, is strong in his opinion that mechanical filters are not as reliable as slow sand filters. His recent statement on the subject reminds one strikingly of the opinion advanced by Hiram F. Mills many years ago. In the early days the water chemists replied to the opponents of alum that the reaction between the aluminum sulphate and the carbonates of the water was so complete that no "alum", as such, passed through the filter. It is now believed that in many places the reaction is not complete before filtration and that not all of the alum is changed to the hydrate of alumina. Just what these side-reactions are has not as yet been fully determined. Apparently the use of alum increases the acid properties of the water, even after the resulting carbonic acid has been removed by aeration. When the new ideas have been fully worked out, a new chapter in the history of water filtration will have to be written.

Another problem of filtration which has received much study is that of the removal of algæ and other microscopic organisms from water. These organisms are sometimes so numerous that they clog the sand rapidly, and the amount of organic matter is sometimes so great that the dissolved oxygen of the water becomes exhausted, — a condition which leads to most unpleasant results. Aeration, double filtration, and intermittent filtration have all been used in the solution of this problem. Aeration has proved itself especially beneficial.

American engineers have given attention to iron removal, water softening, and decarbonation, i. e., the removal of dissolved carbonic acid from the water in the interest of corrosion prevention, but time will not suffice to discuss these subjects here. As filtration has extended to different parts of the country new problems have arisen, until to-day water purification is not the simple process that it was fifty years ago, but is a well established art which involves many processes and combinations of processes.

THE PROBLEM OF THE ALGÆ

Another problem of water purification which has received much study in America is that of the algae and other microscopic organisms which develop in surface waters and some ground waters. The Massachusetts State Board of Health was a pioneer in this study. Important investigations were made by Professor William Ripley Nichols and Dr. W. G. Farlow even before the days of the Lawrence Experiment Station. In connection with this problem the writer may be pardoned a brief reference to his own first researches at the Chestnut Hill Reservoir in 1889, which had to do with the filtration of water through a layer of sponge for the purpose of removing algæ and their accompanying tastes and odors. These experiments, though unsuccessful, aroused his interest in the whole subject of algal growth and the science of limnology and led to the publication of his *Microscopy of Drinking Water* in 1899. In connection with the study of algæ the names of Professor William T. Sedgwick and George W. Rafter should not be forgotten. Desmond FitzGerald was responsible for the founding of the Chestnut Hill Laboratory of the Boston Water Works in which the writer carried on his early studies. This laboratory, established in connection with the supervision of the quality of the Boston water, in which chemical, biological, and bacteriological analyses were made and in which field work was given much emphasis, was the first of its kind in America. In 1897 the writer under the direction of I. M. de Varona, established the now well-known Mount Prospect Laboratory of the Brooklyn Water Works. The work of this laboratory was afterwards extended to cover the entire New York water supply and played an important part in connection with the investigations which led to the construction of the great Catskill water supply project. It was in this laboratory that many of the investigations were conducted for the Committee on Standard Methods of Water Analysis of the American Public Health Association.

The study of the algæ is really a part of a still broader subject, the science of limnology, a science which has received attention here and there, in various universities, but which has never been developed as it should be.   Dr. E. A. Birge, now president of the University of Wisconsin, has contributed much to this science.   His investigations of temperature and dissolved gases in lakes may be regarded as classics.

In spite of all the study which has been given to the algæ, we do not yet know the natural laws which govern their appearance and growth.   The opportunities for investigations in this field are very great.

Although sanitary engineers do not know how to control the growth of algæ and microscopic organisms in reservoirs, they do know how to remove them from water, as well as the odors which they produce.   This can be done by filtration and aeration.   Sometimes double filtration or intermittent filtration is required.

DISINFECTION OF WATER

We now come to the method of disinfection of water by the use of chlorine, a process which has played a most important part in water purification in recent years.   Like the other processes of the art it has its evolutionary history.   It was not long after the germ theory of water-borne diseases was established that scientists began to try to destroy the bacteria in water by the use of chemical disinfectants. Chloride of lime, bromine, and other substances were tried in England with both sewage and water, but little headway was made.   Naturally there was a greater prejudice against the chemical treament of water with poisonous substances than with alum.

In 1902 Dr. George F. Moore brought out his method of dosing reservoirs with copper sulphate to kill algæ and other organisms, including bacteria.   It was found that extraordinarily small doses of copper sufficed for this purpose.   In 1908 George A. Johnson experimented with the use of bleaching powder in connection with the purification of the highly polluted water of Bubbly Creek, Chicago, and a few months later Dr. Leal and Mr. Johnson used this substance for disinfecting the new water supply of Jersey City obtained from the Boonton Reservoir,—the court having decided that the supply as provided by the construction company was not of guaranteed quality, — this new method being cheaper than that of filtration or the removal of the sources of pollution. A new court procedure as to the adequacy of the method of chlorine disinfection led to careful scientific studies, which demonstrated the value of the process. The cheapness and simplicity of the method led to its use in other places, and it was not long before it was taken up by some of the largest cities of the country. About 1910 liquid chlorine began to be used in place of chloride of lime. Several methods of applying liquid chlorine were tried, but at present only one of these is in common use — the Wallace and Tiernan apparatus. The war did a great deal to demonstrate the value of liquid chlorine as a useful and practical disinfectant for water supplies. At the present time the method is used not only as a supplement to filtration, but as a precautionary and emergency method in very many of our large American cities.

Other methods of disinfection than that of chlorination have been tried —notably ozonization. Theoretically sound, its practical difficulties and its high cost have made all attempts to use ozone unsuccessful. The most successful ozone plant which the writer has seen was that being used in Petrograd, Russia, in 1917. Usually these plants when visited are found not to be running for one cause or an other. The use of the ultra-violet ray for disinfection has also been tried, but never employed practically on a large scale. It is not unlikely, however, that in the future these processes may be brought into use where local conditions are favorable.

OPERATION OF FILTERS

In thinking of the subject of water filtration, attention is naturally focused on the methods and designs employed, as they are of the greatest scientific interest. But the safety of a filtered water supply depends not only upon the structure of the filter but upon its operation. A filter plant, with its various appurtenances is a delicate mechanism. It must not be neglected. It needs constant attention and skillful supervision. The art of filtration, therefore, has two co-related parts, design and operation, and a word ought to be said here for the filter operator, for he seldom gets the credit which he deserves. Being a permanent official, or employee, he seldom gets the salary which he deserves. He must be a four-sided man—a chemist, a bacteriologist, an engineer, and an executive. As chemist and bacteriologist he must be able to test the quality of the filtered water; as an engineer he must see that the plant is kept running and in good physical order; while as an executive he must look to the cost of things and supervise the work of the various employees. The filter operator has excellent opportunities for scientific work, and, to an extent not often appreciated, the improvements in the art of filtration in recent years have been due to him.

The water filtration plant very often stands as the prime guardian of the health of the community. Those who have charge of the filter have a grave responsibility. They must not regard it lightly. And no city government can afford to be parsimonious in its treatment of its water filtration plant, or of the men who are employed to design and operate it.

It is of the greatest importance that filter operators be properly educated for their work. It is possible for young men without college or technical school training to acquire experience at a filter plant and ascend to executive control. Such men have their limitations, and in view of the improvements and economies which can be brought about by a well trained filter operator it is to be hoped that the personnel will be kept up to a high standard. The idea of requiring licenses for filter operators has been suggested, but this does not seem likely to solve the problem. There are many places in the country where young men can study sanitary engineering and where courses of study in water analysis, chemistry, and biology, hydraulics, statistics, and accounting are included as a part of a regular program. More and more cities should seek graduates of engineering schools for these responsible positions.

PROTECTION AGAINST POLLUTION

Ever since it became known that polluted water might be a carrier of disease, efforts have been made by public health authorities to safeguard the quality of the water by protective measures. These protective measures have sometimes included the purchase of the entire watershed. Sometimes strips of land around the reservoirs and streams have been purchased and cleaned. Sometimes individual properties have been acquired and nuisances abated. Rules and regulations have been made governing the habits of the inhabitants of the watershed with respect to the disposal of fecal matter. Swamps have been drained in order to reduce the amount of color in the water. Ponds and reservoirs have been deepened in order to prevent the growth of algæ and water weeds. Sewage disposal works have been built to deal with the sewage of communities on the watershed. Diversion sewers have been built. In any discussion of water purification these protective measures should not be lost sight of. Under some conditions they are more effective even than filtration, and they are always useful. Fifty years ago they were practised only to a slight extent.

It has become known also that there are natural agencies which aid greatly in the purification of water. Natural æration is beneficial in ways already mentioned. Storage is a most important factor in lessening the danger of infection, because during storage such bacteria as the bacillus of typhoid fever tend to die out. Fresh pollution is far more to be feared than old pollution. During storage sunlight may not only reduce the color of water by bleaching it, but it may destroy some of the bacteria. During storage also sedimentation may occur. The mere mixing of water in a reservoir under wind action tends to disperse any pollution through large volumes and thus reduce its dangerous possibilities. It is here that the science of limnology comes in. Not all of the natural conditions can be controlled in the interest of water purification, but knowing the natural laws advantage can often be taken of existing conditions.

As people have come to appreciate the need of a clean water supply, standards of purity have risen and there has been a demand for water supplies which are not only safe according to sanitary standards but which are derived from attractive surroundings. In other words, there are æsthetic standards as well as sanitary standards which are coming into demand.

It will be seen, therefore, that there are three main lines of endeavor in safeguarding water supplies — taking advantage of natural conditions, protective agencies against pollution, and artificial methods of purification. Every water supply must be considered as a special problem and those methods of protection chosen which are best adapted to the conditions.

WATER ANALYSIS

Progress in the analysis of water has gone hand in hand with improvements in the art of water purification. Fifty years ago the methods of analysis were crude indeed. Frankland made known his combustion process for measuring the organic matter in water in terms of organic carbon and organic nitrogren in 1867, while about the same time Wanklyn brought out his "free and albuminoid ammonia method." The "oxygen consumed" method, using permanganate of potash in acid solution, had gradually developed a few years before. These tests, together with the determinations of total solids, loss on ignition, hardness, and chlorine, were the leading tests until the late eighties, when other methods such as tests for nitrites and nitrates crept in.

Following the lead of Mallet, Leeds, Nichols, Drown, Mason, and other chemists, the practice of "interpreting water analysis" became common. Then came the applications of bacteriology and microscopy in the early nineties. Practical considerations also came to the fore and quantitative measurements of color, turbidity, and odor became prominent. The adoption of filtration caused a great increase in the number of water analyses, and brought in many new tests. Soon it became evident that standard methods were needed, and in 1899 a committee was appointed by the American Public Health Association to consider the subject. It sat for five years and finally in 1905 issued a report which, with its revisions, has been the American standard since that time.

The history of water analysis is a story in itself and is worth being considered by students of water purification. It is by analysis that processes of water purification are tested and controlled and new processes devised.

RESULTS OF WATER PURIFICATION

What has been the result of filtration and other measures adopted to protect public water supplies during the fifty years covered by the life of the American Public Health Association and in which the members of the Association have played so important a part? First, they have saved thousands of human lives and an untold amount of sickness, with all its consequential losses. Where typoid fever death-rates were 40 and 60 and 80, they are now less than 10, and often less than 5, per 100,000. Other diseases have also been lessened, especially the diarrheal diseases and infant mortality. Second, they have increased human comfort by providing supplies of clean water in place of muddy water, colored water, or water of unpleasant taste and smell. Third, they have tended to raise the sanitary morale of each community where they have been adopted. Efforts to protect water supplies have led to efforts to secure safer and more decent methods of disposing of sewage and other wastes. And almost the best of it is that these community blessings have been obtained at an insignificant cost to each individual. In general it may be said that water purification adds only about ten per cent to the cost of a water supply, and when we think that the annual cost of having running water in our houses is but little, if any, more than what we pay for our daily newspaper, and when we think that the annual per capita cost of filtration is less than the cost of a necktie we realize that this is a small price to pay for the value received from water purification.

PRESENT PROBLEMS

Water purification would not be a growing art unless there was new work ahead, and unless there were new problems which were being studied. A survey of the situation reveals some interesting facts and tendencies.

In the first place, not all of the water supplies of the country to-day are being adequately protected. There are still some places where grossly polluted water is being distributed to the people, although year by year these places are decreasing in number. There are many places where the water is reasonably safe but is not attractive at all times for one reason or another. Fifty years ago, and even twenty-five years ago, the New England water supplies were on the whole better in quality than those in other parts of the country, but to-day filtration has become so common in regions where the streams are naturally muddy that the New England supplies, few of which are filtered, suffer in comparison with filtered waters elsewhere, in so far as the quality of attractiveness is concerned. In New England the policy of utilizing natural storage and preventing pollution in all possible ways was wisely adopted, but these measures have their limits and with increasing populations the filtration of surface waters is likely to become universal. It may even be required by law.

There are many places in the country where disinfection has been adopted without filtration or in place of adequate attempts to prevent pollution. Gradually the weakness of this policy is being found out. Disinfection is very cheap, but cheap disinfection does not accomplish what filtration accomplishes and it ought not to be accepted as a substitute for it or for vigilance in protecting a water supply against pollution.

Now that the typhoid fever-rates of the country have been greatly reduced, consumers are thinking less about the dangers of their water supplies and more about their physical appearance, about their corrosive properties, and about their fitness for industrial uses—that is, they are seeking refinements. Thus a new class of problems, such as water softening with the use of lime and soda, or with permutit, the removal of iron and manganese, and the neutralization of acidity, is receiving the attention of water chemists.

Many of the filters built ten and twenty years ago have been in use long enough to show up defects in practical operation, and experience has indicated where changes can be made to avoid depreciation, reduce repair costs, save money in operation, and get better results. Filter designs are slowly being modified as a result of these findings. It is natural that at the time of installation officials should give greatest attention to construction cost, but as time goes on it is the costs of operation which are scrutinized. The usual lower first cost of mechanical filters is a reason why it is sometimes easier to induce cities to install that type of filter than a slow sand filter, which often costs more to install but less to operate. Higher operating costs, however, make mechanical filters less popular after a term of years. The economics of filter operation can now be studied more exactly than was possible twenty-five years ago, and this is a phase of the subject which is likely to receive increasing attention.

Methods of testing the performance of filters by the use of analyses have not changed greatly in twenty-five years. In the early days stress was laid on the percentage removal of bacteria, color, turbidity, and organic matter. Tests were made to show what the filter was able to do. Now we are more interested in knowing what the filter actually does, and the analyses must serve as a test of the filter operator as well as the filter itself. Dr. Drown used to say, when talking about water analyses, that "a state of change is a state of danger." Now we emphasize the principle that *a state of irregularity is a state of danger*. We want filters operated so as to give a uniform product from day to day and hour to hour. Hence attention is being given to the application of the mathematical theories of probability to filter records. There are great possibilities in this study, appreciated at present by only a few engineers.

At the moment a new impetus is being given to many of the problems of water purification by the use of new and simple methods of determining the true acidity of water in terms of the hydrogen-ion concentration. This and other methods of physical chemistry are likely to clarify many of our ideas in regard to problems of coagulation, corrosion, disinfection, and the growth of algæ.

Bacteriological tests of water have never been as definite as chemical tests. The difficulties have been partly analytical and partly statistical. The test for *B. coli* has been largely used, and on the whole successfully used; but it has many shortcomings. The use of tests for determining the presence of spore-forming organisms is now under discussion, so that water bacteriologists as well as water chemists are active in their researches.

Also in the field of vital statistics there are new ideas coming to the front. The typhoid fever death-rates are becoming so low that they can no longer be regarded as sufficient to measure the healthfulness of a water supply. The so-called Mills-Reincke theorem, which held that for every death from water-borne typhoid fever there were several deaths from other diseases due to water, has been found not to hold universally, although there is much truth in it. Polluted water may cause sickness of one kind or another which does not find record in the vital statistics of the community. Some more careful measure of the effect of water on the health of the community is urgently needed.

Thus it is seen that there are activities among engineers, chemists, biologists, and statisticians in the field of water purification, a fact which is full of promise.

LOOKING AHEAD

And what of the future? It is safe to say that the movement for water filtration will continue until all the surface water supplies are thus treated. By the time the American Public Health Association celebrates its one hundredth anniversary, and possibly by the time it celebrates its seventy-fifth, the filtration of public surface water supplies may be made compulsory by law. Protection against pollution, important though it is, will not be enough. Natural agencies of purification cannot be depended upon alone. Disinfection of water enhances its safety but does not cleanse. Typhoid fever is rapidly decreasing in this country and, therefore, all water supplies, whether filtered or not, are safer now than they were a generation ago, but there must be no lapse of effort lest the ground which has been gained be lost. Furthermore, safety is only one element in the problem. Pure water has a value because of its purity; because people appreciate a clear, colorless odorless, palatable water; and because they instinctively refrain from drinking water unless it appears to be pure. The motive for water filtration is likely to change during the next generation from safety to cleanliness, from health to comfort. Both motives are instinctive and right, and the watchword of the future will continue to be "purity and wholesomeness."

SEWAGE AND SOLID REFUSE REMOVAL

RUDOLPH HERING, D. SC.

Consulting Engineer New York City

WHEN the populations of cities grow to large numbers, and both their liquid and solid refuse materials become greatly increased in bulk, their proper removal from habitations begins to assume serious conditions. Such materials consist largely of organic waste matter, some of which is offensive at the origin, but most of which becomes so when persistently exposed to warmth and moisture.

At first they are easy to remove, dump, and subsequently to be covered when desired, because the distances are short and quantities small. After a certain time such disposal becomes objectionable and nuisances result. Sewage is the first material to give trouble and the first to require better treatment. The solid refuse did not receive regular municipal attention until about fifty years ago.

The collection, removal, and disposition of both liquid and solid refuse, respectively, requires works and treatments of essentially different kinds. Therefore, it is most convenient to speak of them separately.

SEWAGE REMOVAL

The liberal introduction of water into houses for washing and cleaning produced sewage. This was more or less foul, but was allowed to flow away over the surface and in the gutters of streets. The subsequent introduction of water-closets for the reception of excrementitious matter, increased the foul condition of sewage to an extent which soon demanded in many cities an underground removal through sewers. Rome appears to have been the first city to have what might be called sewers (Cloaca Maxima, etc.) which, however, were rather crude in design and construction, and unsanitary. England, during the first half of the last century, provided several of its largest cities with sewers, and later developed the chief principles of their design and construction (Rawlinson), according to which sewers have since been built in all civilized countries.

It is little more than fifty years since we, in America, awaking to the importance of promoting public health, gave proper attention to this subject. Among the most prominent American engineers who introduced modern sewerage were, in order of time, Chesbrough, Lane, Adams, Philbrick, and Davis.

In view of much controversy between the older engineers and Col. George E. Waring, who in 1878 advocated not only the exclusion of all rainwater from sewers, but also the use of very small pipes for sewage removal (4″ pipes for house connections and 6″ pipes for main sewers serving less than 300 houses), the writer was sent abroad by the National Board of Health, to report on the accepted fundamental principles of design of sewerage works that had been established in European cities. The resulting report (1881) set forth those principles and their exemplifications in the best works of Europe. After proper adaptation to our local conditions, those same principles have since been substantially followed by us.

The fundamental requirement was established that: first, we must satisfy the demands of sanitation, by having the design, construction and maintenance arranged so as to prevent any factor injurious to health, and secondly, we must select from among the available sanitary designs the one which costs least per annum, when adding fixed and operating charges.

The essential principles of management and design now advocated by the profession can be grouped under two headings: collection and disposal. The tendency to-day is rapidly and properly in the direction of municipal instead of private ownership, management, and opereration of sewerage works. With an efficient city administration the public health requirements and the demands of the citizens can be satisfied at less cost, than if left in private hands. The municipality therefore should have control and management of the work from the points where the sewage originates to those of its final disposition. At present, however, local conditions may here and there still occassionally suggest a preference for a collection or disposal by contract with the city under efficient supervision.   In Europe such private contracts have been substantially abandoned.

A sewerage system may be either a combined or a separate one. It is combined when the sewers receive domestic sewage, trade wastes and all rainwater.   It is separate when the sewage and trade wastes are taken away by one set of underground channels or sewers, and nearly all of the rainwater, or at least that which cannot flow off on the surface, by another set, usually called drains.   Both systems can be entirely inoffensive, and the preference should be given to the one which under the local conditions is least expensive.

It is generally found that in large cities and densely populated areas the combined system is cheaper.   On the other hand, the separate system will cost less when the area does not require extensive underground rainwater removal, by allowing such water to flow off on the surface or by concentrating it to require but a few drains.   It may also be cheaper when the sewage before its discharge requires expensive purification or pumping, while the rainwater without treatment can be discharged by gravity.

It has been found essential to build sewers with much more care than was customary in the early days.   They should not only be built of durable material, so that the sewage, which is sometimes acid and some times alkaline, will not gradually destroy them, but they should also be so graded and aligned that the flow will be rapid, *i. e·* at least two feet per second.   Junctions and curves should be made so that the flow will be continuous and regular, that no eddies or deposits will form, and that the interior surface is as smooth as practicable to prevent retention of shreds or particles of foul matter, which usually cause the sewer air to become offensive.

To further guard against the generation of foul sewage and foul air, a systematic and frequent flushing should be made an essential part of the sewer maintenance.   This is done in small pipe sewers by automatic flush tanks, which suddenly discharge a few hundred gallons of water into the sewer once or twice a day; and in larger sewers by gates operated by hands, to store sewage above them and to let this stored-up quantity suddenly rush out with a more rapid and therefore cleansing velocity.

Finally, to maintain good air in the sewers they must be ventilated. Artificial ventilation is hardly ever required, because a sufficiently good natural ventilation can be secured simply by providing perforated manhole covers on the street surface and a free and unobstructed passage of air from the street sewers through the house sewers to above the roof. The usually different temperatures at such inlets and outlets will produce a sufficient air circulation. All house fixtures must be securely trapped.

The sizes of combined sewers are determined from the observed maximum rain of greatest intensity falling within five or ten minutes. The sizes of separate sewers depend upon the greatest water supply consumption during the forenoon hours of the day when most of it is used.

The cross-section of combined sewers is usually egg-shaped, because this gives to the comparatively small and otherwise shallow sewage flow a greater concentration, less friction and therefore less deposit, while the circular separate sewers, which carry nothing but sewage and run from one-third to one-half full, give its flow approximtely the desired semicircular section.

The final disposal of sewage became a subject of much controversy about fifty years ago. It was thought practicable and desirable to convert sewage into a valuable manure. It was also thought that even a slight discharge of sewage into our natural water course would be injurious to health, and some believed that even sewage farming, particularly when used for vegetable raising, was unhealthful, although the use of manure was not considered objectionable. These views have since materially changed.

The small rivers and the comparatively concentrated population in England first brought this subject into prominence. The resulting pollution and offensiveness of the rivers demanded the exclusion of most of the sewage or its prior purification.

Land irrigation with sewage was an old and effective process and the first one used for sewage purification. In Great Britain the earliest plant of this type was installed at Edinburgh.   The absence of extended sand beds near most of the British cities however, favored a more intense filtration on smaller areas.   Consequently, an intermittent filtration of greater intensity, through sand, was introduced by Bailey Denton, on the recommendation of Sir Edward Frankland.   It was first successfully tried at Merthyr Tydfil in Wales in 1871.

In order to still further reduce the area of land required, preliminary treatments were adopted to remove the major portion of the suspended particles from the sewage before its application upon the sand. For this purpose various apparatus for screening out the larger suspended particles (up to 15 per cent) have also been used more or less successfully.   Plain sedimentation was introduced, depositing up to 70 per cent and later; in order to increase its effect up to 95 per cent, it was accelerated by the addition of chemicals, such as milk of lime, sulphate of alumina, ferric oxide, and other materials which would precipitate a large percentage, including the finer particles of the suspended matter.   These chemical methods were used for many years, although the results were never quite satisfactory, chiefly because of the offensive sludge which was produced.   It could not be profitably utilized, but required expensive removal.

In 1870 an English commision was appointed to give these questions suitable study, and made several valuable reports.   In 1876, Dr. C. F. Folsom of Boston, Massachusetts, reported the results of the English commission, which indicated that a purification by percolation through land, and chiefly through sand, had given the best obtainable results.

Thereupon, in 1888, the Massachusetts State Board of Health organized an experiment station at Lawrence, and in its classical reports up to 1891 scientifically demonstrated the biological nature of sand filtration.   Thereafter it became possible to design such works with an assurance of obtaining definite results.   A relation was discovered between the size of sand grains, the amount of air required, its temperature, and the quantities of sewage that could be intermittently applied and purified, up to certain definite degrees of purity, per square foot of sand-bed having different depths.   Since then sewage purification by filtration through sand has become an established practice.

To solve the problem where sand was not available, further researches had to be made. The Lawrence experiments proved that the slow movement of sewage in thin films over the surface of sand grains and stone, in contact with air, removed almost all of the organic matter and bacteria contained in the sewage. Coarse materials, such as gravel, broken stone, bricks, and slag were then tried for this purpose in England, where natural sand beds are scarce. In 1893 at Salford, Corbett built the first large filters of this kind, which were afterwards called sprinkling or trickling filters. The sewage was sprayed into the air from jets placed about 12 to 16 feet apart, well distributed over the surface, and then percolated slowly through the bed into subdrains from which the purified sewage was discharged. This system has since been extensively used in the United States and Europe and is generally found to be quite satisfactory.

About the same time so-called contact beds were introduced in England by Dibden and others. They were also built of broken stone, but instead of the sewage being sprinkled over the beds, they were filled with sewage from below, which was left standing in them about eight hours. Then it was allowed to drain away and the beds to remain empty about sixteen hours for oxidation. The results were fair ly good but still not wholly satisfactory either as to the effluent or cost and therefore such beds have been seldom used.

The just mentioned processes are intended to purify and dispose of chiefly the liquids. There has recently been developed in England and America a system of aerating sewage, called the Activated Sludge Process, in which air is forced through and thoroughly mixed with the raw sewage, after the heavier materials have been settled out, producing a quicker oxidation and decolloidization of the fine suspended solid particles and dissolved liquid sewage, than without the added air. The effluent produced can be made very satisfactory, clear and free from putrescible matter, and can be directly discharged without detriment into small streams. The settled "activated" solid matter, or sludge, although richer in manurial matter than ordinary sludge, requires a further treatment, in order to remain inoffensive, and be profitably utilized as manure. Final conclusions regarding the economy and value of the entire process have not yet been definitely reached, although under some conditions it may be found economical.

For a better sludge treatment, septic tanks were suggested by Cameron (1895). The sewage was allowed to remain in the tank long enough (four to six months) to liquefy most of the sludge through the action of anaerobic bacteria. But, besides the generation of considerable foul odor, after being half a year in the tank, there still remained a large quantity of unliquefied sludge to be removed. Except on a very small scale, such tanks are not much used any more.

The sludge problem of sewage disposal is its most difficult part. To reduce the quantity, and to simplify its subsequent treatment, when sewage can be discharged upon land or sand beds, it is customary first to pass the crude sewage preliminarily through grit or settling chambers, and to allow the heavier particles, mostly mineral, to settle out. The contents of grit chambers are small in amount and generally not offensive. The sludge contents of ordinary settling or septic tanks are foul and their disposal has been the chief trouble and expense at such works. The manurial value is almost nil, and does not justify much carting.

In the early days it was thought practicable and economical to convert the sludge into a fertilizer but a satisfactory conversion has not yet been made. The only success so far reached has been the gradual conversion into a material having no offensive odor, which allows it to be used as a filling material or at best as agricultural soil. Such a result can be reached by the gradual substitution of bacteria which produce inoffensive gases for those producing foul gases. So far only three treatments have been successful.

First, when sludge is spread into trenches dug in a dry porous soil about twelve inches deep, and covered several inches with such soil, the sludge is gradually converted into an unobjectionable and non-odorous material. This method, substantially, has been used by J. D. Watson in Birmingham, England, and elsewhere.

Second, when sludge can accumulate in the lower story of an Imhoff tank and be prevented from having any contact with fresh sewage, it becomes unobjectionable in from three to six months. The bacteria producing putrefaction are gradually displaced by those producing chiefly methane and carbon dioxide gases, both of which are inoffensive, as in the conversion of forest leaves into forest soil. When turned upon drying beds made in clean sand, well under-drained, the sludge will dry in a short time, if not withdrawn from the tanks too early. It soon becomes spadeable and resembles soil. These drying beds must be made larger in America than in Europe, because our rainfall is much greater in quantity, which delays the drying. Such tanks are already widely used in Europe and America.

Third, similar sludge results to those obtained with Imhoff tanks have been obtained with covered single tanks, used in rotation, one for settling, through which the sewage passes and deposits the sludge, and one for digestion, through which no sewage passes for about six months, the former corresponding to the upper, the latter to the lower Imhoff tank. Such comparatively shallow tanks are less expensive to build in rocky and very wet ground, but the greater pressure in the lower and deeper Imhoff tank has been found materially to hasten the decomposition.

When there is available a large body of flowing water, sufficient in quantity to dilute the sewage, in such a manner that no putrefaction can thereafter result, this method of disposal still remains the most economical and, if properly arranged, also an entirely satisfactory one for many communities.

Finally, when sewage effluents from treatment works enter water courses to be used below for water supplies, it is now practicable at the works to disinfect such effluents economically.

SOLID REFUSE REMOVAL

After the problems concerning sewage had been satisfactorily solved, those relating to the solid refuse began to demand attention. Until w ithin less than a century, rubbish was dumped at any convenient spot, and garbage was generally thrown upon fields for food of animals and birds, both of which customs are still observed in some places.

As cities grew and the populations became more dense, the solid refuse had also to be removed to greater distances and better dispositions made. It then consisted, as now, of garbage, ashes, rubbish, street manure and sweepings, some night soil and dead animals. Several of these materials could be utilized, garbage could be fed to hogs and chickens, manure and street sweepings could frequently be used as a fertilizer and ashes could be dumped to raise land. Such separate dispositions were satisfactory until the quantities became large and their disposal more complicated. Economy and simplification were required for better service.

Here again Europe led the way. Collections began to be made systematically and the best disposals were carefully studied. Manure and street sweepings continued to be taken to farms and used as fertilizers, some garbage was fed to animals and in some cities the rest of it was buried in trenches. Later, it was thought practicable that most of the garbage, rubbish, and domestic ashes, containing much unburned coal, could be collected and all disposed of by burning in a furnace.

In 1874 Fryer, at Nottingham, England, built the first furnace for effectively destroying such combined refuse. This destructor consisted of a series of cells, which were charged with refuse through hoppers placed above the grates. The results were sufficiently satisfactory that this plan of incineration was followed by other cities. With some substantial improvements it is continued in many cities to this day.

When ashes contain little or no unburned coal, as in some parts of central Europe, they are practically of no assistance to incineration. The garbage therefore was disposed of by burial in trenches or fed to animals, and the rubbish was dumped on land or destroyed by burning, sometimes with some garbage.

In America the means of final disposal developed somewhat differently. Our cities were spread out more thinly over larger areas, thus increasing the length of haul. This afforded also better opportunities for dumping ashes and rubbish at nearby points. The proper disposal of garbage, however, required other methods. It could be taken to near-by farms and fed to hogs or buried in trenches where available. Owing to long hauls and the rapid putrescibility of garbage, hog feeding was not everywhere practised with success.

Furnaces were then built to incinerate the garbage. But on account of the large percentage of water it is not self-burning, and it was necessary to add fuel, such as coal, wood, or oil. The increase of expense caused hereby, required greater saving in the use of such fuel, and consequently the incineration was frequently incomplete and the furnace gave off objectionable odors.

Of such furnaces the first one built in the United States was located on Governors Island, New York City, in 1885, by Lieutenant Reilly, U. S. A. The first municipal furnace was erected in Allegheny, Pennsylvania, by Rider in 1886, and one for Des Moines, Iowa, by Engle. Among American writers advocating incineration at that time, we should mention Morse, Venable, and Parsons.

After these first plants had been built many others were installed in the United States, especially by Dixon and Decairie. Many of them, however, have failed to operate satisfactorily, because they were either improperly designed or operated.

We may add another method long practised, but which we should call a temporary one; it is at present used for the large quantities of refuse in New York City and San Francisco. It is the dumping of garbage, and sometimes also of rubbish, at sea. Such dumping is practised solely for reasons of economy. It is admitted that this method is not wholly satisfactory and permanent, as it exposes the shores near these cities to the stranding of old garbage, much of which floats and drifts ashore. The practice is to be continued only until more satisfactory methods can be established.

Owing to the unsatisfactory conditions of nearly all of the ways and means of disposing of city refuse then customary in this country, the American Public Health Association in 1887 appointed a committee to inquire into the subject and make recommendations. After several years it became evident that such could be made only after a very complete collection of facts relating to the subject, including actual examinations of respective works. The committee acquired much statistical information and studied American and European works. In 1897 it made a report and presented conclusions regarding the entire problem, covering house treatment, collection, and final disposal according to methods which had been found satisfactory. These conclusions placed the subject on a practical basis and have served as a safe foundation for the progress which has since been made in America.

The success of the English incinerators which burn mixed refuse, stimulated the introduction of similar plants during the last fifteen years on this side of the Atlantic. The first successful one was built at Westmount (Montreal) in 1906, the second one at West New Brighton (New York), and the largest plant, burning 300 tons per day, was built in Milwaukee in 1910 at the instigation of Dr. Bading. Since then other plants have been erected with improvements, chiefly in mechanical charging apparatus, in Clifton, New York; Paterson, New Jersey; Savannah and Atlanta, Georgia; Toronto, Ontario; and in other cities. The latter plants, all incinerating mixed refuse, have been fitted with boilers for steam production and can develop surplus power in addition to that required for operating the plant.

Parallel with the introduction of general refuse incinerators, several other systems of garbage disposal were developed in our country. First, in the smaller cities, chiefly of New England, garbage is now being fed to hogs more systematically and under more effective organizations than before, and with the approval of the United States Government. Recent results have been found to be fairly satisfactory when the operation was efficient.

Second, a few cities under favorable conditions have satisfactorily buried their excessive garbage with some success in shallow trenches. In Berlin, Germany, most of the garbage is now buried in this manner in sandy soil.

Third, in many of our largest cities, the garbage has been separately collected and in large works in the suburbs has been reduced to grease and so-called tankage, which latter is used as a mild fertilizer. With sufficient care and the expenditure of sufficient money in the operation, such reduction works can be conducted without causing any nuisance. Due to the fall in value of the grease and tankage within late years, many of the works that were in private hands have been abandoned as losses.

All of these disposal methods can be conducted in a sanitary manner, but their cost differs considerably in different localities. To ascertain their true cost the expense must be reckoned from the house where the refuse is received, to the point where a final disposition has been made of it; in other words, it must include the collection as well as the disposal. It sometimes happens that a smaller cost for collection permits a greater expenditure for the disposal and vice versa, without exceeding the total economical figure in comparison with other methods. Therefore the collection cost must be included in the comparative estimates.

There is no expense to the community at the house. It is more convenient to the occupant to dump garbage and rubbish and sometimes also ashes into the same receptacle. Yet the difference in labor necessary to keep them separated is very slight, and should not control the cost of the method which may be adopted for final disposal.

In many cities there is still a need for improving the collection service, both in its organization and in the coöperation between collector and householder. Regular collections should be made along planned routes, to get the largest load in the shortest time and along the easiest roads. The required frequency of collections should depend on the method of disposal and season. Wagons should be covered and both dust and noise kept at a minimum, and still other details should be attended to for the comfort of the citizens and the reduction of cost. The decision as to the preference between combined and separate collections should be based on the total cost to the city, including the disposal.

The greatest difficulties in solving the refuse removal question, however, do not lie in the collection service but in determining the best method of final disposal. In our country many methods have been tried and many abandoned. What has been satisfactory in one locality was not found best in another. Prices of labor and products have so changed that what was economical at one time is not the cheapest at another. Judgments have varied regarding the preference of having simplicity in the works and in their operation, or having more complex works with more intelligent labor. Opinions have also differed for a long time regarding the preference in certain cities, of conducting the works by contract or by municipal labor.

At the present time, after half a century's experience, it seems that the different judgments regarding the best methods of disposal could be brought closely together by considering the following facts.

After the refuse, particularly the rubbish, has been collected, it has occasionally been customary to reclaim articles at sorting works that had a salable value. This practice has prevailed in some cities in Europe and America. In Europe it is being gradually abandoned, except the picking of unburned pieces of coal from ashes, on the ground that the revenue is small compared with the cost, that the occupation is disagreeable when picking the rejected and often filthy matter for so small a profit, and on account of some danger to the health of the pickers when exposed to discarded contents from sick rooms, which were likely to reach such reclamation stations. It seems probable that the same tendency may show itself also in America. As yet the greater wastefulness here increases the revenue, but it is a serious question how long it will be given a higher value in a civilized country than the abandonment of a filthy and degrading occupation, particularly when such occupation is wholly unnecessary for the health or comfort of the community.

Dumping of garbage or rubbish into the ocean may be economical in some localities, but it is questionable whether a community would not always be willing to pay a reasonable tax to prevent the possibility of city garbage and rubbish, recognized as such when floating, from drifting ashore when the shores are used for habitations and health resorts.

Dumping on land is a satisfactory disposal for ashes, both from the sanitary and economical point of view. Sometimes such dumping under favorable conditions may be employed also for street sweepings and rubbish.

Shallow trench burial, if properly conducted, may be satisfactory for the disposal of garbage and manure, both of which are gradually converted into agricultural soil.

13

Reduction into grease and fertilizer, and also disposal by hog feeding are both satisfactory for garbage, if both are properly conducted.

Incineration, in properly designed and operated furnaces, can be used to convert into steam and clinker-ashes the usual combination of garbage, rubbish, domestic ashes, and manure. Rubbish alone, and also when mixed with garbage, can likewise be burned and even produce steam. The destruction of rubbish by fire is essential because of all refuse materials, it is the one most likely to contain disease germs.

The steam produced from the burning of mixed refuse has been utilized in most European and some American cities, not only to operate the plant but also to generate electricity for lighting a part of the city, and even for storage batteries by the power of which some of the city refuse has been collected from the houses.

The incineration of rubbish alone has been sufficient to create enough heat to incinerate much, and in some cases all, of a city's garbage. It is therefore practicable to utilize this heat for dehydrating at least a large portion of the garbage, thus preventing its rapid decomposition, thereby preserving its food value and permitting transportation to a greater distance.

A few words should be added concerning night soil, dead animals and street sweepings. The removal of night soil from buildings where no sewers are available, requires special apparatus and trained collectors, in order to prevent a nuisance. Odorless excavators for this purpose have been used for a long time on both sides of the Atlantic, and with efficient, conscientious, and well-trained men, no objectionable results occur. The same can be said regarding the removal of dead animals when done in suitable wagons and by competent men.

The removal of street sweepings, after they have been gathered in piles or deposited in bags, cans, or pits, so that no dust can arise, should also be done by specially trained men, with proper tools and in covered wagons. It should be done as frequently as the traffic demands, and at suitable hours, which vary in different cities. The disposal of the street sweepings depends on their composition. If they contain sufficient manure, they may be used for fertilizing, otherwise they may be incinerated if containing enough combustible matter, or dumped if they do not.

CONCLUDING REMARKS

In closing it may be proper to add a word regarding the health conditions of the men who are engaged in the service of removing sewage and solid refuse from a city.

For many years it was thought unhealthful to be engaged in the work of cleaning sewers and in operating disposal works. Ample experience and records, however, exist both in Europe and America, proving that the health of such men does not differ materially from that in other trades. The attendants at the filth hoists of the large sewage pumping stations in London, the most offensive and exposed parts of the system, informed the writer that no one of them had ever been sick, except with colds. The death-rate among the attendants of the large sewage farms in Europe was in fact found to be sometimes lower than the average of that of the respective cities. There is no reason to believe that different conditions prevail in our country. The discharges from sick persons and the wash water from hospital laundries generally reach the sewers. But the delicacy of pathogenic organisms when outside their natural habitat, seems to reduce their virulence, which, according to the prevailing inductive evidence, fortunately safeguards those attending sewage works.

A similar conclusion seems to be justified when considering the health of those connected with the removal of solid refuse. No evidence exists, from the ragpickers in Paris to the rubbish reclamation works in America, to prove that such labor has been deleterious to health. Yet the sorting of rubbish is nevertheless open to the uncontrollable, yet infrequent danger of transmitting disease germs contained in the sweepings, bedding, and discarded materials which may be delivered from rooms where patients with infectious diseases have been confined. So long as this practice continues we should take strong precautions to minimize any danger. No such danger is expected to arise from garbage before it can breed flies, or from ashes.

Evidence collected and reported to the American Public Health Association in 1916 by its Committees on the Sanitary Aspects of Street Dirt and Street Cleaning, (S. Whinery, chairman) after an extended and careful inquiry, concludes similarly that the work connected therewith as conducted in our best managed cities, is but little, if any more, unhealthful than the average of other laboring occupations.

It is gratifying to feel that the supposed health dangers connected with sewage and city refuse removal, which only half a century ago appeared serious, are, under the present advanced methods of design and operation, either no longer in existence or have been reduced to an almost negligible minimum.

STREAM POLLUTION BY INDUSTRIAL WASTES AND ITS CONTROL

EARLE B. PHELPS

Formerly Professor of Chemistry, Hygienic Laboratory, United States Public Health Service

IT is ever a difficult matter to assign definite beginnings to conditions resulting from gradual growth, and the pollution of streams by offensive industrial wastes is a condition of this sort. Historically it doubtless began when the first crudely tanned hides or bark-dyed cloths, or the first family wash was carried to the brookside for rinsing, prognostic of important industries and serious stream pollutions in the future. From these early times down to the first half of the nineteenth century, however, stream pollution does not appear to have caused any real concern. With the introduction of steam power and the consequent rapid development and concentration of industry, conditions gradually arose which, by 1850, had assumed serious proportions. At that time the problem of stream pollution by industrial wastes was definitely recognized, especially in England.

Matters were at first dealt with by the usual resort to the common law, and suits for damages and restraining orders became more and more frequent, while decisions and judgments became increasingly conflicting and unsatisfactory. It shortly became evident that legislation of some sort was necessary, and owing to the magnitude of the interests involved upon both sides of the question a royal commission was appointed in 1865 known as the Rivers Pollution Commission, which, among other things, was instructed to determine . . " . . how far, by new arrangements, the refuse arising from industrial processes can be kept out of the streams, or rendered harmless before it reaches them, or utilized or got rid of otherwise than by discharge into running waters." A second Rivers Pollution Commission was appointed in

1868 to carry on and extend this investigation. The following excerpts from the reports of this commission will show that even at that early date the problem of the control of stream pollution was a real one. Speaking of the rivers of Yorkshire, the great woolen district, the commission said:

> These rivers are indeed subject, in common with those flowing through agricultural districts (as the Thames and Lee), to pollution with the sewage from tanneries, breweries, malting and other ordinary trades, and from exceptional manufacturing such as paper-making, etc.; but beyond all doubt their characteristic peculiarity is that derived from the different processes incidental to the worsted and woolen trade. . . . . In the higher parts of the country . . . . the water is of the purest description; but as it arrives at any point where conditions for the establishment of a woolen mill are sufficiently favorable, so does the character of the water commence to deteriorate, becoming fouler and more foul after leaving each successive mill, till . . . . the stream has to be abandoned as a source of water either for domestic supply or for manufacturing purposes."

The rivers Aire and Calder were found to be polluted with "millions of gallons per day of water poisoned, corrupted and clogged by refuse from mines, chemical works, dyeing, scouring and fulling woolen and worsted stuffs, skin cleaning and tanning." The commission received a letter of complaint written with the water of the Calder for ink, stating among other things: "Could the odour only accompany this sheet also, it would add much to the interest of this memorandum."

The British Pollution Prevention Act of 1876 which resulted from these investigations of conditions was the first general law of its kind to deal in general terms with pollution by industrial wastes. Previously, however, there had been enacted several pieces of special legislation dealing with this subject, among which were the Gasworks Clauses Act of 1847, which prohibited the discharge of gas-house wastes into rivers, the Waterworks Clauses Act of the same year, which dealt with the pollution of streams used for domestic supply, and the Salmon Fisheries Act of 1861, for the protection of certain streams in which the fisheries interest was paramount. The act of 1876 made unlawful. . . . . "the discharge into any stream of any poisonous, noxious or polluting liquid proceeding from any factory or manufacturing process."

Although the passage of the Streams Pollution Prevention Act of 1876 marks the beginning of state control of stream pollution by industrial wastes, it does not appear to have resulted in any immediate beneficial results. According to Wilson and Calvert, from whose excellent work on *Trades Wastes* the foregoing historical resumé has in part been gathered:

> The history of parliamentary action in dealing with trades pollution has been characterized by delay and weakness. Although by the Towns Improvement Clauses Act of 1847, some attempt was made to lessen the pollution of streams by domestic sewage, it was not until 1876 that the much grosser pollution by trades refuse was dealt with, and the restrictions then imposed were such as to give the manufacturer every facility for procrastination and evasion. The reason for this is only too evident, and is well set out by the Right Honorable C. G. Milnes Gaskell in an article in the *Nineteenth Century*, 1903, when he says: "The manufacturers were too powerful a body to be compelled to do their duty. 'Parliament,' I once said to Mr. Gladstone, during the last year of his life, 'has been very lenient to the manufacturer.' 'Say far too cowardly,' replied Mr. Gladstone."

The true reason, however, for the failure of this early effort lies somewhat deeper, as has been shown by subsequent experience. In the first place, legislation was enacted in advance of any suitable study of possible remedial methods and especially of their practicability and costs, and then the enforcement of the law was left to the local authorities. The second of these deficiencies was made good in part when the Local Government Act of 1888 made possible the appointment of Joint River Boards. These are administrative bodies composed of representatives of all the counties in which the drainage area of the stream in question lies, and having jurisdiction over the entire watershed of that stream. These boards made expert studies not only of existing conditions but of possible remedial treatments, and the prevention of stream pollution has progressed just so far as progress has been made in the experimental study of such remedies. By way of illustration, and because this point is of importance to a proper understanding and treatment of this subject in our own country, a moment's consideration may well be given to another waste problem, which at one stage in its history threatened to become a serious stream-pollution factor, namely, the disposal of hydrochloric acid, formerly a by-product in the manufacture of soda.

In the Lablanc process for the manufacture of soda the first step consists in the treatment of common salt with sulfuric acid to form sodium sulphate and hydrochloric acid. The latter had no commercial value in the early days of the industry and was discharged as a gas through the stacks, this resulting in great damage to the vegetation in the neighborhood of the factories and for considerable distances away. Attempts to condense the gas in water and to discharge the solution into the streams were even more disastrous by reason of the effect upon fish life. In 1863, and after it had been demonstrated that the acid could be economically recovered and had important commercial uses, the Alkali Act was passed prohibiting the discharge of waste acid from the soda factories, and placing the enforcement of the law in the hands of a single office at the head of which was placed a man well versed in the practical art of recovery. The effect was immediate and complete, so that within two years the recovery of acid throughout the entire country was over ninety-nine per cent. A capable central authority employing a remedy of demonstrated efficiency had done its work under conditions that were otherwise exactly those under which some years later the Streams Pollution Prevention Act failed. Incidentally, this example illustrates a third factor in the problem which has been and will always be of controlling importance, the possibility of utilization of a by-product. Quite regardless of their relation to stream pollution, waste products are being subjected to an ever-increasing amount of scientific study with a view to increasing the financial returns of the enterprise or to conserving resources. A notable example that has not lacked its proper share of publicity is in the packing industry whose tale of ultimate economy is so well known. A prominent paper manufacturer, who had seen his industry grow from small beginnings, once said to the writer, "Our total profits of today are actually less than the value of the by-products which we now recover and which we once threw away."

Some of the most successful efforts in the direction of protecting streams against pollution have been those in which it has been possible to recover something of value, for even though the value may not be sufficient to justify the cost of recovery by itself, it may often lighten the burden of the cost where stream protection is the essential purpose.

British experience has demonstrated three points of which we may well make note. The satisfactory protection of streams against pollution by industrial wastes must depend upon the demonstration of satisfactory and economical methods of treatment as an antecedent to legislation, upon administrative enforcement of the laws through a competent central authority, and, in part, upon the utilization of by-products.

It would be a matter of interest to follow the details of the development of this subject in England and to show how the resources of chemistry, biology and engineering have been brought to bear upon one after another of these industrial waste problems, either directly or indirectly, after the waste had become a part of the city sewage. The purposes of the present summary will be best served, however, by confining the thought to general principles and administrative procedures rather than to individual cases of scientific investigation.

The history of the subject in continental Europe is of less interest and importance. The protection of the fisheries seems to have been the controlling feature, and little advance has been made outside of Germany where some excellent mechanical devices have been developed, and where elaborate methods have been employed in the removal by chemical means of such toxic substances as cyanides from mine wastes. In Belgium, also, considerable progress has been made through experimental work conducted by the Government.

In the United States our history has been shorter and more diverse. Its outstanding feature is the importance which has been placed upon the laboratory and testing station aspect of the problems as distinguished from the true plant installation, even though the latter may have been experimental in nature.

At the Lawrence Experiment Station of the Massachusetts State Board of Health, experiments were begun as early as 1895, and have been carried on almost continuously since that time. These experiments were for the most part made on a small laboratory scale and had for their primary object the determination of the effect of the addition to sewage of relatively small amounts of the waste in question, upon the various biological processes of sewage treatment. Along similar lines, Kinnicutt and Eddy studied the effect of the acid iron wastes of the local wire mills upon the treatment of the sewage of Worcester, Massachusetts.

In 1902, M. O. Leighton, hydrographer of the United States Geological Survey, read a paper before the American Public Health Association, in which he said:

> The great pollution problem of today is that of the purification and utilization of manufacturing wastes. The opportunity afforded the American Public Health Association along this line is extremely valuable.

At this same meeting, and possibly in response to Leighton's suggestion, a committee was appointed to report upon the present status of trades waste disposal, but the subject seems to have been too large a one to be treated in that manner, and after a single preliminary report the committee seems to have disappeared from view. Perhaps the explanation was unwittingly hinted at in the preliminary report in which it is said:

> As an illustration of the vastness of this field of investigation it may be stated that there are certainly one hundred different forms of industries which produce wastes which make themselves objectionable if not properly cared for. Each one of these industries requires distinct and individual consideration, and while no specific plans can be given for each individual plant, yet there are certain general principles which govern the disposal of these wastes in separate forms of industry which would serve as a basis for determining the requirements in individual cases.

This suggestion of the committee was truly prophetic, for, as will be shown later, there has been developed a general principle, not for the treatment of the wastes but for the capacity of a stream to receive and dispose of organic matter, upon which principle the whole modern theory of stream protection rests. Before taking up this general status of the problem, however, it will be well to note in passing some of the more important of the American investigations, without attempting to make the list at all complete.

In 1905, Leighton again discussed this subject before the American Public Health Association and outlined the various studies of the Geological Survey which were at that time either actually under way or in contemplation. These included the wastes from distilleries, sulphite and soda pulp mills, wool-scouring establishments, bleacheries and other textile mills, and straw-board mills, and the acid iron waste from galvanizing, tube, tin plate and sheet-iron works and from coal mines. This was the beginning of a series of studies which extended over a number of years, a considerable number of which were made in coöperation with the Sanitary Research Laboratory of the Massachusetts Institute of Technology.

The work done at the Institute and the subsequent studies made by Colonel (now General) William M. Black and the writer on the pollution of New York Harbor led to the first attempt to apply in a quantitative way the results of chemical analyses of stream pollution. This quantitative application became possible only after investigation of methods of sewage analysis had led to the virtual abandonment of the older nitrogen basis and the establishment of the present oxygen basis and putrescibility methods. When applied quantitatively analytical results expressed in the latter form give direct and positive indication of the effect of any given pollution upon any known stream. As an example of the accuracy and general utility of this method, a few average figures from the voluminous data now available on New York Harbor may be cited. This is a particularly fortunate case for illustration because the original computations were made for these waters in advance of the analytical determination of the character of the waters themselves. The formulas were derived on the basis of the population distribution in 1910, of the analysis of sewage from certain stations, and of the waters entering the harbor from the ocean and the sound. During 1911, 1870 examinations of harbor water were made by the Metropolitan Sewerage Commission for dissolved oxygen, the results of which were then available for comparison with our computed results. Again, in 1919, the writer made an other but a briefer survey of the harbor, including a series of chemical analyses of the waters, and these results are comparable with those obtained by recomputation with our early formula, modified for a population of 6.5 million. The agreement between the actual and the computed results in 1911 is most striking, and fully confirm the accuracy of the underlying principles upon which the formula was based. In 1919 the agreement is best in the upper harbor, which represents a general admixture of all the polluted waters regardless of the sources of the pollution, while the lack of agreement in the other subdivisions is doubtless due to the assumption of a population distribution in 1919 exactly similar to that of 1910. The figures would indicate a greater increase in the population tributary to the East River and less in that tributary to the Hudson than the assumption of uniform growth in all districts would give.

DISSOLVED OXYGEN IN NEW YORK HARBOR, AS COMPUTED FROM THE BIOCHEMICAL PROPERTIES OF SEWAGE, THE DISTRIBUTION OF POPULATION AND TIDAL STUDIES, COMPARED WITH THE RESULTS OF ACTUAL CHEMICAL ANALYSES OF THE HARBOR WATERS (PER CENT OF SATURATION)

Area	Computed in 1910 for Population of 4,450,000	Found in 1911	Computed in 1919 for Population of 6,500,000	Found in 1919
Upper Bay	65	67	48	50
Lower Hudson	51	55	28	35
Lower East River	62	56	41	24

In 1913, Congress authorized the United States Public Health Service to undertake stream pollution studies, and an extensive investigation of the pollution and self-purification of the Ohio River was begun under the direction of Surgeon Wade H. Frost, with the writer as consultant. In this investigation, which extended over three years, and which is probably the most comprehensive study of the subject ever made, the principles above outlined were employed and the additional factor of reaeration was also studied.

It is obvious that the present condition of any stream is given as the algebraic sum of its initial condition, the effect of pollution and the effect of any natural recovery of which the stream is capable.

The subject of reaeration was treated extensively in the New York Harbor investigation, and the conclusion was reached that in deep and relatively quiescent bodies of water the recovery due to reaeration is a negligible quantity. The agreement between the computed and observed results is offered as evidence of the correctness of this view. On the other hand, in a stream like the Ohio reaeration and self purification are factors of predominant importance. In fact, the Ohio is several times in its course successively polluted with city sewage and industrial wastes, and rejuvenated by natural agencies to a condition approximating its initial condition of purity. This is noticeably the case below Pittsburgh.

In connection with the Ohio River studies two phases of the industrial waste problem were taken up. In the first place numerous studies were made of the actual possibilities of treatment. To this end experimental stations were established at the works and operated for two years or more in the more important cases. In this way there were studied the wastes from two tanneries, a straw-board mill, creamery, canning establishment and chemical works. A more general phase of the work was the study of industrial wastes in general which contributed to the pollution of the Ohio. As quantitative results were required in actual terms of oxygen depletion of the stream, the expedient was adopted of making a careful study of the wastes of one or more typical plants, both the quantity and the oxygen requirement being determined. The product of these, being the total output of the plant in terms of oxygen requirement, was then referred to the output of the major product of the plant — soap, hides, etc. — in such terms that the total pollution effect of the wastes from all similar plants could be at once determined if the output in terms of its major product were known.

The results of what is probably the most exhaustive investigation ever undertaken of a single industry have just been made public in a report by George M. Wisner and Langdon Pearce, Chief Engineer and Division Engineer, respectively, of the Sanitary District of Chicago, upon the wastes of the packing houses. Quantitative oxygen demand methods were employed and the experimental results are capable of direct application to the stream conditions.

Many other investigations of single plants have been made by the states of Massachusetts, New Jersey, Pennsylvania, Ohio, Illinois and Michigan in particular, and by consulting engineers for special industries. Lack of space forbids a more definite enumeration.

If the chief value of history is the lessons it teaches, the purpose of the present résumé would be incompletely served without a summary of present-day practices and tendencies in the light of the past.

With regard to legislation and administrative control experience has repeatedly demonstrated the impracticability of legislation that is in advance of experimental progress. If there are no feasible methods for the prevention of a nuisance that nuisance will in general be tolerated, even though it be a serious one, instead of the industry being destroyed. Moreover, the wisest legislation will be nullified by incompetent and especially by too local administration. The problem is one common to large areas and at best must impose a serious tax upon the industries. Inequality between the requirements of various local administrative bodies is inequality in taxation, a serious matter in an industry where competition is in a healthy state. More dangerous, however, is the uncertainty of court decisions in various local jurisdictions or, from time to time, in the same jurisdiction. The movement in England toward centralized control has led thus far to control by watersheds, a step in advance of practice in this country, where a single important stream may pass through the territory of half a dozen sovereign states. But this has not been sufficient in England, and the last royal commission has recommended a single central control for the whole of England.

The idea of a Federal Waterways Commission for the United States is not a new one, although those who have given the subject the most thought have not had water pollution in mind as the primary object of such unified control. Many years ago Leighton did suggest such an arrangement for the control of stream pollution only, and in later years this item has been included in the larger project of federal waterways control and conservation.

The present writer's views on this subject were fully expressed in his J. E. Aldred lecture at Johns Hopkins University in 1918, a few sentences from which follow:

At present the control of stream pollution rests largely in the hands of the states. Federal authority over navigable waters has thus far and for the most part been restricted to the effect of pollution upon navigation or upon federal property. The federal quarantine powers over the interstate transmission of disease have not, as yet, been extended to the control of pollution in interstate streams.

State legislation is characterized by lack of uniformity among the enactments of the various states and a general evidence of lack of appreciation of the scientific and economic principles that underlie the problem of control.

These characteristics constitute a serious indictment of the principle of state legislation as applied to a general program for stream control. Lack of uniformity not only works an economic wrong in discriminating against the manufacturer in the more progressive states, but it generally results in the tacit or openly avowed exclusion of the great interstate streams from the working of existing state law. Lack of appreciation of the basic principles leads to haphazard and changing legislation, the result of compromise among the various interests affected, providing unenforcible prohibition or ill-defined specific restriction, in place of stream standards and a reasonable economic balance of stream utilization.

State legislation for the most part also recognizes stream control as a public health function, thus bringing it under the extensive police powers of the public health authority, but at the same time limiting it to a single class of nuisance. On the one hand, this limitation may exclude from the proper jurisdiction of the law serious pollution capable of working great economic injury, although of little or no public health significance; on the other, it often results in arbitrary and unnecessary restrictive measures, based upon a too restricted viewpoint and lack of appreciation of all the phases of stream economics.

The public health interest is paramount; but the problem of the control of stream pollution is broader than the public health aspects, and its regulatory and adminis-trative phases require the attention of a higher authority than that of any single interest directly involved.

Whether the question of the control of stream pollution is not so intimately bound up in the broader one of waterways control and development in general as to make it desirable to place this function in the hands of a Federal Waterways Commission with broad jurisdiction over all phases of water control may properly be left for later consideration, but the ultimate solution lies in some form of a national conservation program. There is required for the adequate control of stream pollution in the United States a single jurisdiction, with ample authority vested in the hands of a competent commission or other federal body. This body should apply itself to the formulation of a comprehensive policy of stream restoration, development and control, a policy based upon a thorough scientific study of stream resources, advantageous uses, protective measures, and necessary and feasible restrictions. The development and adoption of such a policy is of greater importance than the immediate enforcement of remedies, for this work looks far into the future. It will be found necessary to mould into form the more difficult existing situations by steady, consistent but gradual pressure, protecting to the maximum all established interests in streams, while enforcing all reasonable and feasible corrective measures.

By the early adoption and effective prosecution of such a program, the United States may not only avoid the difficulties and losses that inevitably result from neglect of remedial treatment until industrial and municipal developments are well established, but in the end will have effected an enormous conservation of the vital capital of the nation.

PROGRESS IN FEDERAL FOOD CONTROL

CARL L. ALSBERG, M. A., M. D.*

Director, Food Research Institute, Leland Stanford Jr. University

THE control of commerce in foods by federal and state governments has been inaugurated and developed to its present degree of efficiency during the fifty years since the American Public Health Association was organized. In 1871 practically no control of the sale of food products was attempted by the federal or any state government. A few municipalities attempted some regulation of the sale of milk and occasionally of other food products, but such attempts were spasmodic and rarely effective. Although little progress was made during the first decade of the existence of the American Public Health Association, the factors that brought effective control later were already at work.

Effective food control has developed principally as a result of three factors. The first factor was the gradual change of the manufacture of food from the home to the factory. Before 1871, except for a few staples like flour, much of the food consumed on American tables was either made in the home or purchased from neighbors, so that the conditions under which the food was produced and the materials from which it was made were well known to the consumers. Gradually, however, more and more food was produced in factories and shipped for longer and longer distances, until the time was reached when city consumers purchased all of their food, and others an increasingly larger portion of their food, after it had been transported for long distances, the consumers being unacquainted with the sources of the food, with the processes it had gone through, by whom it was produced or handled and, in many instances, with its composition.

---

*Acknowledgment is made to Mr. F B. Linton, Assistant to the Chief of the Bureau of Chemistry, for much valuable help in the preparation of this paper.

The second factor in making more effective food control was the development of bacteriology and chemistry. The discovery of the part played by microörganisms in the spoilage of foods, and the development of a technique for isolating and identifying the various bacteria, molds and yeasts that play so important a part in the changes taking place in foods made it possible to develop methods for handling foods in such a way as to more efficiently prevent these changes from taking place, and revealed the danger that might come from disease-producing bacteria.

During the same period chemical methods of analysis were developed to such an extent that the chemist could determine more accurately than ever before the exact composition of food, and the occurrence of adulteration. The development of chemistry also resulted in better methods for the manufacture of food, enabling the factory manager to maintain a more effective control of the manufacturing processes. Thus the development of bacteriology and chemistry provided instruments for both the food control official and the food manufacturer, and at the same time revealed to the public the fact of adulteration as well as the way to lessen it.

The third factor which brought about food control was the educational work carried on by the American Public Health Association and similar agencies. As a result of this educational work, the public was awakened to a consciousness of the prevalence of adulteration, of the dangers to the public health involved in such adulteration, and of the duty of the state to protect its people, since the protection of the public health had come to be recognized as a function of the state. As a result of the operation of these three factors during the first decade of the existence of the American Public Health Association, the states began to consider, and, in a few instances, to enact, legislation for the control of traffic in food.

WIDESPREAD ADULTERATION

During the ten-year period following 1871 the adulteration of food was widespread. Nearly every article of food that entered commerce was adulterated at one time or another in some form. Reports made to the Medical Society of the State of New York in 1879 indicate that adulteration of food was general and that the medical profession was alive to the necessity for taking some means to prevent it. The scope of this paper is too limited to review in detail all the various forms of adulteration that were found and reported at that time, but the following instances show some of the adulterations of the most generally used foods then occurring.

Bread was adulterated with sulfate of copper, with inferior flour, and accidentally with ashes from the oven, grit from the machinery, etc., while butter was found to contain copper, excess water, excess salt, other fats, and starch, and also to be accidentally adulterated with curd. Canned foods were adulterated with copper, tin, chemical preservatives, and excess water, and cheese was found to contain salts of mercury, undoubtedly due to accidental contamination. Ground coffee was adulterated with chicory, peas, beans, acorns, nut shells and burnt sugar, while cocoa and chocolate were found to contain oxide of iron, animal fats, coloring matter, starch and flour. Cayenne pepper was adulterated with red lead, rice, flour, salt, Indian meal and oxide of iron. Alum, ground rice, grit and sand were used to adulterate flour. Turmeric, cayenne pepper and mustard were found in ginger. Lard was found to contain caustic lime, alum, starch, cottonseed oil and water. Mustard was adulterated with chromate of lead, sulfate of lime, flour, turmeric and pepper. Milk was adulterated with water, burnt sugar, yellow dye, sand and dirt. Meat spoiled and infested with parasites was not uncommon. Horseradish was adulterated with turnips, while pickles were found to contain salts of copper. Aniline colors, pumpkin, apples and flour were found in preserves. Pepper was adulterated with flour, mustard, linseed meal, pepper shells and nut shells. Spices of various kinds were found to contain flour, starches and numerous other substances. In vinegar, sulfuric, hydrochloric, and pyroligneous acids, burnt sugar and water were found.

While little progress was made during this ten-year period to prevent such widespread adulteration, the public health forces were at work endeavoring to secure legislation. A model state law to prevent the adulteration of food and medicine was drawn up in 1878-9 by a joint committee of representatives of the New York Academy of Sciences, the New York Academy of Medicine, the New York County Medical Society, the Therapeutical Society, the New York College of Pharmacy, the New York Medico-Legal Society, the American Public Health Association, and the American Chemical Society. The prevalence and danger of adulteration were publicly agitated.

ADULTERATION FOR PROFIT

Food that is intentionally adulterated affects the pocketbook oftener than the body. Most of the intentional adulteration is practised for the purpose of cheapening the food in order to make a greater profit, and the substances that are added to the food for the purpose of cheapening it are usually not harmful. The adulteration that is harmful to health is usually accidental. Zinc, copper, and other metals from the containers or vessels in which the foods are treated sometimes accidentally get into foods during the process of manufacture. Contamination from microörganisms which produce spoilage or produce disease is accidental, since it is usually due to carelessness or ignorance in preparing or handling food. The economic features of food adulteration were early recognized, being reported by Edward R. Squibb in a paper on adulteration of foods and medicines published in the *Transactions of the Medical Society of the State of New York* for 1879:

A very large proportion of the adulterations practised are not attempts at fraud, nor designed to damage health, but are strained efforts to make money. And these efforts are so earnest and so intense, energetic and absorbing as to leave all other considerations in the background. That the public is hurt and cheated is often but an accident rather than a malicious intention.

However, it was the danger to health from adulteration that aroused public sentiment to a sufficient degree to force the enactment of state and national food-control laws. It was the health consideration involved that inspired the American Public Health Association, the various medical associations, the American Chemical Society, public officials and others interested in public health to advocate the enactment of food-control laws.

It was early recognized, as it is to-day, that while the adulteration practiced for the purpose of cheapening food does not usually add substances which are harmful to health, it does sometimes injure the health by reducing for some people the quantity of nourishment below the safe limit. Milk to which water has been added is not harmful, but the child, or invalid, or other person who is getting his chief source of food from milk may be deprived of a sufficient quantity of nourishment if consuming watered milk. It was also recognized at that early date, as it is to-day, that adulteration for the purpose of cheapening foods bears harder upon the poorer classes, who are less able to stand it, than upon others. The wealthier and more intelligent people of a community, by paying higher prices, are more likely to obtain unadulterated foods. The poorer classes, forced to buy at the lowest prices possible in order to obtain a sufficient quantity of food, are chiefly the ones who obtain the foods that are adulterated to the greatest extent, the low prices being due to the fact that foods are cheapened by adulteration.

FOOD CONTROL EXTENDS TO THE STATE

The first attempts at food control were made by local communities, principally by cities where the residents were removed from actual contact with the producers of food, and, as might be expected, were directed towards obtaining a better milk supply. As the food for cities was shipped for longer and longer distances, it became more and more difficult for local boards of health or local municipal officers to maintain an effective control of food supplies, and agitation for state legislation grew in force and volume.

The committee appointed by the various societies of New York, previously mentioned, to draft a model state law for the state of New York expressed the hope that this law, after being enacted by New York, would be adopted in substance by many other states, and thus the beneficent effects of food-control legislation might extend to a large number, if not all, of the states of the Union. At that time, in 1878-79, federal control of interstate commerce in foods and drugs seems to have been considered as unattainable.

State laws which were first enacted usually related to specific products, few covering foods in general. Laws were early enacted relating to milk and other dairy products. Many of these laws were designed primarily for the protection of the dairy industry from the competition of dairy-product substitutes, rather than for the prevention of adulteration and misbranding of dairy products, although many of the state laws included the prevention of adulteration and misbranding as a secondary feature, and a few laws seemed to have had this for their primary purpose. A number of state laws relating to vinegar, wine, oleomargarine and lard were also passed in the early stages of development of state legislation. One of the earliest state laws regarding foods in general was enacted by the state of Illinois in 1874. This was followed in 1879 by a law relating specifically to dairy products.

The efforts of the joint committee consisting of representatives of the New York Academy of Sciences, New York Academy of Medicine, New York County Medical Society, Therapeutical Society, New York College of Pharmacy, New York Medico-Legal Society, American Public Health Association, and American Chemical Society crystallized in 1881 in the enactment of a general food-and-drug law in the state of New York. Food laws were also enacted during that year in Michigan, New Jersey and Illinois. In 1883 food laws, either general in nature or relating to specific products, were enacted in Maine, Nebraska and Ohio; in 1885, in Massachusetts, Maine and Pennsylvania; in 1887, in Virginia; in 1888, in Iowa and Vermont; in 1889, in Connecticut, Kansas, Maine and Wisconsin. From 1890 to 1895 laws, either general or specific, relating to foods were passed in Maryland, New Hampshire, New York, Colorado, California, Georgia, Indiana, North Carolina, North Dakota and Washington. During the decade following 1895 the state legislatures were active in amending old and in passing new food laws.

In a report to the second annual convention of the National Pure Food and Drug Congress held in Washington, D. C., in 1899, Professor J. H. Beale, in making a report for the committee upon the methods of securing uniformity in state legislation affecting the adulteration of food and drugs, the methods of analysis and in the marking of packages containing food products, after reviewing all the state laws then in existence, stated:

In perusing the statutes which have been collected, one is impressed by the wide diversity which they exhibit, both as to the subjects which they treat and in their treatment of the several subjects. While a general similarity can be traced between many of the statutes, showing their origin from a common model, and some are almost exactly alike, very few correspond in all respects, while in many cases the widest diversity exists in the laws relating to the same subjects. In some states the laws are few in number and meagre in proportion, while in others they are voluminous and cover almost every conceivable variety of adulteration, misbranding and sophistication.

It was not until after the passage of the Federal Food and Drugs Act in 1906 that uniformity began to appear in the various state laws. Within two years after the passage of the federal law at least thirty states amended or enacted food laws. Many of these followed the general lines of the federal law, but many differences remained, and the ideal uniformity has not even yet been reached.

FEDERAL LEGISLATION SUPPLEMENTS STATE CONTROL

All federal food-control legislation is based upon the taxing power of the Federal Government, or its power to regulate foreign commerce, or its power to regulate commerce between the various states. Early food legislation was based principally upon the right to tax, and upon the right to regulate foreign commerce. A federal law was passed in 1886 placing a tax upon oleomargarine and regulating its sale. This was amended in 1902. In 1896 the law regulating the taxing of filled cheese was enacted, and in 1898 a mixed-flour law was passed. While these laws were ostensibly revenue laws, they were passed primarily for the purpose of controlling the manufacture and sale of these products.

The application of that clause of the Constitution which gives the Federal Government power to regulate foreign commerce was invoked as early as 1848 for the control of imported drugs. In 1890 a very general law was passed relating to exported and imported foods, but no special provision was made for its enforcement. In 1897 a law relating to the importation of tea was passed and an effective control established. This law not only prevents adulteration, but provides that tea below an established standard may not be admitted into the United States for beverage purposes. The Bureau of Chemistry, of the Department of Agriculture, in 1900 was given authority in an appropriation bill to examine imported shipments of foods and to exclude from the country such shipments offered for entry as were adulterated or misbranded.

The idea of applying that clause of the Constitution which gives the Federal Government power to regulate interstate commerce to the control of the traffic in foods was resisted for a number of years on the ground that it was not the intention of the Constitution that this power should be used for the purpose of performing what might be called the police duties of the state. Proposed federal food legislation, it was stated, was not intended to regulate commerce, but to protect the people from adulterated food. To this argument the reply was made that it was illogical to assume that the Federal Government had the power to regulate interstate commerce, but not the power to regulate it in the interests of the people; that even if the primary purpose of federal legislation were the exercise of police power, it was to be exercised in the interests of the people and came clearly within the provisions of the Constitution.

A meat inspection law was passed in 1891, but this law was not very effective and meat inspection did not become so until 1906, when the present meat inspection law was passed and machinery in the Bureau of Animal Industry provided for its enforcement. In the appropriation bill for the Department of Agriculture for the fiscal year 1903, authority was given to the Secretary of Agriculture to establish standards for food products, but at that time there was no law for the enforcement of such standards.

On June 30, 1906, the Federal Food and Drugs Act was passed and became effective January 1, 1907. This law supplements state control of foods and makes it possible to maintain, by the coöperative efforts of the federal and state governments, an effective control of traffic in foods, whether it be in local, in interstate, or in foreign commerce. The enactment of the Federal Food and Drugs Act was the crystallization of a sentiment developed during a period of approximately twenty years, during which time the question was actively agitated. The cause was ably championed by Dr. H. W. Wiley and others, and when the potent voice of Roosevelt was added in 1906, the long desired measure was enacted into law.

THE ENFORCEMENT OF FEDERAL LAW UNIFIES FOOD CONTROL

One of the greatest difficulties in securing effective food control was due not only to variations in state laws, but also to different interpretations and administrative decisions under laws that were similar. As a result of the variations in the laws, and the variations in the administrative interpretations of the laws, honest food manufacturers were often subjected to annoying and expensive restrictions in the matter of selling their foods in different states, thus tending to bring food control into disrepute, and to increase unnecessarily the cost of doing business, an added cost that is passed on to the consumer. A product that was legal in one state might be illegal in another state. A label that would be considered truthful and correct under one law might be considered as false or fraudulent under another law, or under a different interpretation of a similar law. Foods that were adulterated and could not be sold in certain states that had effective food laws and means for their enforcement might be unloaded on states which either had no effective food laws, or lacked proper means for their enforcement.

Early in my administration of the Federal Food and Drugs Act, I established an Office of Coöperation in the Bureau of Chemistry for the purpose of unifying the action of federal and state food officials and to gradually bring about, in so far as it was practicable, uniformity in state laws, particularly uniformity in the interpretation of laws by administrative officials. Marked progress along this line has been made, although much remains to be done, especially in the matter of securing more uniform state legislation. The Office of Coöperation also established a service for the exchange of information between federal and state officials regarding all matters relating to food control, which has been of very great service to all officials concerned with food and drug control.

The Bureau of Chemistry, under the direction of the Secretary of Agriculture, is charged with the enforcement of the Federal Food and Drugs Act. As a result of nearly fifteen years' experience in the enforcement of the Federal Food and Drugs Act, an organization and a system have been evolved which makes it possible to obtain as effective control of interstate and foreign commerce in foods and drugs as the limitations of the law and the limited organization available will permit. A project system has been developed which enables all parts of the organization to work coöperatively in cleaning up any form of adulteration or misbranding that may be found to exist. The organization, through its districts and stations located in the leading trade centers of the United States, and operating in coöperation with state and municipal food officials, is able to attack the problem in all parts of the United States simultaneously, or in widely different parts, wherever the particular form of violation may be in evidence. Through the drastic power conferred in the seizure action of the federal law, it is possible by means of concerted action of federal, state and municipal officials to seize in widely-separated parts of the United States a large number of shipments of any manufacturer who may be found to be shipping in interstate commerce foods and drugs adulterated or misbranded within the terms of the federal law. This has the effect of making it incumbent upon a manufacturer either immediately to change his practices so as to bring them into conformity with the law, or to go out of business. The usual effect is an immediate change for the better in the product.

The enforcement of federal and state laws and municipal ordinances has produced a marked improvement in the quality of foods and drugs. Probably no commodities regularly sold are to-day as free from adulteration and misbranding as are foods. Practically all the grosser forms of adulteration which were in evidence at the time of the beginning of food legislation have been eliminated entirely, or are only occasionally found, as some dealer attempts to evade the vigilance of the food-control officials, hoping to make a quick and illegitimate profit by the practice of some old form of adulteration which has long ceased to be countenanced by the trade or to be general.

Newer and more refined forms of adulteration, however, are being developed from time to time by unscrupulous manufacturers, and it requires constant vigilance and the development of new methods of analysis to detect the forms as rapidly as they are originated. Most of the new forms of adulteration, as were the old, are for the purpose of cheapening the product, and are not directly injurious to health. There is still need for improvement in the matter of accidental contamination which may be injurious to health, both in the matter of metals which sometimes get into the foods during processes of manufacture, and especially in the matter of accidental contamination with microörganisms due to carelessness or ignorance in the handling of food products. As a result of the work done in the Food Research Laboratory of the Bureau of Chemistry, and elsewhere, marked improvements have been made in methods of handling perishable products, but much remains yet to be done.

FOOD CONTROL OF THE FUTURE

For the more effective control of foods in the future, highly trained, efficient organizations on the part of the federal, state and municipal governments are necessary. In the paper by Edward R. Squibb, above quoted, published in 1879, the following point is made:

"Then the organization necessary to carry into effect any such general and important law of so great necessity and so wide an application must be of exceptional and peculiar fitness, and, therefore, be very expensive, because it must consist of experts of a high order and special training."

The need for highly trained professional men in this class of work has not been fully recognized by state legislatures and the national Congress, which frequently appropriate salaries too low to be attractive to men with the necessary qualifications and training. In the long run it is less expensive to obtain the most efficient men. The total cost of enforcing the Federal Food and Drugs Act, in comparison with the value of the foods and drugs coming within the jurisdiction of this law, is infinitesimal.

Food laws of the future will be more effectively enforced when more work has been done in the establishment of food standards. Food standards are of aid not only to the food official in making it possible for him to secure more uniform and more efficient enforcement of the laws under which he operates, but also to the consumers, enabling them to know exactly what they may expect to get under a given standard, and in addition are of great benefit to the manufacturers or producers of food. The establishment of definite, reasonable, fair standards is one of the greatest factors in eliminating unfair competition, as the trade is coming to see more clearly than ever before.

More work should be done in developing effective methods for the prevention of spoilage, through the better handling of foods in a scientifically sanitary manner from the point of production of the raw materials, through all the processes of manufacture or treatment, and the channels of commerce until the foods reach the consumer's table. Much research work needs to be done in order that we may more fully understand all the factors involved in handling foods so as to reduce to a minimum the danger from contamination, but there needs especially to be a more complete application of the knowledge already available to the actual practice of handling foods.

Education must go hand in hand with federal and state regulation in the future development of food control. As in our public schools, the old system of using the rod freely has long since given way to better methods of teaching, so will the use of drastic legal action gradually become less necessary as an enlightened food industry utilizes better methods for manufacturing, handling and preparing foods. But just as the best results are obtained in schools where some form of discipline supplements the best methods of teaching, so the highest results in the production of pure food in those cases where educational methods alone are not effective will be obtained when there is available sufficient legal power and adequate machinery to administer corrective discipline.

FOOD CONSERVATION

SAMUEL C. PRESCOTT, S. B.

Professor of Industrial Microbiology, Massachusetts Institute of Technology

THE relation of a properly varied and abundant food supply to the health of an individual or the community is too well recognized to require argument. As the source of energy for the human machine, foods of different types — protein, carbohydrate and fat — have long been recognized. It has been known for many years that a suitable variety of foods is essential for well-being, and that when this variety is not obtained, or when certain kinds of food such as fresh vegetables, beef foods, butter fats, and certain portions of cereals are not eaten, the body develops ailments or maladies, such as scurvy, beriberi, rickets, and pellagra, which may be classed as nutritional diseases. In recent years the importance of the character of the food supply in relation to these diseases is recognized, if not fully understood, and a new class of substances, the vitamines, known to be of immense importance to health, is now the subject of special investigation by experts in nutrition.

Knowledge on these matters has been greatly increased in the past fifty years, and whereas these nutritional diseases were formerly of not unusual occurrence among sailors, explorers, and even among the poor in cities and areas of low agricultural efficiency, they are now far less common, and happily seem subject to complete annihilation if intelligent use is made of known facts. In spite of the rapid development of great cities, and the shifting of the mass of population from rural to urban life, with its consequent remoteness from the food-producing soil, proper foods can now be obtained by the great mass of population in a variety and quality not possible a few generations ago. Improved transportation, higher standards of living, and the application of scientific methods to the handling and conservation of food are among the chief factors which have brought about this result. Higher standards of living have led to the demand for better quality and variety of foods; improved transportation has made its acquisition possible, while scientific methods of food conservation have made the products of regions or seasons of plenty available in places of scanty harvest, or seasons of unproductiveness. Food conservation, on a large scale by canning, drying, refrigeration, and other processes, has been a potent factor in health maintenance and improvement, and in making possible the upbuilding of nations not essentially agricultural in character.

It is less than one hundred and twenty-five years since Malthus first propounded the doctrine that increase in population must necessarily be checked because of the inability of the world to maintain a food supply sufficient to meet the demands of the normal increase of population. While this may eventually be true, and while the principle of Malthus may operate in time of general war and disturbance of the normal relations between nations, as seems to have been the case in Europe following the Great War, the ultimate effect of scanty food supply as the chief cause of limitation of population is probably remote, and such an expression of opinion to-day could hardly create a profound impression. The great areas which have been opened up for agriculture during the past century, the possible extension of these areas in the future, the development of scientific farming, the rapid and general communications between nations, all have tended to make starvation less probable and hunger less common. In addition to these, another factor of prime importance suggests itself, namely, the great development of the processes of food conservation which have been brought to a state of commercial success during the past hundred years and which must be considered in any discussion of the food supply of the world.

Ancient Processes. Certain processes of food preservation have long been practised on a small scale, even for hundreds of years. Drying, salting, smoking and preserving by the use of sugar, spices, and condiments have been applied as domestic procedures from early times.

It is within the last hundred years that these processes have been so increased, improved and developed as to form a real commercial food industry and to have an important bearing on the food supply of the world. To the foregoing list must now be added refrigeration, canning, and modern dehydration.

DEHYDRATION

Drying was undoubtedly the first of the food-preserving processes to be used. The origin of the method is lost in antiquity, but it was undoubtedly known to the Egyptians and to the Chinese centuries ago. In our own country drying was practised by the Indians in the preparation of fish, jerked venison, and buffalo meat, and perhaps also with some vegetable products. The colonists dried fruits and berries and prepared "samp" of cooked Indian corn by a similar process. They also establish the first real food industry in America, the drying of codfish, an industry which became and still is of large commercial importance in certain centers of the sea fisheries, such as Gloucester, and along the shores of the British provinces. No marked extension of the method took place for many years, but under the conditions imposed by the Civil War, attempts to prepare dried vegetables for army use were made. These "desiccated" vegetables were produced in compressed form, and were used, although somewhat sparingly, with the intent of improving the army ration from the hygienic standpoint, and especially to prevent the outbreaks of scurvy which appeared among the troops fed almost continuously on salt pork, salt beef, hard bread and the few vegetables which could be secured in the surrounding country. Some of these dried vegetables were said to be good while others were very unpalatable. Among the antiscorbutics issued to the Army of the Potomac in three months in 1864 were 600 pounds of desiccated potatoes, 5,320 pounds of mixed vegetables and over 500,000 pounds of dried apples. Reports of operations show that the desiccated products had been used as early as 1861, although one report adds, "I am informed that the desiccated vegetables are so disagreeable to the taste that the men cannot eat them."

Drying food as a commercial industry, therefore, was confined largely to fish until after the close of the Civil War. Soon after this, however, the fruit-drying industry of California and Oregon had its inception. Here, as in the East, the sun was depended upon to supply the warmth to promote evaporation of the surplus water. In the arid, rainless summer months of the Pacific slope this method could be employed with considerable success, and as a result there developed a large and flourishing industry, until today the dried fruit industry of the Pacific states represents millions of dollars of capital, and a great variety of products, such as raisins, currants, prunes and peaches is prepared. Occasionally a heavy fog or rainfall brings loss of product or inferiority of quality and directs the attention of the manufacturer to the desirability of employing controlled processes in which the proper results may be obtained independent of the vagaries of Nature. Natural drying along the Atlantic seaboard is attended by even greater difficulties, as rains are frequent and often unforeseen, and heavy fog is of common occurrence.

Drying and Dehydration Since 1872

The use of regulated mechanical processes of drying and their application in a comprehensive way to all kinds of vegetables and fruits was first carried out in 1886 by an American, A. F. Spawn, at that time resident in Australia. The industry did not become a large enterprise, however, although products of good quality could be prepared. Ten years later the process of drying vegetables had made some headway in Germany, and products were imported to outfit the prospectors and others who dashed to Alaska following the finding of gold in the Klondike. Some small plants were soon established in Oregon and Washington to meet this demand, but because of lack of intelligent application of the process of drying, the demand for the product soon ceased and the industry languished. With the opening of the Boer War it was again revived, this time in Canada, and millions of pounds of dried potatoes and other vegetables were sent to South Africa for army use. A considerable quantity of this material was never shipped but was stored in paraffined barrels, and fifteen years later, at the outbreak of the Great War, was sent to England and used as a part of the supply forwarded to the British army.

During the past twenty years much thought has been given to the processes of drying, or, as more recently called, dehydration. Many patents on processes and machinery have been issued. By 1910 a few small plants had begun the manufacture of dehydrated vegetables and soup mixtures consisting of shredded vegetables mixed together, generally without meat. The industry was still insignificant, but the soundness of the fundamental principle was recognized, and experimental work was going forward along various lines. With the outbreak of the World War came a demand for large quantities of the dehydrated products for the armies abroad, and the industry grew overnight. With the cessation of hostilities the demand for this type of product again diminished, and many plants, started to meet the war emergency, ceased to exist. A few, however, remained in the business, and will no doubt form the nucleus of what is bound to be a great branch of the food industry. Several different types of dehydration processes have been developed, but all are based on the fundamental principle that removal of the excess water from a food substance renders it immune from the attacks of the microörganisms which cause spoilage and decay while the actual food value is left intact. Since only the water contained in and between the cells is removed, and not the water of constitution, it follows that the food materials, salts, etc., are concentrated in direct ratio to the water evaporated.

Moreover, if the process is carried out promptly and properly, with materials in their prime, the modern dehydrated product may be "restored" by soaking in water and will then have the appearance and the fresh flavor characteristic of the food when prepared from the raw state. If the process is properly carried out, the cells of the substance dehydrated are not ruptured, and there is simply the loss of weight due to the removal of the useless water. The processes in use may be roughly classified under the following heads:

1. Tunnel processes, employing long chambers or tunnels with blasts of hot, dry air.

2. Kiln processes, employing chambers with perforated floors heated by furnaces beneath.

3. Vacuum processes, employing closed exhausted chambers heated by steam.

4. Special types of chambers, using moderate temperatures and regulated humidity and air-flow, and sometimes possessing other technical features, found to be of great advantage in securing high-grade products.

The question as to whether the vitamines are destroyed or diminished is one now receiving much attention, but it seems likely that improvements in method of treatment will soon minimize any danger from this source.

The great advantages of this method of food preservation are too obvious to require explanation, but it may be stated that the processes in which there is the most perfect regulation of temperature, humidity, and rate of air-flow during the period of drying are those which give the most satisfactory results and the ones which are most likely to form the basic processes in the future development of the industry.

Dried Milk, Eggs, etc. During the past twenty years much progress has been made in the drying of other types of foods, normally liquid, or semifluid. Among these may be mentioned especially eggs, milk, cream, and various broths, juices, and soups. The drying may be accomplished either by vacuum, by the use of special types of chambers into which the liquid is introduced in the form of a fine mist by sprayers or by centrifugal force, or the liquid may be distributed upon the surface of heated rolls in a thin film, and the layer of solids deposited after momentary drying removed by a knife edge. Excellent results are possible in all these processes. Vegetable flours may be prepared in the same way. By these methods products of good keeping quality and high food value may be obtained. The success of these methods and the ease with which the dried products may be shipped because of their lightness and reduced bulk give promise of a greatly increased future development. From the standpoint of public welfare, this should be regarded as highly desirable, as thereby the food situation in remote and unproductive regions may be greatly improved. This is especially important in the feeding of babies and growing children, but is also of great advantage in improving the general nutritional condition and preventing the deficiency diseases.

CANNING

The preservation of foods by canning, that is, by enclosing in hermetically sealed containers and then subjecting to the action of heat sufficient to destroy the organisms of fermentation, putrefaction, or decay, dates from the early years of the nineteenth century. The discoverer of this process was Nicholas Appert, who in 1810 was granted letters patent on his process. Appert had experimented for several years previous to the date of his patent and it is probably that knowledge of his methods had become somewhat disseminated, for it is claimed that Saddington, an Englishman, had prepared foods in a similar manner in 1806. The early work of Appert was carried out on a small scale, although later he became the head of a business house which for many years manufactured preserved and canned foods on a commercial scale. The operations of the house of Appert were, however, small in comparison with the great volume of business in these lines in our own day. The use of the Appert method was readily adopted in countries outside France, and small establishments sprang up in England and other countries.

The introduction of canning in America is credited to William Underwood, who in 1821 landed in New Orleans and travelled on foot over most of the eastern United States, settling finally in Boston in 1821, where he established the company which still bears his name, and employed the Appert method in the production of a number of preserved foods, especially sauces, preserved cranberries, and special meat products. In the early days glass containers only were used, but later "canisters" of tinplate, fashioned by hand, were employed. The abbreviation of the word "canister" to "can," as was commonly done in billing and bookkeeping, is undoubtedly the origin of the word *can* as we now employ it, and the process of preservation hence became known as "canning" and the products as "canned goods." Canning in its present form, that is, in tin cans, was first employed by Pierre Angilbert, who was granted a patent in 1823. About 1839 the process was employed in packing oysters by Edward Wright of Baltimore, and in the same year by Upman Treat of Eastport, Maine, in packing salmon. Isaac Winslow in the same year began the canning of sweet corn in Maine, and in 1843 experimented unsuccessfully with the use of steam in sterilization. This method of food preservation developed quite rapidly because of fairly widespread use. Along with it developed the increasing use of the process of preserving with sugar, a method of food conservation of much earlier origin, and one which had been common as a domestic industry for many years.

The commercial development of the industry was hampered by a lack of exact knowledge of the fundamentals of the process. Germs had been discovered, but the work of Schulze, Schwann, and Schroeder and Von Dusch had not been known, and Pasteur had not been born when Underwood came to America. It is all the more striking and significant, therefore, that Appert had so completely and scientifically established the process of sterilization. It is not surprising that in view of the ignorance of microbic life, of spores, and of the significance of anaerobes, there should have been many failures and much spoilage. The use of temperatures above the boiling point of water was not thought of for many years, and as a result of this lack of definite knowledge as to the causative agencies of spoilage, the processes of sterilization were often insufficient, and losses of material were unavoidable and extremely common. The old belief in the action of oxygen or the air as the cause of decomposition was universal, and all processes were based on a belief that the goods would keep if the air were all removed. Accordingly it was the common practice to subject the sealed materials to the action of boiling water for a period of two hours, then to open or "tap" the can and allow the hot air to escape, seal again, heat for two hours, and then repeat the process. Differences in consistency or heat conduction were given no consideration. The wonder is that losses were not more severe and that the industry survived at all.

By 1860 there were a number of firms engaged in the business, and the foods canned had increased considerably in variety. Fish, vegetables and fruits made up the bulk of the product. The outbreak of the Civil War opened a large market for foods of this type, however, and greatly stimulated the business. Meats and fish were now preserved in considerable quantity, although the quality was not always the best. Insufficiently sterilized material was not uncommon and "swells" were numerous. Experience taught quickly, however, that the swelled cans were not wholesome or desirable, but this experience, so dearly bought, gave a certain stigma to canned goods which it has taken a half century to overcome, and vestiges of which still remain. But the needs of the armies outweighed the defects, and experience, as always, taught improvement of method. About this time the "chemical bath" came into use for sterilization. This process, which was guarded with great secrecy and sold as a "secret process" for large sums, was merely the application to food preservation of the fact that the boiling points of solutions may be raised by increasing the amounts of salts dissolved in them. Common salt was sometimes used, but calcium chloride was soon found to be much more effective, as the temperature could be raised many degrees and a correspondingly shorter time of heating employed. Unfortunately the use of the chemical bath added new difficulties to the business, for the hand-made cans, soldered with overlapping joints and ends imperfectly fitted, were unable to withstand the pressure developed within at the high temperatures and losses by bursting or explosion were severe. In short, the process was found to be impracticable and a return to the water-bath method of sterilization was general. In the face of these difficulties, combined with the continued ignorance of the causes of spoilage, it is not surprising that the industry did not make rapid advances.

Modern Canning. About 1870 the use of steam under pressure as a means of sterilization was again introduced. By placing the canned material to be "processed," or sterilized, in strong iron chambers, or "retorts," and subjecting them to the action of flowing steam under pressure, sterilization could be accomplished in much briefer time.

Here there was the distinct advantage over the water bath that the pressure on the can was the same *within* and *without*, hence no bursting or explosion took place if care was used and proper time allowed for the pressure to be applied or released. At first losses were severe, but improvements in methods of making cans reduced the trouble from this source. The whole period from the first discovery of Appert to 1872 might well be regarded as an experimental period, for it was not until the application of steam under pressure as a means of sterilization that canning could be regarded as an established commercial process for treating foods on a large scale. It would be unfortunate to describe the history of the canning industry in America without referring to the application of the process to milk. The first attempts to condense and thus preserve milk were made by Newton in England, who was granted a patent on the process in 1835. Commercially successful condensation of milk dates from 1856, since which time many improvements have been made in the process.

The milk is heated to about 180° F. and poured into large copper vacuum pans after having added to it from 10 to 12 per cent of cane sugar. Evaporation occurs at about 122° F., until reduced to about one fourth the original volume. The milk contains therefore approximately 40 per cent cane sugar. It is then sealed in tin cans, and although rarely sterile it keeps indefinitely, the high concentration preventing the action of the surviving bacteria. Yeasts sometimes produce troublesome fermentation, however. Canned unsweetened milk is also prepared in large quantities, and is commonly sold under the name of evaporated milk. Both these products undergo certain changes as a result of the heat applied, but the industry has been of inestimable value in making it possible for milk to be obtained in a readily transportable form under practically all conditions, and in places where the fresh product is unobtainable. Its use is rapidly increasing, both as food for children and for ordinary consumption.

Other Processes. A number of other processes are in use, among which may be mentioned the vacuum packing of foods, such as dried smoked beef, bacon and peanut butter. This process can be employed with foods which, because of their composition, or because of previous treatment, are but slightly subject to decomposition in the limited period such foods are supposed to be kept before consumption. The use of nitrogen, carbon dioxide, or other inert gases has also been employed and the future is likely to see some development in this field (frankerization, etc.)

In the fifty years that have just passed there has been a great development of the industry. The scope of its application has so greatly increased that it has encompassed nearly all classes of foods. From a few staple vegetables, such as corn, peas, and beans, and a limited number of kinds of fish or meat products, the method has been so extensively applied that there are but few foods which cannot be obtained in canned form — soups, fish, shellfish, meats of all kinds, sausage, baked beans, vegetables single and combined, cereals, poultry, milk, butter and cheese, syrups, fruits, — all these and many other foods now reach the consumer in canned form. Revolutionary changes in the manufacture of cans have been introduced so that in place of a crude, hand-made product, turned out at the rate of a few dozen per day per man, complicated machinery swallows the great sheets of tin-plate at one end of a line and delivers thousands of neat, strong, finished and tested cans to the waiting freight-car to the other end of the factory. Can-making has now become a separate industry, yet so closely allied that the integrity of the product is as dependent on the can as upon the quality of the raw material or the care in the application of the process of sterilization. But improvement in the quality of canned foods has not come about entirely as a result of the mechanical perfection which has been developed in the making of cans. The great losses due to spoilage are not always due to imperfect containers, but may be the result of unscientific sterilization.

The rise of bacteriology has made it possible to investigate this phase of the subject in a thorough manner. The work of Pasteur gave the fundamental principles upon which these studies are based. The discoveries relating to the normal bacteriology of different products; special studies on spoilage by numerous workers; investigations on the conductivity for heat of different foods; studies on the thermophiles and the anerobes, on botulism and food-poisoning; and studies on the effect of different types of containers, and of solutions of different hydrogen-ion concentration have been of incalculable service to the industry.

In the past twenty-five years science has replaced guesswork, processes based on carefully observed data have replaced rule of thumb, exact knowledge is taking the place of ignorance and superstition. Scientific control and the application of our knowledge of the organisms of decomposition has brought the canning industry into an unassailable position as a basic food industry, indispensable alike in war or in peace, — for the product of the cannery, clean, wholesome, sterile, hermetically sealed and safeguarded from contamination, will withstand all climates and may often be kept for years without deterioration. To be sure there are questions as to the effect of sterilization upon those elusive but necessary food accessories, the vitamines, but the test of experience in polar explorations, in the tropics, in war, and in expeditions to remote parts of the earth has given to the canned foods a high place as nutrients which will supply the body with energy, prevent or at least minimize the danger from nutritional deficiencies, and provide the variety and quality which our best welfare demands. Canning may therefore be regarded as a direct aid to public health and in any survey of human welfare deserves consideration.

Pasteurization. A process which has been of immense importance in the prevention of diseases which may be transmitted by milk is pasteurization. The process was first applied by Pasteur in the treatment of wine and beer to insure stability of the product by destroying the non-spore-forming germs which were the causes of "disease." It may be described as a form of partial sterilization. Germs in the resistant form known as spores are not killed, but since these are relatively few in the substances to which the process is applied, the treatment has been of inestimable value, especially when applied to milk. The work of Pasteur was carried out during the period 1860-1864 in the epoch-making series of investigations by which he saved to France the wine industry.

About 1886 the chemist Soxhlet advised the use of heated milk for infant feeding, and soon after 1890 pasteurization began to be practised on an extensive scale in America. Conflicting opinions were expressed as to its desirability. As a result of careful studies by many workers it was found that when temperatures of 140–145° F. were applied to milk for a period of twenty to thirty minutes, its food value was not greatly changed, while the vegetative cells of bacteria, including the types of disease organisms most likely to be transmitted by milk, were destroyed. The value of this process as a public-health measure cannot be overestimated, and at the present time most of the large cities of our country require pasteurization of the public milk supply. The effect of the general use of this process has been to save thousands of lives, prevent much illness, especially among babies and young children, and to render safe the milk supplies of large cities. The process may justly be regarded as one of the triumphs of sanitary science.

REFRIGERATION

Human experience long ago taught that foods may be kept in good condition for extended periods when maintained at low temperatures. Long before knowledge of bacteria or other causes of deterioration or decay of foods existed, the saving effect of cold had been demonstrated. In fact, refrigeration on a small scale and the production of ice by artificial means were known to the ancients. No broad application of the process was made, however, until within comparatively recent times. Experiments with salt solutions were conducted as far back as 1607. In the middle of the eighteenth century investigations were made by Cullen, Fahrenheit, and Lavoisier, but these never arrived at practical fruition. In 1824 a patent was issued to Valauer for a machine in which dry air was passed over water, the evaporation extracting the heat. In 1834 Perkins produced an ether refrigerating machine. Nine years later Dr. Garrie invented a cold-air machine which was later developed by Windhausen, Bell, Coleman, and others. In 1850 Carré discovered the ammonia-absorption process and this was in commercial use in England in 1859. From this time forward progress was rapid and machines of the general types used to-day were developed. Previous to 1872 refrigeration was still in the experimental stage, but it was destined to become one of the most important agencies of food preservation. It has been stated that its introduction has more profoundly affected the economic condition of England, and, to a less degree, of the United States, than any other scientific advance since the establishment of railways and steamboats.

Progress Since 1872. On July 23, 1873, the first cargo of meats, frozen by the Harrison ether machine, was sent from Melbourne to London. The ship arrived at the latter port on October 18, but the meats were in an unsatisfactory condition and unfit for food. In 1875–76 sound frozen meat was successfully carried to England from the United States, and in 1880 the first successful voyage from Australia with a refrigerator ship was accomplished. From this time on refrigerator transportation was recognized as a commercial success and the development since that time has been enormous. While first used primarily for meats the process has been gradually extended until at the present time almost every conceivable form of food substance has been kept for varying periods of time by the preservative action of cold.

Practical experience has demonstrated that different types of foods require different temperatures. While for beef the cold-storage rooms are maintained at approximately 33 to 34° F., for smaller animals, mutton, veal and poultry, lower temperatures are employed. The carcasses are cooled slowly at first to prevent uneven freezing throughout, and the damage due to unequal expansion of the outer ice layer. Fish are generally frozen solid on trays and then maintained at a temperature considerably below the freezing point. Eggs are kept at a temperature just above the freezing point, and special attention must be given to the humidity, as in air laden with moisture moulding and other deteriorations may ensue. Dairy products are kept for long periods in prime condition. Butter is quickly cooled to about 10° F., and at this low temperature it remains unchanged in composition for many months. Cheese, on the other hand, should not be frozen. Fruits and vegetables are in general kept at temperatures just above freezing, although there are some notable exceptions to this. Grapes may have a temperature below 32° F., while lemons and oranges are injured below 36°. Bananas are transported from the tropics in refrigerator ships, but temperatures below 52° are injurious. Since fruits are in general subject to decay as a result of the action of mould, and these organisms are not inhibited completely at temperatures above 32°, it follows that the period of storage of these foods is short, rarely exceeding a few weeks for soft fruits, and a few months for the more stable ones. Altogether, refrigeration may be regarded as a process of inestimable value. The foods so preserved lose little of their flavor, the food values are practically unaltered. As with all methods of food preservation, prejudices have arisen against foods kept in cold storage, but these have been based largely on ignorance or on limited and unfortunate experience. No doubt inefficient methods have often been used, but from a broad standpoint the process has been one of tremendous benefit to mankind.

The fifty years which have passed since the birth of the American Public Health Association have witnessed the development of a new era in food control, and have brought to a high state of efficiency processes which have had a remarkable effect, both from the economic and the sanitary standpoints. The canning industry has been established on a scientific plane; pasteurization has become of general use; dehydration is assuming an importance little imagined a few years ago; refrigeration has changed the food habits of nations. But for these and allied processes, food prices would be prohibitive, health of urban communities would be endangered, and starvation would be imminent in our large cities. The achievements of fifty years are little short of marvelous, and the prediction of Malthus has lost much of its alarm. With new advances of science in these fields, progress is being made daily and the future will undoubtedly witness many new triumphs in food engineering which will find favorable reaction in the health and happiness of the nations.

MILK AND ITS RELATION TO PUBLIC HEALTH

CHARLES E. NORTH, M. D.

Director of the North Public Health Bureau

THE relationship of milk supplies to public health is a world problem. It is world-wide and national in its scope, as well as local in its application. The milk industry has been called the backbone of agriculture and has always played an important part in the economic development of the human race. As a consequence, the point of view of any individual writer on such a vast subject as this is necessarily too narrow and too limited to justly comprehend or state the real relationships of milk to the health of the human race. Any writer is necessarily prejudiced by conditions in the locality in which he lives and works and by the limited experiences which have brought him into contact with milk problems which are local in their nature. In the early seventies family homesteads of both parents of the writer were shipping milk from their dairy farms in Westchester County to the New York City market. Since that time the greater part of the writer's experience has been spent in the study of conditions surrounding the milk supply of New York City. Education under Atwater, Conn, Jacobi, and Prudden gave direction to the studies which he has personally made, and contact with milk supplies of a number of large eastern cities, and a few western cities, has broadened to some extent his point of view toward the principles which should be used in the control of municipal milk supplies in this country. In writing a history of the development of municipal milk supplies in their relationship to public health, the writer, however, is not placing his main dependence on his own experiences but on the able writings of a large number of experts who have participated in the past in the many brilliant epoch-making events that have marked the progress of milk reform and who have recorded the same in their writings.

To do justice to all who have contributed toward the rapid progress made in recent years in the control of public milk supplies is impossible. This is especially true of the numerous technical men who have by their laboratory researches aided in establishing the scientific principles which are now accepted. The omission by me of any names in this history is no indication of their real importance or unimportance, but is due only to the fact that the writer's selection of men and of events marking this history is necessarily biased by natural limitations.

A survey of the writings of medical and scientific men on this subject reveals a most remarkable state of affairs. This is, that writings on the special subject of milk did not begin until the year 1839, and that for forty years thereafter only thirteen writers felt it worth while to write scientific or medical articles on this subject. The year 1879, however, marked an epoch because the number of writers began to multiply, while the year 1889 showed a most decided increase in the number of contributors to milk literature.

In graphic form the number of authors who have written medical and scientific articles on milk is presented in the following chart:

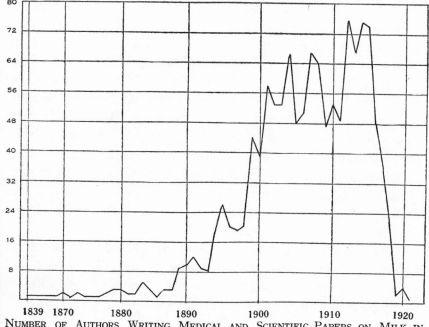

NUMBER OF AUTHORS WRITING MEDICAL AND SCIENTIFIC PAPERS ON MILK IN EACH YEAR 1839 – 1921

The number of these is 1,282. This list is by no means complete, for the reason that many prominent investigators in medicine and science while not writing special papers on this subject have made important contributions in connection with other work. From the tabulation and the graph it is startling to note that the bulk of the work of specialists in the improvement of municipal milk supplies has been accomplished during the short period of forty years ranging from 1881 to 1921.

In general the brief period during which effective work in milk reform has been accomplished may be sketched by dividing the same into several important epochs with which certain prominent men and prominent events have been connected.

The discoveries of Pasteur in 1860 of the fermenting organisms in wine, and of the temperatures at which they were destroyed, gave a great impulse to the study of fermenting organisms in all liquids, including milk.

It was the year 1881 that marked the most important epoch in the history of milk improvement. The real foundation of all the work which has been done since by investigators interested in the improvement of municipal milk supplies was laid in this year by Koch's invention of solid culture media, whereby species of bacteria could be separately isolated and studied. In this same year Hart compiled and reported a long list of milk epidemics, furnishing convincing evidence to the world of the vital relationship of milk to the public health.

The interval between 1881 and 1890 was marked by a series of studies by Koch and his followers using his solid culture media for the isolation of a number of the more important pathogenic organisms. In this same period there was a growing interest on the part of some of the the leaders in the medical profession, including Soxhlet, Jacobi, Caillé, and others regarding the necessity for heating milk for the artificial feeding of infants.

The invention by Babcock in 1890 of a simple and accurate method for determining the percentage of butter fat in milk revolutionized the milk industry economically by enabling buyers to base prices on its composition with respect to its fat content.

Another great epoch, second only to the epoch of 1881, occurred in 1892. In this year the movement toward certified milk was inaugurated by Coit, and the first medical milk commission organized. While this in itself has never resulted in the production of any large quantity of milk of this grade, the principles of dairy farm sanitation, bacterial testing, and bacterial standards have had ever since that time a most profound and far-reaching influence on every branch of the milk industry. Another most important event of this year was the establishment of infant milk depots in New York City by Nathan Straus, under the advice of Jacobi and Freeman and others, for the dispensing of pasteurized milk to the children of the poor. Here again the direct results on the quantity of milk actually dispensed were never through the following years very marked, but the principles on which this movement were based — the value of milk depots in the feeding of infants and the education of the mother, and the necessity of pasteurization have been most potent in bringing not only the industry, but the medical profession and the public, to a recognition of the vital importance of safe milk for infant feeding. Sedgwick and Batchelder in this year made the first bacterial count of market milk in America. Their work attracted a number of followers and inaugurated the methods used since that time for determining the numbers of bacteria in market milk. In that same year Conn began his extensive studies on milk fermentations, resulting in a long series of publications on the bacteriology of milk. In this year also Atwater was carrying on extensive studies of the food value of milk and of the comparative value of foods as determined by the bomb-calorimeter.

In the interval between 1892 and 1900 studies of milk bacteriology were made by numerous bacteriologists. Theobald Smith isolated and identified the germs of bovine tuberculosis, and determined the temperature at which they were destroyed. During this same period Van Slyke and other chemists were conducting extensive investigations of the chemical composition of cows' milk. At this time also the commerical pasteurization of milk by the flash method began to be adopted by the milk industry to a small extent.

The next epoch giving special impulse to milk reform took place in 1900-1901. At this period Chapin coöperated with Conn in the establishment of a medical milk commission in New York City and the production of certified milk. Park began the bacteriological examination of the milk supply of New York City, and aroused great interest among the medical profession by his studies of the bacteria in milk from cow to consumer. A number of other bacteriologists at the same time showed that milk coming directly from healthy cows contains only small numbers of bacteria, and that large numbers were due to contaminations occurring during the period of transit of milk from the cow to the city market. Secret pasteurization by the flash method was considerably extended by the milk industry. Strong opposition to commerical pasteurization was developed, while on the other hand, strong sentiment in favor of home pasteurization of infants' milk was growing. Certified milk commissions in Philadelphia and other cities were being formed. Epidemics of disease from raw milk were multiplying in number. The leading authorities in medicine and public health were being rapidly convinced of the necessity of taking some additional steps for the safeguarding of milk to be sold on city markets.

The work of Rosenau on the thermal death point of pathogenic bacteria and on temperatures necessary for the pasteurization of milk was another epoch-making event that occurred in the year 1906. In this same year North suggested that the flash method of pasteurization be abolished and that milk be pasteurized by the holding method. Experiments conducted by him on the first machine of this new type installed in the largest pasteurizing plant in New York City laid the foundation for the widespread adoption of the holding method of pasteurization which has occurred since that date.

The New York Milk Committee was organized in the year 1907. Its objects were the reduction of infant mortality and the improvement of the milk supply of New York City. The personnel of its organization and its financial support were so strong that at the outset its work gave the greatest impulse not only in New York City, but throughout the United States, to the work of the reduction of infant mortality and the improvement of municipal milk supplies.

In the years 1908, 1909, 1910, the New York Milk Committee established a number of infant milk depots in New York City which proved beyond question their great value in the reduction of infant mortality by the dispensing of clean pasteurized milk and the education of mothers. This Committee also influenced public health authorities to a serious consideration of a complete remodelling of the city ordinance controlling the milk supply. During this same period the Committee undertook the establishment of a large experimental milk station in the country to demonstrate, at the suggestion of North, that by proper supervision and at small expense, the rank and file of dairy farmers could produce milk of the highest sanitary quality.

During this same period the holding method of milk pasteurization was widely extended to all large cities in the United States and Canada.

In 1908, at the suggestion of Evans, the city of Chicago adopted the first ordinance requiring the pasteurization of all milk excepting milk of the highest sanitary character. In 1910 the American Public Health Association established standard methods for the bacterial testing of milk, thereby bringing about uniformity in such testing, laying the foundation for the establishment of municipal and commercial milk laboratories, and bacterial standards for milk.

The National Commission on Milk Standards was appointed by the New York Milk Committee in the year 1911. In its work during that year this Commission announced the principle of grading of milk, which has been so potent a force since that time in model milk regulations. In this same year the first experimental work was begun on vitamines in milk.

In 1912, New York City adopted a new milk regulation providing for the grading system of milk as recommended by the National Commission on Milk Standards, providing bacterial standards for all milk, and for the pasteurization of all milk excepting raw milk of the highest grade.

In the interval since 1912 there has been a constantly growing conviction throughout the United States that the pasteurization of milk is necessary, and while the advocates of raw milk are still evident.

in smaller cities and towns, their voices are growing fainter and fainter since the experience of larger cities furnishes convincing evidence of the value of pasteurization as a public health measure. A study of the list of milk epidemics and of infant mortality shows that the advance of pasteurization has been marked by a rapid falling off in all forms of milk-borne disease. In the period from 1907 to 1910, during which pasteurization was widely adopted by the milk industry, there was a most decided drop in the number of epidemics of typhoid fever, scarlet fever, and diphtheria from milk, and also a great reduction in the infant mortality in cities where pasteurization was established.

Since 1912 the most startling event in the milk world has been the new knowledge of the growth-promoting and protective substances called vitamines contained in milk. The work of the biologists and chemists, among which McCollum is the most prominent, has revealed the fact that no other food is so vital to the welfare and health of the human race as milk. This knowledge has resulted in organized campaigns for a wider use of milk which have greatly increased public interest in this food product. At the same time the milk industry has recognized the increased responsibility attached to its services and has been aroused to the necessity of the fullest coöperation with public health officers in the safeguarding of a food which is a public necessity.

The principles of effective milk control have now been settled to the satisfaction of the scientific world. These principles are sufficiently well understood to form the basis of effective milk legislation and milk regulation. It only remains to educate people of our cities and towns to a complete realization of the food value of milk, and of the correct principles of milk control, to bring about a satisfactory solution of the milk problem in every community. Such a result can confidently be expected within the very near future.

BACTERIA IN MILK

The first recorded observation of bacteria in milk was by Bondeau in the year 1847, who observed such organisms in sour milk through a microscope. He, however, did not connect them with the souring process. In 1857, Pasteur showed that the souring of milk was actually due to the growth of such organisms. In 1878, Boutroux cultivated lactic acid bacteria, as did Lister and Richet. In 1885, Hueppe described an organism which he called *Bacillus acidi lactici*. Conn was the first American bacteriologist to make extensive studies of milk bacteria. He isolated a large number of species between 1890 and 1903, and pointed out a type which he called *Bacillus lactici acidi*, which later on Heinemann showed to be similar to streptococcus. Sour milk bacteria have been made a special study by many bacteriologists since the time of Hueppe (1885) who was the first to apply modern methods to this work. It is now known that there are many species of bacteria which sour milk.

RELATION TO PUBLIC HEALTH

No definite knowledge of the relationship of milk to public health was possible until evidence could be obtained of the causes of human diseases and the sources from which they came. It was not until the period between the years 1815 and 1835 that the microscope was perfected by the invention of achromatic objective lenses, which made possible the observation of the bacteria of human diseases. The studies subsequently made, however, did not for a number of years suggest any relationship between human diseases and milk.

The first milk epidemic of which there is any record was reported by Dr. M. W. Taylor in the year 1857. This was a typhoid epidemic in the city of Penrith, England. Ten years later the same observer reported a scarlet fever outbreak which he traced to milk in the same city. A few epidemics were reported from time to time until the year 1881, mostly by English observers, but these were not sufficient to attract any marked attention by the medical profession or public health authorities, or to result in any efforts to control municipal milk supplies in the interests of public health.

The year 1881, as suggested by Sedgwick, must be recognized as the most important year in the history of milk, in its relation to public health, because it was in that year that two striking events occurred whose influence has molded all of the important researches since conducted by public health authorities in relation to milk supplies. The first of these was the collection of a large list of milk epidemics by Dr. E. Hart of England.   In this list there were included fifty epidemics of typohid fever, fifteen of scarlet fever and four of diphtheria.   The evidence connecting these outbreaks with milk supplies was so convincing that it aroused the medical profession to a realization of the great dangers to the public health of uncontrolled milk supplies.

The second marked event was the discovery by Koch in Germany of solid culture media for the cultivation of bacteria, whereby it was easily possible to isolate pure cultures of different species.   The invention of this culture media constituted a great change from the methods used by Pasteur and his immediate followers, all of whose work had been done with liquid cultures.   Examinations of milk with solid culture media were immediately begun and a long series of important discoveries concerning milk bacteria followed.   These two events laid the foundation for the study of milk-borne infections and of milk bacteriology.   Medical bacteriologists gave special attention to the bacteria causing human diseases.   Another group of workers, later classified as agricultural bacteriologists and milk bacteriologists devoted especial attention to the bacteria causing milk fermentations and other changes in milk.

STREPTOCOCCUS IN MILK

Rosenbach in 1884 first discovered that the streptococcus was found in suppurative lesions.   In 1889 Grotenfeld found streptococci in milk, as did also Weigmaff in 1890, Kruse in 1903, and many other bacteriologists since that time.   The connection of the streptococcus with inflammations of the cow's udder was pointed out by Savage, Stewart, Doane and Buckley in 1905, and by Heinemann, Slack and Trommsdorff in 1906, and by Bergey, Russell and Hoffman in 1907. The studies of these investigators gave rise to special apparatus and methods for the examination of milk for udder inflammation by showing the presence of pus and streptococci. The most recent and simplest of these was devised by Prescott and Breed in 1910. The work of all of these investigators was based on the assumption that presence of pus and streptococci in cows' udders was evidence of inflammation and that such inflammations might discharge material into milk which would be injurious to the health of milk consumers.

SEPTIC SORE THROAT

Since inflammation of the udder in cows is usually caused by the streptococcus and septic sore throat is an inflammation also caused by streptococcus, and many large epidemics of sore throat have been traced to milk, investigators have concluded that the streptococcus causing septic sore throat originates from udder inflammations.

Since 1875 outbreaks of sore throat have been reported in England. A number of large epidemics have been officially investigated there in all of which the symptoms of the disease have been characteristic, and the relationship to the milk supply either suspected or confirmed. Swithenbank and Newman state that, "In all probability these outbreaks are comparatively common. We think it safe to assume that a year never goes by in which there are not outbreaks of sore throat or tonsillitis due to milk or cream. The chief symptoms are local inflammations of the throat and enlargement of the glands of the neck. There are high temperatures, great prostration and numerous secondary inflammations following the primary infection." The first recorded outbreak was in Aberdeen, Scotland, in 1881. About 300 persons were affected, all supplied with milk from the same dairy. The same year it was reported that at Rugby School, England, 90 boys were affected with sore throat. Thirty-one epidemics in all are on record, but the the health authorities believe that this is only a small fraction of the large number that have probably occurred. The Boston epidemic of 1911 affected over 1043 people. The Chicago epidemic of 1911 affected over 10,000 persons. In the Baltimore epidemic of 1912, 602 cases were reported. In the Cortland-Homer outbreak of 1913, 669 cases were reported. The outbreak at Poughkeepsie,

New York, in 1915, is a typical illustration of the origin and spread of such sore throat outbreaks. In this epidemic there were cases in the city of Poughkeepsie and in the Hudson River State Hospital, two miles north of the city, and in the village of Wappinger's Falls eight miles south of the city. All three of these places obtained milk from a milk shipping station receiving part of its supply from a dairy farm on which there were discovered seven cases of sore throat and scarlet fever. Physicians were divided in opinion as to whether the outbreak was one of scarlet fever wholly or of septic sore throat. Physicians at first reported only scarlet fever cases in the three communities and the immediate surroundings, to the number of 212. When sore throat cases were also reported investigation showed that there were 296 of these, making a total of 508 cases in all. The symptoms were of all degrees of severity. Where there were rashes the cases were reported as scarlet fever. Where there were no rashes they were reported as septic sore throat. There were thirty-four deaths. The relation between septic sore throat and scarlet fever is unsettled. Many investigators suggest a relationship between these diseases. The streptococcus is commonly found in both. Milk has been the only source so far discovered for epidemics of sore throat and of scarlet fever. Szontagh in 1912 said, "No sharp boundary line can be drawn between these two diseases. There is no fundamental difference, but merely a difference in degree between simple angina and scarlet fever angina. Malignant scarlet fever is simply the most severe form of ordinary angina."

Keltschmer in 1913 said, "Two persons can easily be affected from the same source, one contracting angina (septic sore throat) and the other scarlet fever."

The question of whether the streptococcus causing septic sore throat is of bovine origin or human origin has been extensively studied. Heinemann (1906) thought the streptococcus in milk in cows' udders identical with streptococcus pyogenes. Savage, Reudiger, Davis and Capps have shown that the garget streptococcus of cows is not pathogenic for man. Smith and Brown (1915) studied streptococcus from epidemics of sore throat in five Massachusetts cities and showed that they were harmless when planted in cows' udders and differed from the streptococcus of udder inflammations. They concluded that strepto-coccus of septic sore throat is primarily of human origin. Krumweide and Valentine (1915) confirmed the work of Smith and Brown, that sore throat infection is of human origin. All investigators are, however, agreed that sore throat bacteria may infect milk in cows' udders and thereby cause sore throat outbreaks.

In the case of septic sore throat we find that epidemics have in-creased rather than decreased since the year 1907. This does not mean that there has been any real increase. Septic sore throat has not been a reportable disease until recently. There have probably always been extensive epidemics of this disease but they have gone unrecognized and unreported. Therefore, the historical record of the many epidemics which occurred previous to 1907 is only fragmentary. There is no reason to doubt that the adoption of pasteurization on a large scale by the milk industry has greatly reduced the number of milk-borne epidemics of septic sore throat as it has reduced the spread of other milk-borne infections.

TYPHOID FEVER FROM MILK

The first typhoid fever outbreak traced to milk was in the year 1857, in Penrith, England. In 1868 a typhoid fever outbreak was re-ported in Dover, England, due to milk, and in 1870 another outbreak occured in Islington. Other outbreaks of typhoid were reported in Eng-land in the year 1872, and six in the year 1873. Outbreaks reported began to multiply in number as soon as physicians became interested in making such observations. Hundreds of typhoid outbreaks have been recorded since the time when Hart read his famous paper on this sub-ject, until all public health authorities at the present time are aware of the fact that municipal milk supplies are frequently the cause of typhoid outbreaks.

In the year 1890 Vaughan isolated the typhoid bacillus from the water and from the milk of a dairy suspected of being the cause of a typhoid outbreak.

In 1902 Reynolds found the typhoid bacillus in Chicago milk. Cultivation of typhoid in milk and its recovery from milk has been noted by a number of other observers.

In 1901 Schuder collected a list of 650 typhoid epidemics and found that 416 of these were caused by water, 110 by milk and 78 by miscellaneous causes.

There has been a great diminution in the number of such epidemics since the year 1907. Previous to that year pasteurization of milk was practiced, but by few cities; subsequent to that time its adoption became very general.

SCARLET FEVER

The first milk-borne scarlet fever outbreak was noted in 1867, in the city of Penrith, England. In 1876 an outbreak was noted in Harmsworth, England of 37 cases. In 1881, 510 cases occurred in Halifax traced to milk. It has been said that while many epidemics of scarlet fever have never been traced to their source, so that their source is unknown, on the other hand, all epidemics which have been so traced have been due to milk. I have listed a number of scarlet fever epidemics in the table following. Again I call attention to the fact that the literature shows a sudden falling off in the number of these outbreaks after the year 1907, and that in my opinion this is chiefly due to the adoption of pasteurization on a large scale.

DIPHTHERIA

The first epidemic of diphtheria traced to milk was reported by Dr. E. J. Jacob in the year 1877, and occurred in Sutton, England. In 1878 an outbreak was reported by Mr. Power in London of 264 cases all traced to the same milk supply. Three other outbreaks of diphtheria which were traced to milk, were reported by Dr. Jacob that same year.

In 1889, Klein cultivated diphtheria organisms in milk. In 1899 Gowhill, Eyre and Klein isolated the diphtheria bacillus from city milk supplies. In 1902 Dean and Todd isolated the diphtheria bacillus from cows' milk and from the throats of people drinking milk.

A tabulation of diphtheria epidemics reported from milk is appended. Attention is called again to the sudden falling off of these outbreaks in the year 1907.

NUMBER OF MILK EPIDEMICS

Appended is a partial list of the numerous milk epidemics which have occurred, gathered from many sources, showing the years in which they were reported.

Date	Typhoid	Scarlet Fever	Diphtheria	Sore Throat
1857	1			
1858				
1859				
1860				
1861				
1862				
1863				
1864				
1865				
1866				
1867		2		
1868	1			
1869				
1870				
1871	1			
1872	4	1		
1873	5			
1874	4			
1875	5	1		
1876	5	1		
1877	7	1	1	
1878	8	1	4	
1879	3	2	2	
1880	9	2	1	
1881	3	6	1	
1882	12	9	1	
1883	13	3	4	

NUMBER OF MILK EPIDEMICS — *Continued*

Date	Typhoid	Scarlet Fever	Diphtheria	Sore Throat
1884	8	1		
1885		4		
1886	6	2	4	
1887	5	8	2	
1888	6	10	3	
1889	11	4	3	
1890	12	2	3	
1891	12	7	1	
1892	15	7	1	1
1893	16	6	1	
1894	14	5	1	1
1895	11	3		
1896	6			
1897	5	2		
1898	6	1	2	
1899	10	4	2	
1900	15	7	1	
1901	12	4	2	
1902	6		1	
1903	7	2	2	1
1904	16	6	3	2
1905	23	4	1	1
1906	20	2	2	
1907	12	4	3	
1908	4			
1909	4			
1910	1			
1911	1			2
1912				4
1913	2			1
1914				
1915	9		2	1
1916	6	1		2
1917	5	2		6
1918	7	1		
1919	1			
1920			1	
Total	375	128	55	22

BOVINE TUBERCULOSIS

The bacillus of tuberculosis was discovered and isolated by Koch in the year 1882. This was the bacillus of human tuberculosis. In

1884 Bang cultivated the germs of bovine tuberculosis from rabbits. In the same year Stein cultivated them in guinea pigs. Ernst, Mc-Fadden and many other observers studied the germs of bovine tuberculosis by the infection of guinea pigs and rabbits during the following ten years.

In the year 1896 Theobald Smith announced that the germs of bovine tuberculosis were a different species from those of human tuberculosis. In the year 1901 Koch announced that bovine and human tuberculosis were two separate diseases and that the bovine species could not infect human beings. This was disproved by Ravenel, who had isolated from the mesenteric glands of a child, tubercle bacilli which were fatal to calves and a grown cow, the first recorded experiment of the kind. Subsequent observations in this country and abroad have confirmed this work and demonstrated beyond question that the bovine type is infectious for human beings, especially children. A collection of observations made by Park and Krumwiede in 1910 showed that in children under five years, 27 per cent of the cases of tuberculosis were of the bovine type; in children 5 to 16 years, 25 per cent were of the bovine type, and in adults over 16 years, 1.3 per cent.

Tuberculosis has always been a disease of cattle more or less widespread. Accurate knowledge of its extent was impossible until the tuberculin test was devised. Tuberculin was discovered by Koch in the year 1890. When properly controlled, injection of this material into a tuberculous animal gives a reaction which is considered diagnostic.

Veranus A. Moore states that tuberculosis is one of the oldest diseases of cattle of which we have record. Under the Mosaic laws, there were rules that the flesh of animals which suffer from wen or scurvy should not be used as food. In the ninth century French ecclesiastical laws were passed against the eating of flesh of cattle and swine affected with tuberculosis. In 1730 the sale of such flesh was forbidden in Munich, and 1843 in Wurtsburg. In 1783 the Berlin Board of Health passed regulations for meat inspection. In 1847 Klencke stated that there is a positive connection between the milk of scrofulous cows and scrofula in children. In America the first conference on bovine tuberculosis was held in 1879 by Dr. Noah Cressy, who held meetings among farmers in the western part of the state of Massachusetts in country districts, starting an agitation against this disease. In January, 1881, the Cattle Commissioners of Massachusetts referred to bovine tuberculosis for the first time. In 1889 the report of the Massachusetts Cattle Commissioners states: "Should the diseases materially increase where milk is produced for town or city markets, as a measure to guard the public health it may become the duty of the Commissioners, or the local Boards of Health to cause the inspection of herds producing market milk, and the removal therefrom of all animals exhibiting the slightest symptoms of this disease."

Melvin, chief of the Bureau of Animal Industry, stated in 1908 that it is estimated that about 10 per cent of the dairy cattle of the United States are infected with bovine tuberculosis. In 1893, Russell in Wisconsin reported that from one-fifth to one-sixth of the herds of the state had been tested for tuberculosis and that not over 5 per cent were tuberculous. Tests made in North Carolina on native cows in 1909, after three years' work showed that only 0.1 per cent were tuberculous. In Savannah, Georgia, 47 herds were tested in 1914 and in 19 of these positive reacters were found. In Hawaii, in 1910, according to Parker, every dairy on the island of Oahu was tested and 7.8 per cent reacted. Under my own supervision, over 1,000 cows were tested in Cortland County, N. Y. in 1910 and 273 reactors were found, or 27 per cent. In 1906 Anderson tested the milk supply of Washington and found in 233 samples of milk, 6.7 per cent contained bovine tubercle bacilli. In 1909, Hess tested New York milk and of 107 samples, found 16 with bovine tubercle bacilli. Tonney in 1910 testing the milk supply of Chicago, found in 144 samples of milk, 10 which contained tubercle bacilli. Goler reports 5 per cent of samples of Rochester with bovine tubercle bacilli. Rosenau states the average of tests in all cities collected by him shows 8.3 per cent. The practice of tuberculin testing of dairy cows has become widespread in the United States. Under the auspices of State Departments of Agriculture, State Departments of Health and Municipal Health Departments, these tuberculin tests have been conducted, and in those parts of the country where dairy herds are out doors most of the year the percentage of reacting animals is very small, being not more than 1 per cent, while in those parts of the country where animals are kept in the stable a large part of the time, the percentage of reactors may be very large.

INFANT MORTALITY

For centuries the world has taken it for granted that a large percentage of infants born must die during the first year of life as a matter of course. In the animal world the larger percentage of the young perish very soon and only a fraction of those which are born reach the adult stage. In the human race the death of infants during the first year of life was generally considered a matter of constitutional weakness and inherited disability to endure the climate or to properly digest nourishment. It has always been recognized that infant deaths were greater in number during the hot weather and the summer season. No accurate knowledge of the total deaths or of the seasonal variations was obtainable until the civilization reached a point where public health authorities began the tabulation of mortality statistics, including birth-rates as well as death-rates. The keeping of such mortality statistics is considered to be one of the highest marks of the development of intelligence by civilization. That such development is still incomplete is obvious from the large portions of the United States which are still outside of the registration area, and from the numerous nations in the world which also fail to keep such vital statistics. Before the activities of health authorities were directed toward the prevention and reduction of infant mortality, more than half of the infants born perished during the first year of life. Even during the last twenty years the records show many large cities of the world having death-rates of more than 400 per every 1,000 infants born.

The census report of the United States in the year 1900 shows eight cities having death-rates ranging from 300 to 419 per 1,000. The records of France and Germany show a wide variation during the same period; in most cities the death-rates being lower than in American cities. Cities in hot climates show higher death-rates than those in cold climates.

All authorities are agreed that the principal cause of infant deaths has been diseases of the intestinal tract. The terms "cholera infantum" and "summer diarrhea" of infants have been popularly used to designate such diseases. Harrington states that the average death-rate in 42 German cities in 1906 was 198 per 1,000, and that infant diarrhea was responsible for more than 80 per cent of these deaths. The records from the city of Leipsic for the year 1900 show a death-rate of 55 per 1,000 due to diarrhea, but of 430 of every 1,000 for the month of August.

The Registrar General of England reports for the year 1906, from 76 cities in England and Wales, that 50 per cent of infant deaths occur during the months of July, August and September.

Deaths from infant diarrhea are commonest among infants which are artificially fed. In 1900 Planchon in Paris reported that more than six times as many artificially fed infants died as those which were breast-fed. Harrington reports figures from Berlin, for the year 1904, showing ten times as many artificially fed infants died as breast-fed. Schereschewsky stated in 1907 that between 75 and 85 per cent of deaths from infant diarrhea were among infants artificially fed. Rosenau stated in 1917 that from a study of 44,226 deaths under one year in New York, Chicago, Boston and Philadelphia, 28 per cent were due to acute gastro-intestinal diseases, and that the New York City Department of Health reported 85 per cent of such deaths were among artificially fed infants; that in Great Britain 75 per cent, and in Germany 86 per cent, of such deaths were among infants artificially fed.

The above evidence hints only briefly at a great mass of material which has been compiled since health records have been kept, all of which points strongly to the fact that artificial feeding and summer heat play the most prominent part in the causation of infant diarrhea, and that infant diarrhea is by far the most important cause of infant death.

The direct connection between infant mortality and milk has been noted by observers at least since 1825, when Casper reported the high death-rate among children in Norway and Sweden who were fed cow's milk instead of mother's milk. Medical men in France and Gemany seem to have been the first to study systematically the relationship of milk to infant mortality, and to take the steps necessary to prevent milk infections from injuring the artificially fed infant. The principles established by the pioneers in this work have now been adopted in other civilized countries.

Local and national associations have been established for the reduction of infant mortality. In the United States there is now an American Child Hygiene Association, a Federal Children's Bureau, and numerous infant welfare societies in the cities throughout the country.

The statistical report of infant mortality published by the American Child Hygiene Association shows the record of infant mortality of the United States for the year 1920 for 519 cities. In cities having a population over 50,000 those having the lowest and highest infant death-rates are as follows:

Cities with Lowest and Highest Infant Death Rates in the United States, 1920

Lowest		Highest	
Tacoma, Wash.	37	Nashville, Tenn.	203
Houston, Texas	37	Savannah, Ga.	166
Berkeley, Cal.	45	Fall River, Mass.	134
San Diego, Cal.	52	Kansas City, Mo.	129
Seattle, Wash.	56	Birmingham, Ala.	125
Portland, Ore.	60	Saginaw, Mich.	123
San Francisco, Cal.	62	Johnstown, Pa.	120
Spokane, Wash.	71	Pittsburgh, Pa.	110
Oakland, Cal.	72	Buffalo, N. Y.	104

For this same year the infant death-rates in the largest cities in this country were as follows:

New York City	85
Philadelphia	89
Boston	101
Baltimore	104
St. Louis	77
Pittsburgh	110

(Chicago records are not given because infant births are not recorded.)

Food Value of Milk

The use of the milk of domestic animals for human food is as old as the human race. The wandering tribes of Asia used their flocks and herds not only as a source of clothing and of meat, but habitually used their milk as a most important element in their diet. The ability of the domestic animals to make use of vegetation as food enabled the wandering tribes to support life through the medium of such herds in territory where agriculture was impossible.

Without the aid of the chemist it would always have been logical to assume that a food obviously produced by nature for the nourishment and growth of the young must be possessed of superior characteristics. The English scientist, Saleeby, states with reference to milk, "Search earth and sky and you will find that only once has Nature set out to make a food — something which exists in order to be a food and for no other purpose." It was no accident that made the ideal land for the tribes of Israel a land flowing with milk and honey.

Until the bomb-calorimeter was invented by Berthelot it was impossible for chemists to accurately compare the amount of energy present in different foods. Atwater was the pioneer chemist in America to pursue studies which compared the value of milk with other foods by the combustion of measured quantities in the bomb-calorimeter. The calorie, being the amount of heat necessary to raise one liter of water one degree C., was used as the unit of measurement. Atwater found that 145 grams of milk would create 100 calories. The respiration calorimeter devised by Atwater, Rosa, and Benedict, permitting experiments on the oxidation of foods by human beings, was a further development of this same system of comparison.

The period from 1900 to 1910 was marked by a long series of important experiments by food chemists for the comparison of food values by the determination of calories and digestibility. The conclusion of all observers was that no other animal food is to be compared with milk from the standpoint of nourishment, energy, and cheapness. For example, Holt states: "There is no food as economical at present prices for the nutrition of infants as milk. For children between the ages of two and six years, the daily ration of milk should be one pint per day as a minimum." Lusk states: "Milk is the most important single food for adults. It is more economical to produce than meat. If it were a question of one or the other, I think it important that a man have milk rather than meat." * * * "Milk is the cheapest form of protein you can get. It is the most complete and efficient food that can be had. Around the dairy farms centers the proper nutrition of a nation." Sherman states that people can afford to pay twenty cents a quart for milk if they can afford to pay twenty-five cents a pound for beef.

Rosenau states that a glass of milk is equal in food value to two large eggs, or one large serving of lean meat, or two moderate-sized potatoes, or five tablespoonfuls of cooked cereals, or three tablespoonfuls of boiled rice, or two slices of bread.

A study of the results of chemical tests shows that one quart of milk is equal in food value to the following: 3/4 pound of lean beef, or 8 eggs, or 3 pounds of fresh codfish, or 2 pounds of chicken, or 1 pint oysters, of 4/5 of a pound of loin of pork, or 3/5 of a pound of ham.

The United States Department of Agriculture states: "Two facts stand out prominently as reasons for increased production and use of milk: First, that milk as purchased on the market usually supplies food material together with growth-promoting elements more economically than either meat or eggs; second, that the dairy cow is the most economical producer of human food. One great law of food conservation is to turn inedible foods into edible foods. The dairy cow will utilize coarse materials inedible by humans, such as grass, corn stalks, hay, etc., and will turn them into milk which is suitable for human food."

Sherman states that the average income of families in the United States during normal times is less than $800 per year. Not over 45 per cent of the income is spent for food. This amounts annually to about $7,000,000,000. The national expenditures for food in the United States annually are as follows:

17

	About	About
Meats, poultry, fish	$2,800,000,000	40%
Eggs	400,000,000	6
Milk	500,000,000	7
Cheese	50,000,000	1
Butter and other fats	500,000,000	7
Grain products	1,000,000,000	14
Sugar, molasses, etc.	500,000,000	7
Vegetables	500,000,000	7
Fruits	300,000,000	4
Nuts	50,000,000	1
Miscellaneous	400,000,000	6
	$7,000,000,000	100

A study of the daily diet of 92 New York families by Sherman showed that their expenditures for food were as follows:

Per cent total food cost

Meat, fish, poultry and shellfish	33.19
Eggs	5.55
Milk and cream	9.08
Cheese	1.13
Butter and other fats	8.14
Grain products	17.85
Sugar, molasses, etc.	3.80
Vegetables	9.12
Fruit	6.03
Nuts	0.35
Miscellaneous	5.76

As compared with this, Sherman recommends because of its nourishing qualities and cheapness that milk be used to a much larger extent, and that meat and fish be reduced. He practically recommends that the meat bill be cut to one-third and the amount of milk be multiplied by three. The expenditure for an ideal diet for the American family recommended by Sherman is as follows:

Per cent total food cost

Meat and fish	12%
Eggs	6
Milk	30
Cheese	3
Butter and other fats	11
Bread and cereals	13
Sugar	3
Vegetables, fruits	17

Lusk states: "We cannot expect a good community dietary if that community uses less than one-half quart of milk per capita per day." He further says: "No family of five should buy meat until they have bought at least three quarts of milk." The actual quantity of fluid milk consumed in the United States at the present time is about two-fifths quart per capita. Much of this is used for cooking purposes. It is also very unevenly distributed, rich households using much more, and poor households using much less. McCollum states that one quart of milk daily should be the allowance for every growing child and that adults would be greatly benefitted physically and mentally by the drinking of one quart of milk daily.

Recent investigations have revealed an alarming percentage of undernourished children. In one school in New York City, Copeland states that 70 per cent of the children are undernourished. Extensive examinations in other cities of the same nature have shown that the widespread prevalence of undernourishment is chiefly due to lack of milk in the diet. The remedy is plainly to provide more milk for the feeding of these undernourished children. The city of Seattle has taken the lead by establishing milk dispensaries in all public schools. Six years' experience has already resulted in a most marked improvement in the physical and mental condition of Seattle children. Recently, in the city of Rochester, N. Y., the Board of Education has taken steps to establish milk dispensaries in all public schools. A strong movement is taking place throughout the United States for the establishment of such milk dispensaries for school children. The problem of undernourishment in school children is recognized as an emergency problem. Copeland in New York proposes the establishment of nutritional clinics to be operated under the auspices of the Department of Health for the physical examination of children for undernourishment and for prescribing for their treatment. Such prescription must necessarily mean more milk.

VITAMINES

Previous to the year 1900 food chemists believed that all food products could be divided into four classes of substances, namely; proteids, carbohydrates, fats, and salts.

In 1906 the original experiments on vitamines were performed by Professor Hopkins, a chemist of Cambridge, England. He took two sets of rats about the same age and weight, feeding the first on protein, fat, sugar and salts, and the second on the same substances plus a very minute quantity of fresh milk. The first set lost weight and became sick, while the second set remained well and steadily gained in weight. After 18 days Professor Hopkins reversed the diets, with the result that the first set now gained in weight and recovered from their disease, while the second set lost weight. The only difference whatever in these diets was the use of a very minute quanitity of milk.

In 1909 Stepp, a German, found that rats fed on bread and milk increased in weight and reproduced normally. On the other hand, when the bread and milk was extracted with alcohol and ether and then used the animals lost weight and failed to reproduce.

In 1912 Professor Hopkins published his experiments extending over several years showing that rats grew very well on foods in a crude condition, and failed to grow when these same foods were purified, but that a small daily allowance of milk added to purified food made them grow. Hopkins' experiments really marked the beginning of an appreciation of the importance of what he termed, "the accessory factors to the diet."

In 1913 McCollum and Davis found that rats were unable to grow on artificial rations of purified food stuffs, but that the material extracted from butter and eggs supplied the missing food factor necessary for growth, while on the other hand lard and olive oil were unable to do so.

In 1913 Osborne and Mendel reported that when butter was substituted for lard in the diet of rats their normal rate of growth was resumed.

In 1914 Funk (who originally coined the word "vitamine") and Osborne and Mendel, and in 1915 and 1916 McCollum and Simmonds examined numerous fats and oils and found that there was a growth-promoting substance present in animal fats such as butter, cod liver oil and beef fat, but that this substance was absent from oils of vegetable origin.

As a result of the experiments mentioned above, it was generally believed that there was only one vitamine, or growth-promoting substance, and that this existed in butter fat and in cod liver oil, and to a smaller extent in beef fat. But in the year 1915 several workers, including Funk and McCollum, showed that in some cases young rats even when fed butter fat and cod liver oil in addition to purified foods not only rapidly declined in weight, but died, and some showed symptoms of a disease called "beri-beri." The addition of yeast to the diet of these rats was followed immediately by recovery and growth. This proved the existence of a second essential dietary factor distinct from that found in fats.

The credit of making this discovery belongs to McCollum and Davis in 1915, and their announcement was as follows: "There are necessary for normal nutrition during growth two classes of unknown accessory substances; one of these is soluble in fats, and the other soluble in water and apparently not soluble in fats." To these substances they gave the names "Fat Soluble A" and "Water Soluble B." They showed that Fat Soluble A is present in the fat of milk and that Water Soluble B is present in the water of milk.

All investigators now admit the indispensability of these two factors, Fat Soluble A and Water Soluble B, for the growth and nutrition of the animal organism.

A child cannot grow normally unless the milk from its mother's breast contains vitamines. Breast milk will not contain vitamines unless the mother's diet or food contains vitamines. The human mother is able to store up a certain amount of vitamines in her body fat. During the siege of Paris in 1870 young women were able to nurse their infants for considerable periods even though they themselves were partly starving through the shortage of food supply. Lack of vitamines in the diet of cows, or in the diet of human mothers, causes debilities in infants which may not be recognized as disease. Cows fed on certain pastures produce milk which is deficient in vitamines. When the forage is improved, the condition of the cows and the milk is improved. The summer pasture of cows rich in green feed furnishes the maximum of anti-scorbutic vitamine. Cattle which are stall-fed or fed on dry grains produce milk deficient in vitamines.

The nursing mother's diet should include a plentiful supply of milk — at least a quart a day. If the mother's milk is not produced from a diet adequately supplied with vitamines, the breast-fed baby may suffer more than the artificially fed baby.

Butter fat can even be heated with steam without losing its vitamine content. All three vitamines, however, are susceptible to heat. Water Soluble C is the most susceptible; Water Soluble B the least.

There are three vitamines so far discovered. The first is *Fat Soluble A*. This is present in abundance in milk, butter, egg yolk, and to a lesser extent in beef fat, and in vegetables, including lettuce and spinach, cabbage, carrots, and beets. It is present in green leaves, absent from lard, vegetable oils, and cereals. Steenboch has observed that it is always associated with a yellow pigment. It promotes growth in the young and maintains health in adults. It also prevents rickets. It is probably synthesized by plants. It is stored by the body in association with the fat. Milk, cream, butter, and cod liver oil form the basis of treatment of malnutrition and tuberculosis. Too much exposure to the oxygen of the air and high heat may destroy this vitamine, as in some processes of drying milk. Rickets is caused by an insufficient supply of Fat Soluble A, also a disease of the eye which if untreated may lead to blindness. To prevent rickets, children should be fed milk fat. Sweetened condensed milk is undesirable for the reason that the degree of dilution required by the high sugar content renders the food deficient in fat. In order to insure calcification of the teeth and effective growth up to the eighteenth year, this vitamine is necessary. Three-fourths of the infants in such cities as New York show signs of rickets. In Vienna in one community which included many breast-fed infants, rickets was diagnosed in 50 per cent of the infants up to five months old. Hess found among negro women in New York City, whose children almost always suffer from rickets, that these women live on a diet derived from wheat flour, corn meal, polished rice, tubers and meat.

McCollum and Simmonds showed that Fat Soluble A is not found in mother's milk unless it is present in the diet. McCollum and Simmonds are more cautious regarding the relation of Fat Soluble A to rickets than English authors and state: "We are not now willing to hazard any statements in regard to the factors operating to produce rickets in the child or the experimental animal. It might seem that the cause of these diseases lies in a deficiency of Fat Soluble A, or calcium in the food, or a disturbance in the metabolism of these factors."

Water Soluble B. This is more abundant in Nature than the other vitamines, nearly all natural foods containing some of it. Yeast, milk, and orange juice are especially rich in this vitamine. Heating with alkalis destroys it. Attempts to extract it have been partly successful with Fuller's earth, and by chemical processes. The evidence shows that animals cannot synthesize this vitamine. The plant kingdom is the primary source. It is affected by prolonged heat, such as that used in condensing milk.

Water Soluble C, or the anti-scorbutic vitamine. This is contained in most fresh fruit and fresh vegetables. Oranges and tomatoes are the best sources. Cow's milk, even raw, is not rich in the anti-scorbutic vitamine. When heated or dried the amount present in milk is still further reduced. To avoid danger, all infants whether fed on raw or on pasteurized milk should receive extra anti-scorbutic material such as fresh orange juice, or tomato juice, even from canned tomatoes. Grape juice contains this vitamine but is not so powerful as orange juice. It is most important that both pregnant and nursing women should consume daily an adequate supply of anti-scorbutic food.

The potency of milk depends almost entirely on the fodder of the cow. Cows fed experimentally for three weeks on fodder devoid of anti-scorbutic vitamine produced milk almost devoid of this factor. This raises the question whether winter milk is a well-balanced food. Summer pasture milk is much richer in the anti-scorbutic factor than winter milk. Even silage made from well matured corn and partly dried before putting into the silo did not greatly increase the quantity of this factor in the milk. One author fed guinea pigs with milk from cows fed on dry fodder, and from cows fed on fresh grass only. All guinea pigs on dry-fodder milk developed scurvy within twenty-one days, and died of scurvy within fifty-six days. Animals receiving pasture milk were still alive after one hundred and twenty days. Two of these, however, showed mild signs of scurvy. The spray processes of drying milk are more destructive of the anti-scorbutic vitamine than the other processes.

While other foods contain various vitamines in various quantities, milk contains all three vitamines. On this subject McCollum states: "The best sources of Fat Soluble A are whole milk, butter fat, and egg yolk fats, and the leaves of plants. Milk and the leaves of plants are to be regarded as protective foods and should never be omitted from the diet. Milk is a better protective food than are the leaves when used in proper amounts."

MILK SANITATION

At the Paris Exposition in 1900, fresh milk and cream in bottles were shipped every two or three weeks from farms in Illinois, New Jersey and New York. This milk kept sweet with no precautions except cleanliness in its production and cold in its preservation. No other country except France tried to show natural milk or cream at this Exposition. French exhibits of milk and cream were in striking contrast to the American, since not a single sample kept sweet one day after reaching the grounds, while the American products were still sweet a fortnight after bottling.

Cleanliness in connection with milk is not a new idea. Washing and scalding of milk utensils was known as desirable to the ancients. Cleanliness in the cow stable was recognized by Shakespeare, who characterized one of his heroines by the statement, "She can milk, look you, a sweet virtue in a maid with clean hands."

The importance of cleanliness in milk production and milk handling became more evident with the discovery of the relation of bacteria to the cleanliness of dairy operations. The first bacteriologist to undertake the testing of milk for numbers and kinds of bacteria present, quickly discovered a close relationship between the abundance of bacteria and the abundance of dirt. The first bacteriological examinations, which followed the invention of solid culture media in 1881 by Koch, showed that milk samples taken directly from the udder of healthy cows contained small numbers of bacteria, while the exposure of milk to stable dust and unclean utensils resulted in large numbers of bacteria.

In America, in 1892, Sedgwick and Batchelder were among the first to discover that milk fresh from the cow contained from 500 to 1000 bacteria per c.c. In 1893 and 1894, Conn studied the sources of bacteria causing milk fermentations and suggested that these came from stable dust. In 1896, Russell found from 5,000 to 20,000 bacteria in milk fresh from the cow. The same year, Moore showed that bacteria were more numerous in the milk first drawn from the udder than in the milk last drawn. In 1901, Park reported that milk fresh from cows contained only from 400 to 6,000 bacteria, while market milk contained millions. He also showed that in New York City during cold weather, the average number of bacteria in milk was 300,000, while in hot weather it was 5,000,000.

These studies led to the realization by all investigators that the initial contamination of milk takes place in the dairy barn after it is drawn from the cow. This resulted in a campaign to bring about improved sanitary conditions at the dairy, which was greatly stimulated by the work of medical milk commissions in the production of "certified" milk, referred to elsewhere. It was obvious that the bulk of the milk supply for cities must come from ordinary dairy farms which could not afford the expense of equipment and methods used by certified dairies. Consequently during the years following the preliminary tests made on milk by the bacteriologists mentioned, the activities of the pioneers in milk sanitation in America were directed toward the finding of those improvements which the rank and file of dairy farmers could be expected to adopt, and which would be most effective in protecting the milk produced on such farms against serious contamination.

As stated by Chapin, in 1902: "What is wanted is a plentiful supply of fresh milk in the same condition as when it left the cow's udder. This is possible anywhere at a trifling advance in price by improved methods of handling. Counting the number of bacteria will tell whether milk has been properly cared for or not. Few bacteria mean sanitary conditions and cold milk, large numbers of bacteria mean dirty conditions and milk not properly cooled. Costly stables are not necessary. One cent per quart above the market price is enough to pay for the cost of producing milk equal to certified milk."

In 1903, Stocking showed the advantages of using small mouthed milking pails to keep dirt out of milk during the milking process. In 1906, Pearson suggested a set of standard methods to be adopted by dairy farmers to keep their milk in sanitary condition.

Dairy score cards were devised as the best means for educating the dairy farmer in dairy sanitation and for the use of milk inspectors in determining the sanitary condition of dairy farms. Woodward, of Washington, in 1904, devised a sanitary score card for dairies. Pearson, in 1905, proposed another such card, and Lane in 1906 drafted a card of another type. All of these gave a list of dairy equipments and operations but made no attempt to lay emphasis on one group as against the other.

In 1908, North suggested the splitting of the score card into two divisions, equipment and methods, for the purpose of laying especial emphasis on methods. This suggestion was submitted to the Official Dairy Inspectors Association which had appointed a committee to draft an official score card. The card finally adopted contained this division, and has been extensively used since that time in improving sanitary conditions of dairy farms.

Special emphasis on methods, as contrasted with equipment has been of the greatest value in educating dairy farmers to understand that the personal element is the vital factor in clean milk production.

After several years' trial the city of New York has abolished the use of score cards giving a numerical score, on the ground that they are misleading to the dairy farmer and have no direct relation to the sanitary character of milk. As a substitute the city furnishes its dairy inspectors with a report blank itemizing the methods and equipment considered necessary for clean milk production, and which are positively required by the Department of Health.

CERTIFIED MILK

This term is used to designate milk produced under the supervision of commissions composed of physicians appointed by medical societies. The object of such supervision is to secure raw milk of the very highest sanitary character, from healthy cows handled by healthy employees, so that such milk will be available for clinical purposes, — especially feeding of infants.

The idea of producing an exceedingly pure and safe raw milk, under the supervision of a Medical Milk Commission, originated in the mind of Dr. Henry L. Coit of Newark, New Jersey, in 1890. At that time Dr. Coit secured the coöperation of forty physicians of the Medical Society of New Jersey in an effort to get the legislature to pass laws that would improve the milk supply of the state. Failing in this effort in 1892 he submitted a plan to the Practitioners' Club of Newark, New Jersey, for an organization of a Medical Milk Commission to supervise the production of clean milk. This plan had previously been submitted by him to Professor A. R. Leeds, Dr. T. M. Prudden and Dr. R. G. Freeman, and met with their approval. In June 1892, a Medical Milk Commission appointed by the Essex County Medical Association of New Jersey, made a contract with a dairyman for the production of milk under their supervision. Dr. Coit coined the word "certified" milk because the Commission issued a certificate to the dairyman. In his original paper Dr. Coit says the character of this milk is indicated:

1. By the absence of large numbers of bacteria and the absence of pathogenic varieties.
2. By resistance to fermentations and by its keeping qualities.
3. By constant nutritive value and chemical composition.

Dr. Henry Dwight Chapin, at a meeting of the New York County Medical Society, in October 1901, recommended the appointment of a commission to supervise the production of certified milk in New York City. Between 1892 and 1906 twenty-seven medical milk commissions were organized in the principal cities of the United States. In 1907 in Atlantic City a National Association of Medical Milk Associations was organized. Through this Association national standards for certified milk have been established. A number of states have passed legislation prohibiting the use of the term "certified," excepting for milk conforming to the national standards and under the supervision of authorized medical milk commissions.

The movement for certified milk, started in 1892, gave a great impulse to the interest of the medical profession in the dairy industry, the improvement of the sanitary character of all milk, and better control over the health of dairy cattle and dairy employees. All classes of milk have been improved by the certified movement, and all milk legislation since 1892 has been strongly influenced by the standards for certified milk.

On the other hand, the total quantity of certified milk produced is less than half of 1 per cent of the fluid milk consumed. The retail price ranges from 10 to 15 cents per quart above the price of market milk, thereby greatly limiting demand. The tremendous success of the campaign for pasteurized milk has almost removed the necessity for a raw milk even of the certified class from the minds of the leading public health authorities. As a matter of fact the danger of infection even in such a high-class raw milk still exists. Several serious outbreaks of infection which have occurred from such milk, and the discovery of tuberculosis on a large scale among certified dairy herds, have convinced a majority of public health authorities that there is no secure safeguard excepting pasteurization.

The certified movement created a powerful impulse towards expensive barns, cow stables, and milk houses, and expensive barn and dairy equipments. Sentiment was strongly towards the idea that only model dairies could produce milk of high sanitary character, and that because model dairies were out of reach of the rank and file of dairymen, the rank and file could not be expected to produce a very sanitary milk.

During the decade beginning 1900 extensive studies were made of the possibilities of producing sanitary milk on ordinary farms. Chapin and Park reported successful production of milk with extremely low bacterial counts on numerous ordinary dairy farms shipping to New York City. The many reports from bacteriologists of the freedom of milk from bacteria as it leaves the udder made it seem feasible, by simple means, to prevent contaminations from occurring from cow to consumer. In agricultural experiment stations in Virginia, Wisconsin, New York, and elsewhere, workers in the United States Department of Agriculture made extensive studies of dairy sanitation. Sentiment was rapidly forming in favor of the proposition that clean milk could be made under commercial conditions in ordinary barns.

In 1908, North suggested a method of milk production for ordinary dairy farms, and succeeded in interesting the New York Milk Committee in his plan, which resulted in the establishment of a large milk-shipping station at Homer, New York. Here for ten years, from ten to twenty thousand quarts of milk have been produced daily, by between one and two hundred farmers, which laboratory tests have shown to contain remarkably small numbers of bacteria. This demonstration, lasting as it has over a period of years, under the daily control of the Bacteriological Laboratory, has shown conclusively that a large group of dairy farmers of the ordinary type can produce milk under sanitary conditions to satisfy all the demands of decency and public health, at the lowest possible expense.

As further evidence of the fact that methods and not equipment are the primary factors in producing clean milk, North transported ten dairy farmers from their homes into a new dairy district, where in ten barns of the ordinary type, entirely strange to them, with no changes in equipment, these men produced milk within the limits of the certified standards for bacteria of 10,000, compared with milk containing many millions of bacteria produced in the same places the previous day by the owners of the premises.

The method of milk production adopted at Homer has been established at many other places, and the principles have been adopted by many of the largest milk companies. Most of the Grade A milk marketed in New York City, Philadelphia, Baltimore and other cities, is now produced by this system.

The work of North was confirmed by Harding, the United States Department of Agriculture, and many others. There remains no longer any doubt that any dairy farmer with even the poorest barn and poorest equipment can produce clean milk by clean methods, under practical working conditions.

The establishment of this principle did much to stimulate the adoption of bacterial standards and the grading system of milk, based on bacterial tests by municipal authorities.

PASTEURIZATION

The studies made by Pasteur from 1860 to 1864 revealed the fact that the diseases of wine were caused by yeasts and bacteria, and that these could be killed by heating to a temperature from 50 to 60° C. for a few minutes. In 1868, under Pasteur's direction a cargo of heated wine was sent around the world on a ship without any spoilage. In 1870, Pasteur studied the diseases of beer and found that the organisms causing these were destroyed at temperatures from 50 to 55°C. In 1886, Soxhlet, in Munich, recommended that all cows' milk fed to infants should be boiled or sterilized for at least 35 or 40 minutes to kill the germs contaminating the same. He states: "During the process of milking particles of manure and other forms of dirt get into milk, and during transportation and general handling fermentation sets in, so that much of our milk is really unfit for consumption before it gets into the stomachs of infants and children. Mother's milk on the contrary is taken directly and would undoubtedly be equally contaminated and frequently injurious to infants if it suffered the same manipulation as cows' milk." He quotes the well-known fact that calves fed on milk from a trough frequently suffer from diarrhea. Soxhlet recommended and described a set of utensils for sterilizing milk for infants in the home, consisting of five ounce bottles with stoppers of rubber and glass, and trays in a water vat for performing sterilization. On his recommendation this apparatus was widely adopted in Germany and Austria.

In 1888 Dr. A. Caillé of New York City visited Germany and witnessed the work of Soxhlet. On his return he published a statement advocating the adoption of Soxhlet's methods, in which he says: "Dr. Soxhlet reports his experiences in preparing and feeding sterilized milk, and describes an apparatus by means of which the procedure can be practically carried out in every household. This work does not seem to have attracted attention on this side of the Atlantic. I have never heard it spoken of and have never seen a press notice on the subject in any of our journals."

Jacobi as early as 1873 read a paper before the Public Health Association of New York in which he said: "Cows' milk ought to be cooked at once in order to keep it as long as possible from turning sour. It ought to be preserved in a cool place if not in the ice box. Pour the whole amount of boiled and skimmed cows' milk the infant is to have through the day into a number of two or four ounce bottles. You avoid the development of fungi by this plan and prevent decomposition. This end will be obtained still better by heating the milk in the bottles before corking."

In 1889, Jacobi referred to the Soxhlet apparatus for the boiling of milk. Writing in 1895 he says: "To remove the dangers of intestinal disorders and the sources of excessive mortality and invalidism, nothing has been more successful than the widespread practice of sterilization and pasteurization of cows' milk. Both are the logical development of the plan of treating milk by boiling which I have persistently advised for these forty years at least. There can hardly be a doubt that if raw milk could always be had unadulterated, fresh, and untainted, and as often as it was wanted, it would require no boiling, but such ideal milk cannot be had so long as cows are tuberculous: scarlet fever and diphtheria are met with in the houses, about the clothing, and on the hands of dairymen and women; and typhoid stools are mixed with the water which is used for washing utensils." Jacobi, who must be recognized as having occupied for many years a position at the head of the medical profession as a specialist in children's diseases, always advocated the bringing of cows' milk to a boil before feeding to children.

In 1892, Jacobi and Freeman advised Nathan Straus to adopt the Soxhlet method for sterilizing milk in the infant milk depots he was about to establish in the tenement house districts of New York.

Flügge, in 1894, created a decided reaction in the minds of the medical profession regarding the advisability of heating milk, by reporting harmful results to the milk, and to infants fed thereon, due to destruction of lactic acid bacteria and the multiplication of putrefactive and toxic-producing organisms remaining. This attitude was strengthened by the advent during the same period of the movement for the production of certified milk, and the feeding of infants on raw cows' milk which was fresh and clean. It was the constructive work of a large series of investigators during the following years that restored the pasteurization of milk to the secure position which it now occupies.

Budin and Chovane, in 1894, reported successful results in Paris in the feeding of infants on sterilized milk.

Freeman, in 1898, showed that milk heated to 68°C. for thirty minutes and kept cold was suitable for infant feeding.

Theobald Smith, in 1899, reported that the germs of bovine tuberculosis were destroyed by heating to a temperature of 60°C. for twenty minutes. This was confirmed the next year by Russell and Hastings. On the other hand, the objections to pasteurization were strengthened by the reports of Koeppen, in 1897, and the American Pediatric Society, in 1898, of cases of scurvy resulting from the continued feeding on sterilized and pasteurized milk. To counterbalance this, however, Straus and his advisers were reporting yearly favorable results from the feeding of heated milk to infants in New York, and many European observers were reporting favorable results from sterilized milk.

In 1901, Maygrier reported the results of feeding sterilized milk to 590 infants, with no cases of diarrhea. Denmark had already in 1898 passed a law requiring the heating of all milk fed to calves to a temperature of 85°C. to prevent the transmission of infection.

There is no doubt that this was a transition period, and that medical men and scientists were gradually drawing apart into two camps: those on the one hand who favored the use of raw milk for infants and for municipal supplies, those on the other who favored the heating of milk for both of these purposes. Meantime the multiplication of milk epidemics was making the necessity for some definite action to control municipal milk supplies and milk for infants more and more evident. Those who advised the heating of milk were uncertain as to the temperatures which should be used. These ranged all the way from a minimum of 60°C. for fifteen minutes, advised by Hesse, in 1900, to 70°C. for thirty minutes, advised by Oppenheimer, and to such high temperatures as 85°C. as adopted by Denmark for the pasteurization of cream.

A great impulse was given to the adoption of pasteurization by the work of Park and Holt in 1903, in the feeding of tenement house babies, in which the groups fed on raw grocery store milk fared so badly with a high mortality, while those fed on pasteurized milk showed such favorable results. In 1905, Freeman called attention to the decline in . infant mortality in the United States due to the increase of pasteurization.

The movement towards the adoption of the processes of heating milk called "sterilization" and "pasteurization" had up to this time been chiefly limited by its advocates to the consideration of the use of these measures in the home, with small and simple apparatus which could be handled by any housewife. There was decided antagonism even by the most ardent advocates of the heating of milk to the adoption of this measure by the milk industry itself. Such opposition existed, of course, to an even greater extent among the advocates of raw milk for infant feeding and for the general public. From the broad standpoint of public health, it was obvious to men of vision that if milk infections were so serious a menace to both infants and adults, and if the prevention of such infections was a public health measure of such importance to municipalities, the pasteurization of milk in the home by consumers themselves was a remedy wholly inadequate to secure the results desired. Only a small fraction of the population could be expected to attempt to use this process, and even when used it must necessarily be accompanied by intermittence, irregularity, and unreliability.

Consequently the more far-sighted of public health authorities turned their eyes toward the milk industry, in the hope that reliable methods for pasteurization of the entire milk supply of cities, or at least the major portion thereof, could be carried out in a reliable way by dealers so that infections would be checked before they could reach the homes. As early as 1880, in Germany, milk was pasteurized in a small way by commercial concerns. In Denmark between 1880 and 1890 apparatus was perfected for heating milk on a large scale. The Danish commercial machines of that period permitted a continuous flow of large quantities of milk, and heated the same momentarily to the required temperatures, followed by rapid cooling. This method of quick momentary heating was designated the "flash method," and was soon adopted in Germany.

During the decade 1890 to 1900 a few of these Danish heaters reached the United States and in a small way in several places milk dealers made use of flash pasteurization. By 1900 a considerable number of dealers in large cities were pasteurizing milk by various types of flash heaters, but such pasteurization was for the most part secret and unrecognized by the health authorities or the medical profession. Its adoption by the industry was chiefly because of the commercial advantages in the preservation of milk against untimely souring. The fact that this was practised in secret and the milk marketed without any label indicating that it had been heated was entirely due to the strong sentiment against pasteurization by the dealer. In 1901 one of the largest milk concerns was actually marketing in the same wagons milk labelled "Pasteurized" at nine cents per quart, and milk with no label at eight cents per quart, to consumers who purchased these two grades of milk in the belief that the eight cent milk was raw, while as a matter of fact, the entire supply of this concern was pasteurized. The emphasis with which the consumers stated their ability to distinguish between the taste of these two grades of milk illustrated very well the deep seated popular prejudice against pasteurization.

Unfortunately, the machinery for pasteurizing commercial milk by the flash method was uncertain in operation, and this coupled with the opposition to the process by the medical profession and the majority of health authorities, held back the milk industry from the establishment of commercial pasteurization on a large scale.

Rosenau, in 1906, gave a new impulse to the importance of pasteurization and the necessity for its adoption, by the publication of the thermal death point of the bacteria of tuberculosis, typhoid fever, and diphtheria, showing that all of the organisms of diseases commonly transmitted by milk are destroyed when heated to a temperature of 60°C. for twenty minutes. In the same year North showed that the taste of milk and the rising of the cream in the glass bottle was not affected by temperatures below 65°C. for thirty minutes.

The temperature of 60°C. for twenty minutes advocated by Smith, Russell and Rosenau could not be adopted by the milk industry under commercial conditions because at that time there was no machinery manufactured capable of performing such a process.

In 1905, J. H. Monrad in his book on pasteurization stated:

In view of the assumed necessity of keeping the milk or cream at high temperatures for twenty or thirty minutes if it is to be sold and not manufactured, and in view also of the difficulties of heating all the milk in a body when we have to handle large quantities such as must be handled at milk shipping stations if pasteurization is ever to be introduced generally, I have suggested the following plan: Use any continuous heater which you find best, but instead of running the milk directly to the cooler, run it into a storage tank which should hold one-third of the hourly capacity of your heater and cooler if you desire to keep the milk for twenty minutes at the high temperature; or one-half if you want to keep it thirty minutes. . . . By having one partition in the tank and two attached to the cover the milk is compelled to go to the bottom first, then up, then down, and at last up and out to the cooler, and I challenge bacteriologists to show any reason why this arrangement does not solve the problem of combining a continuous apparatus with the strictest bacteriological demands.

One manufacturer in Philadelphia in that same year actually made a crude form of apparatus for holding milk hot twenty minutes according to the suggestion of Monrad. Unfortunately this suggestion passed unnoticed both by the milk industry and by scientists until 1906, when North called the attention of the manufacturers of machinery, as well as some of the largest dealers, to Monrad's suggestion and urged the construction of commercial pasteurizing apparatus which would hold milk in tanks at the temperatures and for the period of time recommended by Rosenau and others. The largest manufacturer of milk machinery immediately adopted this suggestion and produced such a tank, in which milk was automatically heated to the required temperature and held for the required time, and this was installed in the pasteurizing plant of the largest milk company at that time pasteurizing milk.

The tests of this new process over a period of months by North in 1907 demonstrated conclusively that large quantities of milk could be pasteurized under commercial conditions with no impairment of taste or appearance, and at a temperature which the bacteriologists had shown was necessary for the destruction of the pathogenic bacteria found in milk. This event marked the birth of the process since known as the "holding method" of pasteurization, and was followed by its adoption by all large milk dealers, not only in America but in Europe. While numerous modifications of the apparatus have been developed since that time, the principle of the holding method has remained the same. The medical profession and the public health authorities, while skeptical at first, soon were compelled to recognize that the standards demanded by the authorities in bacteriology had been fully met by the milk industry, and that under commercial conditions and the supervision of health authorities, the holding method of pasteurization was so reliable that commercially pasteurized milk deserved the confidence of the public. This conviction led to the widespread adoption by states as well as cities of definitions of pasteurization in laws, ordinances, and regulations, establishing standard temperatures and standard length of time for this process.

The perfection of the commercial process has almost entirely supplanted the use of the small home pasteurizers and heaters recommended by Soxhlet and his followers. The fact that the milk industry, as well as the leading public health and medical authorities, became satisfied that the holding process of pasteurization was reliable has not been sufficient, however, to secure all of the popular recognition which this process deserves. The feeding of commercially pasteurized milk under the auspices of the city of New York to many thousands of infants at the baby health stations constituted the most extensive infant-feeding experiment the world has ever seen, and demonstrated conclusively that such milk was entirely satisfactory as a safe and wholesome food for infants.

While many large cities followed the lead of Chicago in the adoption of regulations requiring the pasteurization of milk, there are still many cities of the second, third, and lower classes in the United States where opinion is divided and the merits of pasteurization are even at the present time debated as they were among the pioneer investigators thirty years ago.

There is no question, however, that pasteurization of the bulk of the milk supply has outgrown the experimental stage and has come to stay. The results of this measure in the reduction of infant mortality from all forms of disease transmissible by milk has been so marked that public health authorities are now practically unanimous in their opinion that the bulk of the milk supply of all cities should be pasteurized in the interests of public health.

In this connection the statement of the National Commission on Milk Standards very well represents the prevailing opinion:

The Commission thinks that pasteurization is necessary for all milk excepting Grade A raw milk. The majority of the Commissioners voted in favor of the pasteurization of all milk including Grade A raw, but since the action was not unanimous, the Commission recommended that the pasteurization of Grade A raw milk be optional. . . . Experience with the pasteurization of milk by the use of the time and temperature recommended by this Commission has justified in every way the selection of the time and temperature which were recommended in the year 1917, which was as follows: That the pasteurization of milk should be between the limits of 140° F. and 155° F. At 140° F. the minimum exposures should be twenty minutes. For every degree above 140 the time may be reduced by one minute. In no case should the exposure be for less than five minutes. In order to allow a margin of safety under commercial conditions, the Commission recommends that the minimum temperature during the period of holding be made 145° F. and the holding time thirty minutes.

INFANT MILK DEPOTS

The first infant milk depot in the world was established in the city of Hamburg, Germany, in the St. Gertrude District, in 1889. The second infant milk depot was established in the Good Samaritan Hospital, New York, by Dr. Henry Koplik, also in 1889. These were followed in 1892 by the establishment in the Bellevue Dispensary of Paris of an infant milk depot by Dr. Variot. The Straus milk depots were begun in New York City in 1893. The Riverside Hospital in Yonkers established an infant milk depot in 1894. The first municipal milk depot in America was established by the city of Rochester, New York, in 1897. During the period from 1898 to 1905, numerous other cities followed their example not only in the United States but in England, France, Germany, Italy, Spain, Switzerland, Africa and South America. In France three types of milk depots were developed:

1. Mutualité Maternealle, for the education of mothers.
2. Consultations de Nourrisons, attached to obstetrical clinics for instructions in nursing and artificial feeding.
3. Gouttes de Lait, dispensing milk and advising mothers.

In America there have been two types of milk depots, as follows:

1. Preparing milk according to formulas for infant feeding in the nursing bottles, pasteurizing the same at the depot, with instructions to mothers for its use.
2. Milk dispensaries distributing milk in quart bottles, sending nurses into the homes, instructing mothers in its preparation and in the care of the baby in the home.

The Straus milk depots are good examples of the first type. Depots operated by the New York City Health Department are good examples of the second type.

Dr. Rowland G. Freeman was one of the earliest physicians to be identified with the establishment of infant milk depots of New York City, and favors that type of milk depot where milk is completely prepared in nursing bottles and pasteurized before distribution. He states that 60 per cent reduction in infant mortality can be expected in a city district patronizing an infant milk depot, and that this has been repeatedly demonstrated in French and also in American cities where milk depots have been established.

In 1912 he proposed the establishment of an endowment fund of five million dollars to pay the cost of operation of a sufficient number of infant milk depots in New York City to place good milk within reach of every infant. Nathan Straus was a pioneer in the establishment of infant milk depots and the use of pasteurized milk for infants. Though engaged in large business enterprises and a man of great wealth, he devoted a large part of his time to the establishment and operation of infant milk depots in New York and in other cities, and in advocating not only in America, but also in Europe, the use of pasteurized milk for the reduction of infant mortality. He first established infant milk depots at his own expense in 1893 for the distribution of pasteurized milk to infants in New York City. He states that in the months of July and August alone in 1890, 1891 and 1892, there died 13,201 children under five years of age, of which 6,122 died from infant cholera. Wherever Straus milk depots were established infant mortality was greatly reduced. Twenty-six years, or until 1919, Mr. Straus continued at great personal expense to pay the cost of the operation of at least nine infant milk depots in New York City, and of milk dispensaries for adults during the hot weather, and also presented the equipment for infant milk depots to numerous other cities in the world. The vigor with which he advocated the operation of such depots must be recognized as having been a great force in the world in influencing cities to undertake the reduction of infant mortality by such means.

The New York Milk Committee gave a great impulse to the work of reduction of infant mortality in New York City. This Committee was established in 1907 by the Association for Improving the Condition of the Poor. The average infant mortality for the previous ten years in New York City was 153 per thousand. The Committee announced as its chief object the reduction of infant mortality, and as a secondary object the improvement of the milk supply of New York City. It was composed of a number of prominent philanthropic men and women who freely gave of their time to its work. During the first year of its existence this Committee established four infant stations which it operated at its own expense. These stations dispensed milk in quart bottles, and sent nurses into the homes to instruct mothers how to prepare milk and how to care for infants. During the following years the Committee increased the number of infant milk stations until 1911, at which time it operated thirty-one. A demonstration of the wonderful results in the reduction of infant mortality in the neighborhoods patronizing these stations so convinced the municipal health authorities of their value that in 1912 the city officials agreed to operate under their own auspices all of the stations established by the New York Milk Committee, and arranged to increase the number as circumstances required. During the period of the Committee's milk depot work, extending over four years, the infant mortality of the city was reduced from 153 per thousand to 111. At the present time, under the auspices of the Department of Health of the City of New York, there are 68 infant milk depots in operation. Private health agencies are operating in addition 25 infant milk depots. The number of babies enrolled at the Department of Health stations is 27,059; at the stations operated by private agencies 6,172 — a total for the city of New York of 93 infant milk stations with 33,231 babies enrolled. The death-rate among infants enrolled at these stations is less than 50 per thousand births. The death-rate among infants in the entire city for the present year up to October 1, is only 76 per thousand births.

Infant milk depots have passed the experimental stage. A reduction of infant mortality of 60 per cent among the infants patronizing such depots is not uncommon. A question often asked is this. "Is such a reduction due to milk or to the education of mothers?" Dr. Rowland G. Freeman in 1912 answered this question by quoting the work of Park and Holt, who, under the auspices of the Rockefeller Institute, fed large groups of infants on different milks with the following results:

Milk	Mortality
Condensed Milk	20 %
Store Milk	19 %
Good Bottled Milk	9 %
Milk Depot Milk	2.7%

He also pointed out that the Association for Improving the Condition of the Poor, in 1911, equipped one Assembly District of New York City with doctors and nurses who held clinics and visited more than 116,000 families purchasing milk from grocery stores. The result was a decrease in infant mortality of 11 per cent, while in the same year, in the rest of the city, the infant mortality increased 4 per cent. From his studies of the work of infant milk depots Freeman concludes that 15 per cent of the reduction of infant mortality is due to education of the mothers, while 45 per cent is due to the dispensing of good milk. On the other hand, Dr. S. Josephine Baker, chief of the Bureau of Child Hygiene, of the New York City Health Department, concludes from her study of the operation of milk depots that 20 per cent of the reduction of infant mortality is due to pure milk and 80 per cent to the training of mothers. This difference of opinion may be due to the fact that the type of infant milk depot studied by Freeman completely prepares the infant milk in nursing bottles at the depot, while the depot studied by Dr. Baker prepares the milk in the home under the direction of nurses who instruct the mothers in such preparation.

The value of good milk is unquestioned, and it is not necessary to consider the education of the mother independently, since a large part of such education must consist in teaching mothers to recognize the value of good milk, the proper methods of its preparation, and care in the feeding of infants.

The results achieved by infant milk depots in the numerous cities where they have been established are sufficient evidence that there is no institution which will so quickly bring about a reduction of infant mortality, and that cities having large infant mortality rates can quickly reduce the same by the establishment of such milk depots.

LABORATORY TESTING OF MILK

The necessity of testing milk to determine its quality was not sufficiently felt to result in the invention of laboratory methods for such tests until the factory system of manufacturing cheese was developed about 1850, and for manufacturing butter about 1870. The volume of milk handled in such factories was so great and the financial aspect so dependent on honest milk that the owners were compelled to devise methods which would indicate the quality of milk brought by their patrons. The earliest methods used were physical, and consisted of cream gauges, or glass tubes in which milk was allowed to stand, the quantity of cream rising to the surface being observed. This method of testing was followed by the better method of determining the weight, or specific gravity, by hydrometers adapted for milk, which were then designated lactometers. Churn tests, oil tests, pioscopes, lactoscopes and lactocrites were all early forms of apparatus for testing physically the amount of fat in milk. Soxhlet, Wanklyn and Adams devised methods for the chemical determination of fat too complicated and impractical for use under commercial conditions. Up to 1888 there was no apparatus which would determine the fat in milk accurately, easily, cheaply, and quickly. From 1888 to 1890, a number of chemists worked on quick and simple methods for fat determination, among these being Dr. S. M. Babcock, of the Wisconsin Agricultural Experiment Station. In 1890 Babcock published a method which used a single reagent, sulphuric acid, and simple glassware, which could be understood and effectively carried out by any intelligent superintendent. The value of this simple and accurate test was quickly recognized, and its adoption by the milk industry, because of its far-reaching importance in controlling the composition of milk sold by producers and dealers, marked an epoch in the history of milk control. The food value of milk, since 1890, has been determined chiefly by the use of the Babcock test supplemented by the determination of total solids. There is no other test which has been so far-reaching in preserving high standards of food value in municipal milk supplies. While more refined tests such as the Rose-Gottlieb method are used for special purposes, the Babcock test is still universally considered as the standard test for fat both by the milk industry and by public health authorities.

Tests for Bacteria. The invention of solid culture media by Koch in 1881 was soon followed by its use for determining the numbers of bacteria in milk. The first record of such work is that of Von Geuns, who made counts of pasteurized milk in Amsterdam in 1885. In 1889, Claus reported the numbers of bacteria in raw milk in Wurtzburg, as did also Hohenkamp, and Knof counted the bacteria in the milk of Munich. In 1891, Renk made such tests of the milk of Halle, and in 1892 Uhl made bacterial counts of the milk of Gessen.

The first bacterial counts of milk in America were made in 1892 by Sedgwick and Batchelder on the milk supply of Boston. Rolland tested the milk in London in 1895, and in 1896 Frey tested the milk in Buffalo. In 1900 Pakes reported bacterial counts of the milk supply of London, and in 1901 Park made counts on the market milk of New York City. In 1903, Goler tested the milk of Rochester; in 1904 Burns and Berger, the milk supply of Philadelphia, and Jordan, the milk supply of Chicago. Up to this time all of these tests were looked upon as experimental in character and the reports were received as curiosities by the medical profession and by public health authorities. They were not used in a practical way either for the control of milk production, milk handling, or the regulation of milk sold on city markets. Freeman, Ravenel, and others, had been practising since 1892 such tests as this for the control of certified milk, but such milk was considered to be outside of the regular milk supply, and neither the milk industry nor the medical profession had yet recognized that the bacterial count of milk should be adopted for the control of the entire milk supply of any city. Park in New York, in 1901, suggested the control of the city supply by bacterial test, but was unsupported by the municipal authorities and opposed by the milk industry. Goler made a similar attempt in Rochester in 1903 but was unable to enforce a regulation based on such test at that time.

One of the greatest draw backs to the recognition of the bacterial test of milk was the fact that no standard methods for preparation of culture media, or other steps in the process of bacterial testing had yet been recommended, and each milk bacteriologist was a law unto himself. Similar methods were being used for determining the numbers of bacteria in water, and water bacteriologists were also in disagreement as to standard methods for performing such tests.

In 1905, Prescott suggested that a committee of the American Public Health Association be appointed to study the methods used for bacteriological examination of milk and to recommend uniform procedure. At Atlantic City, in 1907, this committee presented a preliminary report and a progress report was made at the annual meeting in 1908. This went into sufficient detail to bring about a great reform in the laboratories throughout the country, so that for the first time the same methods of testing milk were generally adopted. To the American Public Health Association, Laboratory Section, must be given the credit for having brought about the standardization of the methods for the bacterial testing of milk, so that at the present time not only public health laboratories, but those of the milk industry can all use methods which make their results comparable.

The confidence in the reliability of bacterial tests has steadily increased until many state and municipal health authorities have incorporated bacterial standards for the control of public milk supplies in their laws and ordinances. The technique for performing bacterial tests by the plate and microscopical methods, can be found in the publications of the American Public Health Association. It is difficult to estimate the value of such tests from a public health standpoint. Their relationship to sanitary conditions on the dairy farm is so close that they are now regularly used in country milk laboratories to determine the care exercised by the milk producer. The accuracy with which they show the efficiency of pasteurization has made it necessary both for the milk industry and public health authorities to apply such tests to all machines used for pasteurization since they so clearly show whether or not the operation has been properly performed.

The relationship of the numbers of bacteria to the care exercised in the transportation of milk, and to cooling, refrigeration and prompt delivery to the consumer, have resulted in the use of such tests on samples of milk as retailed on city markets, to determine whether the milk dealer has properly performed the duties entrusted to his care.

The Commission on Milk Standards after more than ten years consideration of the value of bacterial tests of milk says in its last annual report:

Among the present available routine laboratory methods for determining the sanitary quality of milk the bacterial count occupies first place, and that bacterial standards should be a factor in classifying milk of different degrees of excellence.

The adoption and enforcement of bacterial standards will be more effective than any other one thing in improving the sanitary character of public milk supplies. The enforcement of these standards can be carried out only by the regular and frequent laboratory examinations of milk for the numbers of bacteria it may contain. An opinion concerning the reliability of laboratory tests for numbers of bacteria had been reached, based on voluminous statistics secured for the most part by groups of observers working together, as well as by individuals. The results of extensive study justify the Commission in the conclusion that the analysis of duplicate samples of milk made by routine methods in different laboratories may be expected to show any average variation of about 28 per cent, with occasional samples of wider variation. In some good laboratories the variation may not be greater than 10 per cent. If five samples of the same milk are tested, the results may be relied upon as fairly accurate, and always sufficiently accurate to place any particular milk supply unhesitatingly in grade A, B, or C. The object of bacterial tests of milk samples for the numbers of bacteria should be primarily to determine the sanitary character of the milk supply from which the sample is taken, rather than the character of a single sample of milk. It is strongly urged by this Commission that no grading of milk should be made upon the analysis of single samples, and that no prosecutions or court cases should be brought upon the bacterial analysis of a single sample of milk.

MILK REGULATIONS

The history of milk regulations has followed closely the history of scientific knowledge of the relation of disease to milk. As early as the fourteenth century there were laws in Europe against the sale of diseased meat, but it was not until 1860 that the first English milk law was passed, and this only prohibited the dilution of milk with water. In 1866 a large dairy company of London voluntarily adopted sanitary regulations for the control of dairy farms.

In 1856 the first milk law was passed by the State of Massachusetts prohibiting the adulteration of milk. In 1859 the first milk inpector in the city of Boston was appointed to enforce a regulation against the use of distillery slops in the feeding of dairy cattle. In 1864 Boston prohibited the use of milk from diseased cows.

The city of Washington in 1863 passed a law declaring insanitary cow yards to be a nuisance, and a law against adulteration of milk in 1871. In 1873 the first dairy inspector was appointed by the city of Washington. In 1874 regulations against the skimming of cream from milk were passed. The city of Boston in 1859 authorized the collection of samples of milk for examination. In 1870 the city of Providence also authorized the collection of milk samples, and was followed by Washington in 1871 and by Syracuse in 1877. New York City did not authorize the collection of milk samples or laboratory testing until the year 1895, followed by Batimore in 1896 and Indian-apolis in 1897.

The city of Newark authorized the inspection of dairies in 1882. Dairy inspection was established in Washington, D. C. in 1895, in New York in 1902, and in Chicago in 1904. The growth of municipal activity in the control of milk supplies is indicated by the summary taken from the records of seventy-seven cities, compiled by Parker as follows:

	COLLECTION OF SAMPLES	INSPECTION OF DAIRIES
Dates	Number of Cities	Number of Cities
Prior to 1885	4	1
1885 — 1889	8	1
1890 — 1894	7	1
1895 — 1899	6	7
1900 — 1904	13	6
1905 — 1909	18	36
1910 — 1914	20	9
Total	76	61

The first city to make any regular bacteriological examination of milk as a part of the work of the public health officer was Montclair, N.J. under Parker, in 1900. The bacteriological examination of milk has been developed in American cities as a municipal function since the year 1900.

Bacterial standards for milk were first suggested for New York City in 1901, and the standard proposed was 1,000,000. This, how-ever, was found impractical at that time. In 1905, the city of Boston proposed a standard of 500,000 for its milk supply, and in 1907 Rochester proposed a standard of 100,000.

While the chemical examination of milk was placed on a sound foundation by the work of Babcock in 1900, and numerous municipal laboratories have regularly carried out chemical tests since that date, the bacteriological testing of milk was not placed on a sound footing until the establishment of standard methods by the American Public Health Association in 1910.

A survey in 1910 of milk regulations of American and European cities showed plainly the greatest variation not only in their extent but in the character and standards of their requirements. It was natural that this should be the case because of the transitional phases through which such questions as dairy sanitation, pasteurization, and bacterial testing had gone up to that time. The uncertainty of public health authorities as to correct standards for milk, and the lack of agreement on the part of medical and scientific authorities, was so great that each municipality was a law unto itself, and no standard milk regulations worthy of the name were in existence.

The evidence regarding the frequency of epidemics of milk-borne disease and the close relationship of unsanitary milk to infant mortality convinced the members of the New York Milk Committee that an effort should be made to bring about an agreement among the leading authorities on milk sanitation and public health. In order to accomplish this, a conference was called in December, 1910, in New York City by the New York Milk Committee of a large number of leading medical and public health authorities as well as milk scientists, and an unanimous resolution was passed in favor of the appointment of a national commission to consider the establishment of uniform standards for milk. In accordance with this resolution, from a list of over two hundred names submitted, twenty men were selected to compose this commission. Under an arrangement with the New York Milk Committee to provide financial support for the necessary expenses of its meetings, this Commission met for the first time in May, 1911, and has held meetings annually, and occasionally semi-annually, each year since that time. Reports of the agreements reached unanimously by members of this Commission have been regularly published by the United States Public Health Service, and have covered such subjects as chemical and bacteriological standards for milk and its principal products, and have recommended a system of grading of milk into at least three grades according to its sanitary character.

The principle of grading was recommended by the Commission as the best means for securing efficient control over the sanitary condition and safety of milk by the health officer, and for the marketing of milk according to its quality and price. This grading system and the standards proposed were first adopted by New York City in the year 1912, and have been modified and improved by that city since that time. They have been adopted in principle by the state of New York for all of its cities and towns, by Newark, N. J., Jersey City, N. J., and the state of California, and all the cities and towns therein, and by many cities in other states.

The recommendations of this Commission have been endorsed by the American Public Health Association and numerous other public health organizations.

As a result of an extensive survey of existing municipal milk regulations in the United States, North has compiled in regulations written by him for the city of Kansas City, Mo., 1921, the following list of subjects to be included in a model municipal milk regulation:

Organization, Personnel, and Laboratory
Milk and Milk Products (Definitions)
Sale of Adulterated Milk and Cream Prohibited
Applications and Procedure
Fees
Permits
Exclusion of Source of Milk or Milk Products Supply
Milk, Skimmed Milk and Cream shall Conform to Grades and Requirements. Other Milk Products shall Conform to Requirements Related thereto.
Requirements for all Grades of Milk
Standards and Requirements of Grade A Raw Milk, Skimmed Milk, and Cream
Standards and Requirements of Grade A Pasteurized Milk, Skimmed Milk and Cream for Infants and Children
Standards and Requirements of Grade B Pasteurized Milk, Skimmed Milk and Cream for Adults
Standards and Requirements of Grade C Pasteurized Milk, Skimmed Milk and Cream for Cooking and Manufacturing Purposes only
Cream
Cows and Other Bovine Animals
Cow Stables
Milk Utensils
Milk House
Methods
Employees
Water Supply.

Removal of Refuse
Toilets
Employees
Buildings
Machinery and Equipment
Processing
Storage of Milk and Milk Products on Undesirable Premises
Water Supply
Hot Water
Cleanliness of Buildings and Vehicles
Animals Barred from Premises
Smoking and Spitting Prohibited
Tasting of Milk
Delivery Wagons and Trucks
Sale of Dipped Milk Prohibited
Milk Tickets
Drinking Milk from Covers Prohibited
Milk Cans shall not be left on Sidewalks
No Water Preservatives or Adulterants to be upon any Wagon
Removal of Milk from Railroad Platform
Sale of Milk in Restaurants
Delivery to Quarantined Homes
Returned Bottles
Bottles to be Returned to Owners
Shelters for Cans
Sale of Milk in Stores
Storage of Milk in Stores and Restaurants
Ice Cream and Ice Cream Plants
Buttermilk Manufacture and Labeling
Permit necessary for Vehicles other than Milk Wagons Delivering Milk
Pathogenic Bacteria
Misbranding
Violations Reported to City Counselor
Penalties
Enactment
Repeal

THE HISTORY OF CHILD WELFARE WORK IN THE UNITED STATES

PHILIP VAN INGEN, M. D.

Clinical Professor Diseases of Children, College of Physicians and Surgeons, Columbia University; Attending Physician, Children's Service, Bellevue Hospital; Chairman Executive Committee, and President, 1919–20, of American Child Hygiene Association.

FIFTY years ago there was practically no child welfare work as we understand it to-day being carried on. In fact, before 1872 the child had hardly been discovered. What efforts were being made in his behalf consisted in providing him with food and shelter when he was deprived of his natural protectors, caring for him when sick, and punishing him if he broke the law. Even these efforts in his behalf were very inadequate. Orphan asylums and foundling institutions did exist. For the child whose mother was obliged to work, we know of six day-nurseries which existed prior to 1872. Usually he was left to the care of his little sister or a convenient neighbor. The hospital facilities for children were utterly inadequate and special hospitals for children were almost unknown. The first one to be established was in Philadelphia in 1855. Two years later the Nursery and Child's Hospital in New York City was opened, and Dr. George T. Eliot, describing the reason for its existence, said in his address: "This is the only hospital in this city where children during the fatal years of life are received — unless very exceptionally." Small special hospitals for children were opened in Chicago in 1865 and in Boston in 1869. Some slight attention was being paid to the fact that the child was being exploited in industry and deprived of an education thereby. Little was done, however. Somebody noticed, too, that children were dying by the thousands in summer time in New York tenements and for a short time there was considerable activity.

An important event occurred, however, in 1866. That was the establishment of the Society for the Prevention of Cruelty to Animals, modeled after a similar organization which had been in existence in England since 1823. It is interesting to note the relation of this organization to child welfare, as described by Payne in his intensely interesting book, *The Child in Human Progress.* A mission worker in the slums of New York came upon a child who had been adopted at an early age by two disreputable individuals who were treating her with great cruelty. Being unable to get action through her own efforts, she called upon the Society for the Prevention of Cruelty to Animals! The matter was taken under careful consideration and referred to the counsel of the Society, who decided that "the child being an animal," the Society would act. So much attention was called to the Mary Ellen case and so many demands for action were made in similar cases that the Society for the Prevention of Cruelty to Children was established April 27, 1875.

From that time on, progress was more rapid, but the basis of practically all child welfare work up to the beginning of the twentieth century was providing shelter and the prevention of cruelty. The protection of the health of the child is the development of the twentieth century.

It is impossible to give a chronological account of the development of this work. Various problems have been called to the attention of the medical profession and of the laity, and each problem has been studied and the methods of combatting it developed without regard to other activities. This has led to a tremendous specialism in child welfare work, as well as to much waste of effort and resources. The older child, who was more in evidence than the baby, received the first attention and it has only been as years have passed that we have gradually begun to realize that we must start early if we are to insure a healthy, intelligent, efficient race.

In looking back over the past twenty years, seven events stand out as milestones marking incidents, which in themselves may seem trivial, but which have had a tremendous influence in the course of the development of this work: —

1. The publication, in 1906, by the Census Bureau, of the *Mortality Statistics* for the five years 1900–1904. Vital Statistics had

been published before by local communities, but it would be hard to find any report which paid much attention to the child mortality. A few local reports would give the number of deaths under two years of age, but that was all. Statistical methods varied in different communities according to the interest and object of the compiler. It was these accurate and systematic statistics from the Census Bureau which first called the attention of the country at large to the appalling loss of human life during infancy and childhood.

2.   The establishment in New York City, in 1908, of the Division of Child Hygiene. This was the first official admission by a great municipality that child hygiene was a matter worthy of, and requiring special attention from, a health department. To the credit of the city, it may be stated that it has consistently increased the opportunities for work by the Division, and to the credit of its director that she has made steady and rapid progress in developing the almost untilled field of preventive public health work among children.

3.   The Conference on Prevention of Infant Mortality called by the American Academy of Medicine in New Haven in 1909. For the first time an imposing and overwhelming mass of evidence was presented to the public showing the enormous and unnecessary waste of infant life, and the claim was made that it was largely preventable. As a result of this conference, the American Association for the Study and Prevention of Infant Mortality was organized and, as the American Child Health Association, has continued its work of studying the problem and the best methods of meeting it.

4.   The formation of the Federal Children's Bureau in 1912. This was the recognition by the federal government of the rights of the child and the advisability of special machinery to study and protect him. It was more than that, for it was an important step in arousing the interest and activity of the lay public in meeting a situation which had been considered to be the function and responsibility of the medical profession.

5.   The establishment of the Division of Child Hygiene in the New York State Department of Health. This was the first state division authorized by law and, what is more to the point, provided

with the necessary support to carry on an active campaign for child welfare.

6. The establishment of the Birth Registration Area and the publication of birth statistics for 1915. For the first time birth statistics, on which are based all infant mortality rates, were available for a considerable area and were compiled in a uniform manner.

7. The formation, in March, 1920, of the National Child Health Council and, in December of the same year, of the National Health Council, composed of organizations of a national scope, whose object is to bring about better coöperation through better understanding of each and thus coördinate the work which is being done.

In the following pages a very brief and incomplete account of the development of certain phases and methods of child welfare work will be found. To discuss this subject fully would more than fill this entire volume, had it been possible to secure information. In practically all forms of this work will be noted the ever increasing prominence given to four principles: Personal, individual contact; education in simple and attractive form; concentration on the mother or future mother; and the availability and success of non-medical persons in carrying out plans founded on a sound medical basis.

CHILD LABOR

Interest in the working child was one of the earliest of child welfare activities. This interest at first was aroused from its connection with education — or lack of it, although a small group of people were active because of the cruelty to the child. The Puritan doctrine that the best way to keep a child out of mischief was to keep him at work still had a strong hold on a very large number of people. Also economic conditions seemed to demand, according to many, that the child should do his share. In 1836 the first law touching upon child labor was passed in Massachusetts, which required that no child under fifteen should be employed in any manufacturing establishment unless he had attended some public or private day-school taught by a "legally qualified teacher" for at least three months of the preceding year.* In 1842 Massachusetts made a still further advance by restricting the hours of labor for children under twelve to ten hours a day.

Connecticut, in 1855, refused to allow any child under nine to work in mechanical or manufacturing industries, and the following year increased this age limit to ten. These laws were, however, practically dead letters, as no adequate machinery for their enforcement was provided. A constant, though intermittent, agitation was kept up on the subject until about 1888, when Massachusetts passed a law more drastic than any existing at the time, forbidding all children under thirteen to engage in any manufacturing, mechanical, or mercantile occupation and likewise in any indoor occupation, during the hours that public schools were in session, and, also, forbidding the employment of such children in any manner unless, during the preceding year, twenty weeks of schooling had been completed. The history of child labor legislation from that time is a long one. Much progress was made, but the majority of the laws which were passed were seen to be ineffectual. Constant investigations were being made, and opposition was encountered from various sources, including the more unscrupulous business interests and those who objected on the grounds of interference with personal liberty and parental control. In 1904 the National Child Labor Committee was formed and has been a very active and effectual agent in spreading knowledge and arousing sentiment against child labor.

H. H. Hart, in an unpublished memorandum, said of conditions fifteen years ago,

Many states had no laws regarding child labor; others had laws which could not be enforced; and a few had laws which could have been but were not. Less than ten states had anything like an adequate method of meeting the increasing problem of child labor. . . .†

The extent of child labor is very difficult to estimate. Our only extensive sources of information are from the census figures, but these are very inaccurate, owing to the impossibility of including seasonal occupations. In the 1910 census, for instance, only eighteen children

*School Attendance and Child Labor, Ensign, 1921.
†A Quest of Constitutionality," Fuller, Child Labor Bulletin, Nov., 1918.

under fifteen were reported as working in the cranberry bogs, but in the fall of that year, 347 under fourteen were found at work in the bogs of one company in New Jersey. There are plenty of other examples even more striking. In spite of that, the figures for 1910 showed 1,990,225 children from ten to fifteen engaged in gainful occupations. To-day this number has probably been greatly reduced. The 1920 census figures are not as yet available.

To-day every state in the Union has a child labor law of some sort, although they vary to a great degree in their character. Three times an effort has been made to secure some legislation by the national government. As early as 1907 a bill was introduced in the Senate to use the interestate commerce power to prohibit child labor, but the bill was never acted upon. In 1916, however, a bill utilizing this power was introduced and passed and became effective in 1917. In 1918 it was declared unconstitutional by the Supreme Court. In 1919 another law was passed imposing a heavy tax upon the products of child labor. This law has again been assailed and is now before the Supreme Court for decision as to its constitutionality. The fight is still on and probably will be on for many years to come. The efforts of those interested are now being directed not only toward the exclusion of the young child from work, but to provide adequate substitutes to occupy his mental and physical activities. The problem is further being studied with the idea of trying to find a way by which the adolescent may enter an industry for which he is both mentally and physically fitted. The period of adolescence in both sexes is one of extreme importance for the health of the individual, and child labor interests are attempting to improve the health conditions under which they work.

DELINQUENT CHILDREN

A very great change has occurred in the attitude of society toward the criminal and especially so in the case of the child who has had a misunderstanding with the law. Much less than fifty years ago, he was treated exactly the same as an adult and was either acquitted or convicted. No constructive work was being done. In 1852 a Massachusetts law declared the county jail an appropriate place for the truant and put the limit of confinement at one year! Massachusetts, however, was the first to make provision for the hearing of children's cases apart from those of adults and a few other states made similar provisions. It was not until 1899 that the first children's court was established and to Illinois belongs the credit. This law established the principle that a delinquent child is not to be regarded as having committed an offense for which he must be punished, but is the subject of the state's special attention and care.

In 1919, in a study made for the Children's Bureau,* it is stated that all but two states had definite laws on the subject and that these two had special provisions in the law for handling such cases. Three hundred and twenty-one specially organized children's courts were found to be in existence in forty-three states and the District of Columbia. All but one state provided probation officers for dealing with the children in the court. In some few psychiatric examinations are made and the mental status of the child is receiving more and more attention in this connection.

While the laws provide probation officers in almost all the states, the number is utterly inadequate and much assistance is being rendered, especially in the larger cities, by volunteer organizations. The most successful of these are the "Big Brothers" and "Big Sisters." These organizations are doing valuable and very-little-heard-of work. Appreciating the importance of the subject and the need of better methods and understanding of the problems, forty-five groups have formed the Big Brothers and Big Sisters Federation, and its membership is stated to be about ten thousand.

MEDICAL INSPECTION OF SCHOOL CHILDREN AND CORRECTION OF
PHYSICAL DEFECTS†

The history of medical inspection of schools begins in 1892, when the first public medical school officer in the United States was appointed

---

*"Probation in Children's Courts," Children's Bureau Publication No. 80, 1921.

†Much of this material is taken from Gulick and Ayres' *Medical Inspection of Schools*, 1908, and "Over a Century of Health Administration in New York City," Department of Health, Monograph Series, No. 13, March, 1916.

by the city of New York. As in so many other cases, this accomplished little, and the first real beginning of this work occurred in 1894, when the city of Boston appointed fifty physicians for the fifty school districts, to inspect school children for the detection of contagious and other diseases.

In 1895 Chicago divided the city into nine districts and appointed an inspector for each district. As each district covered approximately twenty square miles, the efficiency of the work done may be imagined.

In 1897, five years after its lone medical school officer had been appointed, the city of New York appointed 134 medical inspectors, who were to visit each school daily for the purpose of excluding infectious diseases.

In 1898 Philadelphia's Board of Health ordered that fifteen medical inspectors be appointed, each to visit one school a day.

By a state law, Connecticut made the first move to go further than the exclusion of infection from the school, by requiring that the sight of every child in the public schools be examined during the fall term each year, and that parents, or guardians, should be informed in writing of the exact abnormal conditions found. Again is seen an example of the absurd character of many of such regulations, for all this work was to be done by the superintendent, principal, or teacher in the school.

In 1902 New York City appointed a staff of Municipal school nurses. This was the first effort to use nurses in this form of preventive health work.

In 1903 the New Jersey Legislature authorized the board of health to employ physicians as medical inspectors for the schools. Vermont passed the first law requiring the annual examination of the eyes, ears and throats of all school children.

New York City in 1905 inaugurated a system of examination of every child for uncorrected physical defects.

The most extensive and far-reaching law as yet passed was that of Massachusetts in 1906, in which every town and city was required to establish and maintain a system of medical inspection, with competent physicians for the detection of contagious diseases and to examine for non-contagious physical defects. It also required testing of the vision and hearing by the teachers.

By 1908 some system of medical inspection of school children existed in seventy cities besides those in Massachusetts.

There has been a rapid development of this work, as already indicated. Starting from an effort to exclude contagious diseases, the work gradually extended to the detection of physical defects, at first the most obvious, and later to a more thorough examination for all defects. At first the authorities seemed to feel their responsibility ended with discovering these defects and informing the parents, but to-day efforts are being made in many localities by persistent follow-up work to secure the correction of these defects. Owing to the enormous amount of work to be done — judging from the prevalence of adenoids and diseased tonsils (statistics of which, however, must in many cases be accepted with caution), many communities have made efforts to provide the means of correcting them. New York City established, in 1912, the first school children's clinic for the treatment of adenoids and diseased tonsils. During the first year, five such clinics were established. They were discontinued in 1915, owing to the opposition aroused in many quarters. During those four years, 1720 children were operated upon.*

Rochester, New York, is attempting the very thorough and widespread correction of easily remediable physical defects, through the activities of its Dental Dispensary. After a careful survey of the schools, a campaign was started which is attempting to reach every child needing operation on tonsils and adenoids. During seven weeks in 1920, 1,470 children were operated upon.†

Dental treatment is now occupying a very prominent part in school health programs. Beginning at first with the correction of existing defects, following the ideas of Dr. Fownes, of Bridgeport, the prophylactic care of the teeth through the use of dental hygienists has spread like wildfire. In almost every large city in the United States

---

*"Free Municipal Clinics for School Children," N. Y. City Department of Health, Reprint Series No. 41, Feb., 1916.

†"The Tonsil-Adenoid Clinic of the Rochester Dental Dispensary," Oct., 1920.

and in many small ones, dental clinics for school children are being carried on. I know of no form of child welfare work which has met with such immediate and universal appreciation as prophylactic dental work.

DAY NURSERIES

The first day nursery of which we have any definite record was established in 1858. Before 1872 five others had been established, and their increase was very rapid during the eighties. They were originally founded to provide shelter and food for the children of "worthy mothers" when these mothers were away at work. As early as 1885 it began to be realized that the problem was a big one and that much would be gained by exchange of ideas and discussion of problems. That year a group of managers assembled in New York to informally discuss plans. In 1892 regular conferences of a more formal nature were inaugurated, and in 1898 the Federation of Day Nurseries was organized. This Federation has held nine national conferences, the last in 1919, at which sixty-three nurseries from forty cities in eighteen states were represented.

It is interesting to study the development of the work from the printed proceedings. The discussions at the early conferences largely centered upon such problems as the type of child to be admitted and the duties of the managers. The health of the child as a problem was touched upon mainly in considering whether the children should wear their own clothes in the nursery, or not, and as to the safety and advisability of giving a daily bath. This is not entirely true. Occasionally physicians were asked to address these conferences, but the general attitude was that a doctor was unnecessary if the children were not sick.

However, in 1897, Miss Love, of the Fitch Crèche in Buffalo, called attention to the fact that the nurseries were neglecting to care for the mouths and teeth of children, and the following year Dr. Jessie E. Shears urged that "more attention should be given to the care of the teeth than is usually deemed necessary."

In 1892 at the Grace Church Nursery in New York a physician visited three times a week.

When the health authorities began to take an interest in the management of day nurseries and to formulate rules and regulations, there was at first considerable opposition, but to the credit of the day nurseries it may be said that, as soon as the matter was explained, the majority not only bowed to the inevitable, but have faithfully tried to carry out regulations.

The problem of the child of pre-school age is one which is difficult to solve, and many of the nurseries are realizing the opportunities they have to meet it. As an educational force these opportunities are great. Before 1890, the Fitch Crèche, in Buffalo, established a training school for nursery maids. In 1892 Dr. Alexander Lambert, in addressing the conference, called their attention to their opportunities in the early care of eye, ear and throat conditions in children before they reached a serious stage. To-day there are a number of nurseries all over the country, which are doing real health center work, keeping track of the children after they pass from their daily control and carrying on classes and meetings for mothers, which are of the greatest value. A rule of one of the Chicago Day Nurseries is, "One child cannot be taken unless all of the children of the family can have care provided for them out of school hours and during the mother's absence from home."

During the War a number of industrial nurseries were started and some of them were most excellent, especially that of the Cheney Brothers in Manchester. Most of these have, however, been discontinued. In Los Angeles special effort has been made to link up the school with the day nursery so that the children of working mothers who are attending school may be cared for after school hours by the nurseries. There are also several which have changed their purpose to a certain extent by not taking children of mothers who are *obliged* to leave them, but by *persuading* the mother to send the child away from its home all day in the interests of its health. Such an institution is the Chelsea Day Nursery, New York, where children from families where tuberculosis exists are kept all day, thus cutting down the chances of infection to a considerable extent.

To-day there are about 550 day nurseries in the United States. There are few agencies for child welfare whose opportunities for work are so great. The weak point in our chain is the pre-school period, and these children are the very ones for whom the day nursery was organized.

NUTRITION WORK

Probably no phase of child welfare work has been so utterly neglected as that directed toward correcting the vast amount of malnutrition existing to-day among the children of this country. Its practical beginning was made with the school lunch movement. In New York City, this was started in 1908, but its primary object was to feed the underfed child and not the improperly-fed child. In 1909 Emerson, of Boston, started the first class for delicate children. With the onset of the War and the possibility of food shortage and serious malnutrition, the work advanced with leaps and bounds. Classes are now held, under varying names, in hundreds of cities, many of them by public authorities. They have stimulated much needed study of standards of nutrition, and much valuable material has been published. The entrance into the field of the Child Health Organization of America has had a great influence in stimulating this work. With the nutrition class has come an increase in school lunch work. In Milwaukee, in twenty schools milk and crackers are given to the children and follow-up visits to the home are made by the nurse. In Seattle, in nineteen public schools, hot-lunch rooms are provided and any child may receive a bottle of milk a day. The Memphis General Hospital established the first nutritional clinic in the South last year for children from two to twelve years of age. Chicago has an industrial clinic for undernourished children applying, or intending to apply, for work papers. In New York City, the Department of Education is now providing hot school lunches in twenty-six public schools and is feeding 3,000 children a day. Food is charged for and the receipts pay for its cost. Forty-nine thousand dollars is available for the administration and equipment.

HEALTH EDUCATION

No more striking example exists of the change, both of program and of methods, which has occurred in child welfare work, than that in health education. Fifty years ago there was none. Our energies were expended in caring for the sick, relieving poverty and distress, the latter often due to ill health, and giving babies milk. To-day health education is the fundamental principle of the practice of medicine, public health work and all welfare work. Instead of mopping up the floor, we are trying to keep the pipe from freezing.

And the method has utterly changed. Compare, for instance, the present health literature distributed by the ton, in attractive form and simple language, with the book which was the "most popular seller" fifty years ago, Chavasse's *Advice to a Mother*. It was arranged in question and answer form. Part of the first will suffice:

Q. I wish to consult you on many subjects appertaining to the management and care of children. Will you favor me with your advice and counsel?

A. I shall be happy to accede to your request and give you the fruits of my experience in the clearest manner I am able and in the simplest language I can command — freed from all technicalities . . . .

And so on for a full page.

CHILD HEALTH AGENCIES

No longer are medicine and physiology surrounded by mystery. No longer are diseases and conditions, knowledge of which is essential for health, considered improper subjects to mention. No longer are facts about health, which must be learned in childhood to bear fruit, taught in such ways that there is no chance of arousing the interest of the pupil. To-day health is a game, a story, a play, or a "movie." It is impossible to do more than briefly mention a very few of the most active and valuable agencies engaged in this work.

Child Health Organization of America. No organization has more realized the importance of arousing the interest and enthusiasm of the child than the Child Health Organization of America. Its motto, "Health in Education — Education in Health," and its attractive seal showed at the very start that this side was appreciated. Organized and starting work in June, 1918, it has made a tremendous impression all over the country.   Its program is:

A scale in every school.
Time allowed every day for teaching health.
Hot school lunches.
Teachers trained in all normal schools to teach health habits.
Every child's weight to be taken and the record sent home each month.

Early in its career a plan submitted to the Federal Bureau of Education for stimulating health education of school children was approved by the Secretary of the Interior and a very close relation has existed between these two organizations.   In fact, the Child Health Organization has produced practically all of the literature on this subject which has been issued by the Bureau.   To bring home the lesson they are trying to teach, characters were invented, the best known of which is "Cho Cho" — in the literature a health sprite; in life, a professional clown, whose coming is awaited with interest and excitement by every school to which he goes.   His name has become a household word.   Another character is the "Health Fairy," who travels about with her portable house which "the Children" have built for her. Every time they learn to drink milk, they have added a brick to her cottage.   These characters have turned vegetables into living people. For these children "Paddy Spinach," "Tommy Turnip" and "Charlie Carrot" are friends.   The campaign develops the child's ingenuity. They write and produce health plays.   It has also tended to stimulate the ingenuity of the teachers.   A school teacher in the Primary Department of a school in Waterford, Pennsylvania, Miss McCray, was stimulated to see what she could do without any equipment except a pair of scales.   She drew a picture of a coffee-pot on the blackboard and, at the other end, a picture of a cow.   Under this she wrote, "We drink Milk," and each day the names of those who were drinking milk regularly were added.   The same way she drew a picture of a tooth-brush, under which were inscribed the names of those who used it at home.   In this way she taught some of her children not only health habits, but addition and subtraction.   Health poster contests by the school children have been suggested, and in Trenton last year 15,000 school children each presented an original poster.   A competition with a cash prize was carried out in New York City, the winning posters being exhibited in the Metropolitan Museum of Art. In the schools of Newton, Massachusetts, this health education has been carried out to a remarkable degree. The teaching of health is an integral part of the regular school work. The children write health jingles as part of their composition. They make health posters during the hand work periods.

Health Crusaders. This method of education in health is a very recent development and its appeal has been very striking. The attempt is made to teach children health habits by bringing in the element of play, ceremony, organization and routine. For its ceremony it falls back upon the customs of medieval chivalry. Each child is required to do certain health chores every day and eventually becomes a knight, or a knight banneret. The plan is capable of adaptation to various special needs and various ages. It can be continued for a number of years, with varying ceremonies and activities. The first "chore" record was published in 1917. To-day crusade work is being carried on in schools in every state. The state boards of education have officially adopted or recommended its inclusion in the curriculum in nine states — Maine, Alabama, Tennessee, Kentucky, Missouri, Iowa, Wyoming, Utah, and Idaho. In the schools of Washington, D. C., it has been made obligatory from the third to eighth grades and optional for the other grades. It is stated that for the thirty-week course, with all insignia and records, the cost is from five to ten cents per child. Already over six million children have been reached through the crusade.

Girl Scouts. This excellent activity was organized in 1912 and was incorporated as a national organization in 1915. Special attention is given to personal health, home nursing, and child care. Beginning with girls who have completed their tenth year, its activities continue almost indefinitely. When accepted as a Scout, the girl begins as a "Tenderfoot," and various and quite extensive accomplishments in health knowledge, as well as scout craft, must be acquired before she can become a "Second Class Scout." Among these may be mentioned that she must keep her health record, which is similar to that of the Health Crusaders. There are various special decorations which she may acquire, all of which are for distinct health activities. Among these are Home Maker, Child Nurse, First Aide, Home Nurse, Health Guardian, and Health Winner. There are other badges of proficiency. To become a "First Class Scout," she must have qualified as Home Maker, First Aid, Home Nurse and in two others of the special tests. This organization in its brief existence had, September first, 1921, 210 local organizations, with troups of Scouts in every state in the Union and in about 1500 towns. The total Scouts enrolled were 102,030.

Boy Scouts. The Boy Scouts have a very similar organization to that of the Girl Scouts, with their three grades and necessary tests. "A Scout is taught to know and obey the laws of hygiene. He learns how and why to keep his body fit, clean and healthy, which means also keeping a fit, clean and healthy mind and standards of conduct." There is hardly a town of any size in the country that does not have its quota of Boy Scouts, who are enrolled to the number of 409,000, with 110,000 men associated with them as Scout Leaders and other officials.

Camp Fire Girls. The Camp Fire Girls is an organization similar to the Girl Scouts. It "aims first to develop the home spirit and make it dominate the life of the entire community . . . . Every Camp Fire Girl regards her health as a sacred thing. Special health honors are given and habits of health developed." One of the honors is obtained by caring for a baby for an average of an hour a day for a month. There are 123,000 Camp Fire Girls and 7,000 Guardians in the United States.

Little Mothers' Leagues. The New York City Department of Health started Little Mothers' Leagues in 1908. They were primarily originated to teach the fundamentals of infant care to little girls in the public schools, much of whose time — especially in the summer — is spent in caring for the baby. The idea was to arouse an interest and pride in the child's somewhat tiresome occupation. Any child twelve years of age was eligible. They met in the school buildings, usually in the summer time, and were given a series of talks and demonstrations by the medical inspectors and school nurses. When they enrolled they received a badge naming them as volunteer aids of the Health Department. After they had been through their course they were given an examination, chiefly practical, and those who passed were given certificates. Especially capable children received a silvered or gilded medal in addition. This movement has spread with great rapidity. In many localities so great is the interest that the leagues have developed into health leagues or clubs, are open to both sexes, and continue throughout the year. Very many of these leagues were organized throughout the country as a result of Children's Year.

Infant Welfare Work

Long before the baby received much attention, considerable work was under way for the benefit of the older child. One of the earliest evidences of public notice was the discussion of the deaths of babies in the tenement houses in New York in 1874, which resulted in a simple leaflet on the care of the baby being prepared and distributed widely. In 1879 the State Legislature required the Board of Estimate and Apportionment to appropriate $10,000 to be spent in sending a corps of physicians into the poor homes in the tenement districts to treat sick babies and advise on their care. The first point that was brought to the attention of the medical profession was the enormous number of deaths from diarrheal disease. Milk naturally was credited with being the cause. About this time the modification of cow's milk to approach the composition of mother's milk was receiving a great deal of attention and pasteurization was first coming into vogue.

In 1893 Nathan Straus established the first milk stations for babies in this country. Much milk had been distributed by relief organizations for sick children. These stations, however, were intended for all children and a series of formulas was prepared. Milk was pasteurized and then dispensed, the formula being prescribed according to the age of the child. A number of other cities followed the example after several years, the earliest ones being Yonkers, New York, in 1894, Rochester, New York, in 1897, Pittsburgh in 1898, Cleveland in 1899, and Chicago, Philadelphia and Baltimore in 1903.

It was soon found, however, that, while this method of meeting the problem did some good, it had many faults. In the first place, as Dr. Caroline Hedger has expressed it, "you cannot feed babies by the carload." It was found that almost as much damage could be done by good milk improperly modified as by bad milk.

Further, it was stimulating artificial feeding from the false security roused by this simple process of changing cow's milk into mother's milk. The mother was given the baby's food in individual bottles. She learned nothing. Moreover, it was extremely expensive. That these lessons were being learned, and learned fairly quickly, may be seen from what happened in Cleveland. In 1902 the Milk Fund Association was started to supply modified milk to babies who were brought to the central station and examined by physicians who prescribed the formulas. Little attention was given to the instruction of the mother and no attempt at home-visiting was made. After two years of experience, the Association procured a farm where they produced their own certified milk, substituting for the wholesale distribution of modified, their own whole milk. In 1906, with the coöperation of the Visiting Nurse Association, an infant clinic was formed and home-visiting for instruction and advice was carried on.

With experience, the tendency increases everywhere to place more emphasis on trained supervision and educational work. At the outset these centers, or stations, were open only during the summer months, the idea being to reduce the most obvious cause of infant mortality, summer diarrhea, but it soon became evident that to accomplish definite, permanent results, the work must be kept up all the year round.

In 1907 the Public Health and Marine Hospital Service made a study of infant milk depots* and found that out of 143 stations in twenty cities, only fifty-four of these were open the year round. In fourteen cities all milk was dispensed modified to a set formula. In five it was all pasteurized, in six in part, and in nine not. The education of the mother in the care of her child by personal instruction by

---

*"Milk in Relation to Public Health," Public Health and Marine Hospital Service of the U. S., Hygienic Laboratory, Bull. No. 41, 1908.

a trained nurse was the most important development in the whole work. In 1915 the Children's Bureau made a detailed study and discovered 539 infant welfare centers, as they were beginning to be called, in 142 cities in thirty-two states. In 198 cities, 926 infant welfare nurses on full or part time were working, not connected with these centers. A total of 287 cities were found doing some amount of child welfare work.

Prenatal Work. By this time people were beginning to really pay attention to, and study the problem of, infant mortality in a more thorough way. The annual report on mortality statistics by the Census Bureau was throwing much light upon the situation. It was found that a very large percentage of the deaths of babies occurred from conditions vaguely classified as "prematurity" and "congenital debility." In New York, Mr. George H. F. Schrader became interested, and provided the Association for Improving the Condition of the Poor with funds to carry on work among expectant mothers. He also provided a home in the country where they could go and rest with their babies after they were born. This was really the first consistent effort in prenatal work.

In 1908 the Pediatric Department of the New York Outdoor Medical Clinic undertook the prenatal supervision and instruction of all women applying at the Obstetric Department for care. The following year, in 1909, the Committee on Infant Social Service of the Women's Municipal League of Boston organized an experiment along these lines. Pregnant women were visited once every ten days, and oftener if necessary, by a specially trained visiting nurse. They were instructed in the general hygiene of pregnancy, preparation for confinement, the value of maternal nursing both to mother and child, and taught how to prepare themselves to perform this function. The urine was examined at each visit and the blood pressure was also taken. This important work was somewhat limited in its field, owing to the fact that the better class of poor mothers were sought out and the effort was made to make the work as nearly self-supporting as possible. Only women who were to be under the care of physicians or maternity hospitals were accepted.

In 1911 a very extensive demonstration of the importance of infant welfare stations in reducing infant mortality was carried out in New York City by the Department of Health, the New York Milk Committee, the Diet Kitchen Association and several other organizations.   The results of this investigation were very carefully studied from a statistical standpoint, and it was found, as might have been expected, that very few babies came to the station before they were a month old.   A study of the death records for the city showed that approximately forty per cent of all infant deaths occurred during this first month.   A plan was then worked out for carrying on an intensive experiment as to the effect of prenatal work along lines similar to those of the Boston experiment, but of broader scope.   It was determined to find out what could be accomplished in reducing the stillbirth rate and the mortality under one month by careful prenatal work among the poorer class of people.   Districts were selected in various parts of the city where conditions of living were at their worst, where the ignorant midwife and the unskilled physician were most abundant. Each district was in charge of a specially trained nurse who made visits on every case every ten to fourteen days.   The urine was examined, but the blood pressure was not taken.   Every effort was made to secure the birth of a full term baby, and, through the coöperation of the relief organizations of New York, much needed rest for the mother during the last months of her pregnancy was urged.   If the woman was determined to have a midwife, she was more carefully watched and advised on this account.   After the birth of the baby, mother and child were visited until the baby was a month old and then both were transferred to the nearest welfare center.   Among 2,644 women thus cared for the deaths of babies under one month were 27.9 per thousand, while the rate for the Borough of Manhattan as a whole was 40.   The stillbirth rate was 39.8 as against 47.5.   The stillbirth figures, however, are not fair for comparison, as among the 2,644 women, "the loss of the product of conception at any period of gestation" was called a stillbirth and most of them occurred at a very early period.

For the year 1910, for the first time, the Census Bureau published in its Mortality Report tabulations showing the deaths at special ages under one year. As yet we had no Birth Registration Area, but these figures showed a decrease of 4.5 per cent in the total deaths at all ages under one year, but an increase of 15.6 per cent in deaths under one week, during the three years 1910–1912. The results of the experiments carried on and the publication of the facts brought out by these mortality statistics aroused great interest and stimulated rapid increase in the work. The maternity hospitals began to attempt to do something along this line in a few places, notably Boston and St. Louis. Dr. Holt said, in 1912, "In maternity hospitals infants are tolerated as one of the unavoidable incidents of obstetric practice."

In April, 1918, the Maternity Center Association was formed in New York City — to provide for every woman proper prenatal care, and to try to secure for her adequate medical and nursing care. The Borough of Manhattan was divided into districts, and centers for examination by obstetricians were established. Visiting nurses were provided for prenatal care and, through coöperation of the Henry Street Nurses Settlement, for postpartum care. The results of this work show a rate of mortality among mothers 60 per cent lower than that of the City, and a 50 per cent lower mortality among babies during the first month of life.

Work Among Foundlings. The foundling asylums had long been recognized, in many places, as providing a comfortable place of death for a very large portion of their charges. It was, however, claimed that this was unavoidable, probably on account of the poor condition in which these unfortunates were when admitted. In San Francisco, the Association of Collegiate Alumnæ was interested in a foundling home in the city and were horrified to discover in 1907 that 46 per cent of the babies admitted died during the first year, and in 1908 almost 60 per cent. The home was closed and all foundlings were boarded out with foster mothers. Supervision was provided by trained nurses and certified milk provided to the foster mothers, the difference in cost from ordinary loose milk being paid by the Association. From 1909 on, the mortality among these babies was 12.5, 8.5, 5.3, 5.8 and 3.3 per cent.

Experience has proved that, as a rule, these children do much better when boarded out than in an institution. On the other hand, Washington, D. C., and the Hebrew Orphan Asylum in New York have shown that with enough room, enough help, and enough individual attention, even in institutions a much lower death-rate can be secured.

Midwife Problem. Another phase of the campaign in reducing the "natal" and "neonatal mortality," using the term adopted by Ballantyne to cover stillbirths and deaths during the first month of life, has been the increasing attention to the problem of the midwife. It was found that, in some of our cities with large foreign populations, anywhere from 25 to 40 per cent of the confinements were attended by midwives. Unlike the attempted careful training and supervision practised in Europe for many years, almost nothing was being done in this country to regulate what is generally admitted to be an unsatisfactory situation. To the late and revered Abraham Jacobi belongs much of the credit for demanding that we do not try to eliminate the midwife by legislation when the demand for her services will for many years be great, but, as it were, to educate her to death — that is, adopt standards which she must live up to, thus eliminating the most unfit, and educating the people to demand such good obstetrical care that the demand for midwives will be decreased.

In 1913 the trustees of Bellevue Hospital, in the face of considerable opposition, established the first school for midwives in this country, where training was given, both theoretical and practical, under medical supervision, candidates having both hospital and outdoor training. In 1907 the New York City Department of Health had been empowered to regulate and supervise the practice of these midwives and had adopted fairly stringent rules, the enforcement of which in one year reduced the number of practising midwives nearly 50 per cent. With the formation of this school, to the regulations was added the requirement that the candidate must be a graduate of a recognized and approved school for midwives.

The regulations in force in various states and cities vary, Massachusetts not recognizing the existence of the midwife, although in some of her industrial cities the larger proportion of births are attended by midwives. Many states to-day have laws requiring registration of midwives, while few provide for their supervision, and up until recently almost none for their education. In the Southern states the colored midwife is a big problem. In 1914, Jacksonville, Florida, passed an ordinance forbidding midwives to practise without having passed an examination, and the State Board of Health was required to provide instruction in the simple principles of midwifery. South Carolina last year in one remote rural community established a temporary open air clinic, twelve colored midwives being summoned by the county nurse and given their instructions. In North Carolina county conferences for midwives have been organized. In New Jersey there are six teaching centers.

Comparison of the results obtained by midwives with those by the medical profession as judged by analysis of birth and death records has not always been to the advantage of the profession. It has been felt for a long time by many that education in obstetrics has been woefully neglected and of recent years efforts have been made to improve the standard. Ballantyne's remarks in 1902 that antenatal pathology is an almost untilled field is unfortunately almost as true to-day.

Medical Education. That child welfare work is an integral part of preventive pediatrics is being gradually appreciated, and practical and didactic instruction in what is to-day popularly called "social pediatrics" is being gradually included in the curricula of certain medical schools. In the Albany Medical School for two years a considerable amount of time has been required in this work.

A committee of the American Pediatric Society was appointed two years ago to draw up a schedule of instruction in child welfare work, which program has been approved by the Society and distributed among all medical schools. The beginning is being made in the College of Physicians and Surgeons, Columbia University, this year (1921).

Results of Infant Welfare Work. The infant mortality rate being dependent upon the number of births reported during the same year, it ought to be easy to get a fairly accurate estimate of results. Unfortunately, interest in birth registration has only recently received much attention, and figures for a large area are available only since 1915. To compare the relative results of work among babies under one month, and from one month to one year, it is only necessary to take any state figures, for the error will apply to both groups. In the following table these facts are presented, based upon the reports from six states, — Massachusetts, Minnesota, New York, Ohio, Pennsylvania and Wisconsin. Until these states were admitted to the Birth Registration Area, state figures of births were used; after admission, those of the Census Bureau. All deaths were from the latter source.

| | INFANT MORTALITY RATE | | AVERAGE FOR THREE YEARS ENDING WITH YEAR UNDER WHICH LISTED | |
	Under 1 Month	1 Month to 1 Year	Under 1 Month	1 Month to 1 Year
1910	46.5	80.1	. . .	. . .
1911	45.7	65.7	. . .	. . .
1912	46.6	63.4	46.3	69.7
1913	47.4	65.1	46.6	64.7
1914	45.4	56.0	46.5	61.5
1915	44.3	53.4	45.7	58.2
1916	43.8	54.8	44.5	54.7
1917	43.2	51.8	43.8	53.3
1918	44.2	59.6	43.7	55.4
1919	41.5	46.7	43.0	52.7

From the above it will be seen that there is a marked change for the better during the period one month to one year, ever since accurate birth registration was established, while there has been comparatively little change in the rate under one month. This is probably because prenatal work has been done only for a few years and is not generally carried on. At the earlier age there has been a reduction of only 7.1 per cent as against 24.4 during the later period, based upon the three-year "progressive averages." The high figures in 1918 were due to the influenza epidemic.

DEVELOPMENT OF NATIONAL GOVERNMENT ACTIVITIES

Twelve years ago practically nothing had been done by our national government. The Hygienic Laboratory of the Public Health

Service had made a study of milk and had published in 1908 a report on milk stations existing in 1907. It was not, however, until 1912 that the child was considered as requiring attention from his government.

Children's Bureau. In 1912 a law was passed creating, in the Department of Labor, a Children's Bureau, to "investigate and report. . . . upon all matters pertaining to the welfare of children and child life among all classes of our people and . . . . especially investigate the question of infant mortality, the birth-rate, orphanages, dangerous occupations, accidents and diseases of children, employment, legislation affecting children in the several states and territories." The original appropriation of the Bureau was $25,640, and by the end of the year a staff of fifteen was at work. The first activities of the Bureau were a series of studies of infant mortality in various localities, of which eleven have been made.

It was very soon evident, as has been noted on many other occasions, that people are less interested in repeated assurance and evidence of their failings and shortcomings than in what to do to correct them. In other words, in medical terms, the patient is less interested in pathology than in therapeutics. The purposes for which the Children's Bureau was organized are so broad that the activities of the Bureau have gradually and naturally increased. Excellent literature in simple language has been published, which has been of great help to many thousands of mothers, such as the pamphlets on Prenatal Care and Infant Care. Up to date eighty-six publications, largely studies of various problems in child welfare, have been issued by the Bureau. By 1915 the staff had been increased to seventy-six and the appropriation granted by Congress to $164,640.

In 1916 the Bureau began to stimulate activity in local communities in a more definite way. Through coöperation with private organizations, especially those composed of women, a National Baby Week Campaign was started. The purpose was to arouse local interest in the problem of child welfare and attempt to cause the establishment of definite work. This work was carried out in various ways with celebrations in 2,083 communities.

With the entrance of the United States into the War, and the staggering figures relating to physical disability shown by the draft, the country was aroused as never before to the need for health protection. In the middle of 1918 — again through the coöperation of many and varied local organizations — Children's Year* was inaugurated. State Committees were organized in forty-six states. The four aims of this drive were:

1. Public protection of maternity and infancy.
2. Mothers' care for older children.
3. Enforcement of child labor laws and free schooling for all children of school age.
4. Recreation for children and youth, abundant, decent, protected from any form of exploitation.

An enormous amount of work was done throughout the country in arousing interest. The Bureau estimates nearly 17,000 local committees organized and composed of eleven million women. The first and most extensive piece of work done was the weighing and measuring and physical examination of children of pre-school age. The extent of the work done is hard to estimate. There is also no question that a great deal of it was badly done, but it did arouse a tremendous amount of interest and did bring home the lesson Children's Year was trying to teach. As an example of how vast an amount of work was done, the figures from California are impressive — 53,462 children weighed and measured, of whom 40,000 received complete physical examinations. And California was only one of forty-six states at work. Not only is it difficult to tell the amount of work done, but equally difficult to estimate the results obtained. That they have been great is without question. It is interesting to note that in 1919 the infant mortality rate in the Birth Registration Area reached a new low mark.

In 1919 the Bureau organized a series of conferences to determine minimum standards for child welfare and has published a very valuable contribution on that subject.

---

*"Children's Year," U. S. Department of Labor, Children's Bureau, Publication No. 67, 1920.

In order to stimulate interest and activity in the most neglected parts of the country — the rural districts — in 1920 the "Child Welfare Special" was sent to various localities at the request of state health authorities to conduct a series of examinations of children.* The parents were given a card showing the height and weight of the child and what it ought to be. Their attention was called to irregularities — in diet, for instance — and advice as to better hygiene was given. If any physical defects were found which needed correction, a statement thereof was also given, with the advice to refer it to their local physician. An amusing incident in connection with this work was the activity of one of the county agents making local arrangements. Being impressed with the lack of cows in the district he started an "Own a Cow" campaign. It is stated that ten car loads of cows were imported and sold.

The appropriation for the Bureau for the fiscal year 1921 was $271,042.60. The personnel consisted of 108. The Bureau has been a force of inestimable value in the child welfare campaign. It has presented facts of great value to those who are looking for facts. It has stimulated interest in all parts of the country as it has never before been stimulated and, most of all, it has enrolled the interest of the lay public in a problem which needs the interest of the entire country.

United States Public Health Service. This is the oldest government activity directed toward the health of the country, but, until 1915 very little work was done other than of a scientific nature. In 1908 the Service published a volume on *Milk in Relation to Public Health*† containing a report on milk stations showing the location of all known at that time, and it has also from time to time published the reports of the National Commission on Milk Standards. In 1915, however, it began active field investigations in child hygiene and conducted a sanitary and medical survey of the rural schools of Porter County, Indiana.

Probably its most valuable contribution has been the work which is now being carried on in the State of Missouri.‡ True to its tradi-

---

*"Health on Wheels," Frances Sage Bradley, *Mother and Child*, vol. I, no. 1.

†Public Health and Marine Hospital Service of the United States, Hygienic Lab., Bull. No. 41, 1908.

‡*Public Health Reports*, 1920, vol. 35, no. 53.

tions of trying to fill gaps, when the Missouri Legislature created a Division of Child Hygiene and failed to appropriate any money to carry it on, or even organize it, the Public Health Service, at the request of the State Department of Health, assigned several of its personnel to assist in the formation of the division and to work out a plan for its activities. Assistant Surgeon Knight was made director of the division and he secured the active coöperation of the Southwestern Division of the American Red Cross, Missouri Tuberculosis Association, University of Missouri, Parent Teacher's Association, Women's Christian Temperance Union, local child health organizations, and many members of the medical and dental profession. It was planned to make a survey of all cities except the three largest ones, which survey would include a study of birth registration, infant mortality, prenatal problems and studies in the subject of school hygiene. This later involved the weighing and measuring of all school children, physical examinations, correction of defects, formation of nutrition clinics and health centers, this work to be inaugurated throughout the state, placed on a permanent basis, and carried on at local expense. By October, 1920, the school survey had been completed in twenty-five cities; in twenty-one health centers had been, or were being, established; twenty-five nurses were being employed for school work; in four counties temporary county health units had been organized and were working; in two counties, in addition to the original program, surveys of rural schools were made. As a result of this work, to-day practically 100,000 school children are under health supervision in the State of Missouri.

· *Bureau of Education.* The work of this Department in child welfare is of recent origin, having first taken up, in 1918, the subject of health education in the schools. A close relation exists between the Bureau and the Child Health Organization of America. A number of excellent pamphlets on standards in health of school children and methods of improving their health have been published and have established new standards for government publications. The program which the Bureau of Education is emphasizing is to secure:

Weighing scales in every school.
Time allowed every day for teaching health.
Hot school lunches.
Teachers trained in all normal schools to teach health habits.
Every child's weight to be taken and the record sent home each month.

With its tremendous field and widely distributed contacts, the influence of the Bureau of Education should be very great.

Department of Agriculture. Through its Extension Service in Agriculture and Home Economics, with agents in every state, this Department has done considerable work, chiefly along nutrition lines. The home demonstrations have assisted in stimulating child welfare campaigns.

STATE AND MUNICIPAL CHILD WELFARE ACTIVITIES

The Louisiana Board of Health in 1911 presented a report, urging the formation of a state division of child hygiene. No action was taken by the Legislature, but the following year a subdivision of child hygiene in the Division of Hygiene was created by the Board. No funds, however, were provided for its special activities. The Board at once proceeded to publish bulletins of instruction on the hygiene of children and the care of infants, which were used in the schools and distributed widely through the state. In 1913 a health train was utilized for spreading broadcast information and advice regarding the health of the school child.

In 1912 the New York State Department of Health appointed a consulting pediatrician, without salary, and two years later, as a result of the recommendation of a special commission appointed by the Governor, a Division of Child Hygiene was created by law and funds provided for carrying out its work. This division immediately proceeded to action with the former consulting pediatrician as director. An investigation in the state showed that there were only twelve localities with established infant welfare work and that these were all larger cities. A campaign for stimulating child welfare activity, especially in the prevention of infant mortality, was immediately started. Exhibits were sent throughout the state and the "county fairs" were utilized, thus reaching a large number of the rural population. As a result of a four months' summer campaign, thirty-five infant welfare stations had been established in twenty-two different localities.

In 1915 divisions of child hygiene, or their equivalent, were established in Kansas, Ohio, New Jersey and Massachusetts. In 1917 Montana and Illinois came into line and, in 1918, Pennsylvania, Florida, North Carolina and Minnesota. The effect of Children's Year in arousing interest in the subject — and one of its purposes was to stimulate the formation of divisions of child hygiene — may be seen from the fact that, in 1919, twenty states joined the twelve which already existed. In 1920, four were added and, in 1921, two, so that to-day thirty-eight states have divisions of child hygiene — only New Hampshire, Vermont, Maryland, Iowa, Tennessee, Oklahoma, North Dakota, Wyoming, Nevada and Oregon not having established them.

Of course the activities of these divisions — many of which are so new that they have hardly had time to get into line — are greatly hampered by insufficient, or even absence of any, appropriations. Missouri, however, has shown its ability to carry on a tremendous piece of work without special appropriation by calling into united action all forces existing in the state and obtaining the assistance of the United States Public Health Service. The states with large rural populations have naturally concentrated their efforts on this most neglected part of the population. At least five have made use of automobile exhibits, or clinics, in reaching distant areas.

The activities of state authorities have by necessity been largely in stimulating local communities to organize and maintain efficient work. Eleven are engaged upon a campaign for the establishment of county health units. Pennsylvania this year is asking for an appropriation of $700,000 to establish such units in every county in the state.

Methods vary in different communities. Many send a special baby book to every mother upon the registration of the birth. Louisiana and New York started this in 1914. In Kansas, Massachusetts,

North Carolina, Texas and Michigan, through coöperation with other organizations, letters are sent to every expectant mother who can be reached. At least twenty-six states have prepared, and circulate widely, special literature on the care of babies. Twenty-five have travelling exhibits and five have made use of the motor or rail exhibit, or clinic. The dental work is becoming more and more prominent. North Carolina has nine dentists in field clinics during the summer.

In cities, child welfare work is being carried out with a varying degree of intensity in a very large number. In going over many bulletins and reports from the health authorities, seventy-five per cent reported some activity. As already mentioned, in 1874 the subject of infant mortality was discussed in New York and an educational leaflet was circulated. In 1879, $10,000 was ordered appropriated to send the doctors into the tenements to treat needy, sick babies. It was not, however, until 1908 that the first real child welfare work was organized under city control. New York's Division of Child Hygiene started the ball rolling and has been alert to adopt every useful method proposed elsewhere as well as very active in starting new movements. In 1909 Detroit established a Division of Child Hygiene and in 1910 Buffalo, Philadelphia, Nashville, Tennessee, and Los Angeles followed suit. To-day we have records of the establishment of fifty-two such divisions, in twenty different states. It is impossible to give a résumé of city health department work. Much of it is described in other parts of the brief review.

DEVELOPMENT OF CHILD WELFARE WORK IN PRIVATE ORGANIZATIONS

While fifty years ago it might almost be said that the child did not have a friend, to-day he seems to be the most important part in the programs of almost all national organizations engaged in social and health work. In the recent summary of activities of national organizations doing child welfare work, published by the American Child Hygiene Association, sixty national organizations are listed who do, or claim to do, some child welfare work. The first national organization to be formed whose sole purpose was encouraging methods for saving the lives of babies was the American Association for the Study and Prevention of Infant Mortality, organized in New Haven, Connecticut, in 1909, as a result of a conference called by the American Academy of Medicine to discuss the problem. It did not take long for the Association to find that the prevention of infant mortality was only part of the big problem of child welfare, and that to promote the work having only the infant in mind was to promote duplication of effort. Its field has gradually and naturally extended to cover the whole period of childhood. To better express its purpose, its name has been changed to the American Child Hygiene Association, and it is doing valuable work. It publishes a monthly magazine, *Mother and Child*.

The National Tuberculosis Association has gradually and naturally changed its field of activities. Its work among children at first consisted largely in protecting the children of tuberculous parents. To-day it is responsible for the Modern Health Crusaders and most of its work is directed toward the prevention of tuberculosis through the promotion of healthy infancy and childhood.

Organizations of another type, especially those composed of women — the National League of Women Voters and the Federation of Women's Clubs especially — have, largely through the influence of Children's Year, become deeply interested in the problem and have adopted programs for child welfare work.

DEVELOPMENT OF COÖPERATION

As has been mentioned elsewhere, the various problems connected with the welfare of childhood and infancy have been recognized so rapidly that efforts for their solution have been disjointed and have led to a tremendous amount of specialism and, therefore, wasted effort. To-day the pendulum is swinging in the other direction and we are seeing ever-increasing signs of coördination of all these various activities. The nursing profession engaged in public health work — and to-day there are approximately 11,000 public health nurses — has realized this situation and is attempting to adjust things within its own ranks.

In the fall of 1919 an informal conference of representatives of those agencies doing child welfare work was held and resulted in the formation of the National Child Health Council, whose purpose is by coöperation to bring about the coördination of all child welfare activities. A few months after the formation of the Council, the great national health organizations met informally and, similarly, organized a coördinating agency, the National Health Council. In this bigger movement the National Child Health Council is included.

In smaller activities the same thing is being seen. Work is being definitely defined and divided and each group not only confines its major activities to its own field, but coöperates with the others in working out well rounded programs. The splendid work being done in Missouri, Minnesota and many other states in carrying out health programs, the wise decision of the American Red Cross to try to supplement existing work rather than start new work, the establishment of the East Harlem Health District in New York, where a dozen or more local organizations have joined forces to carry on a definite intensive constructive campaign, — these all show the way the tide is running.

From being a neglected, almost friendless member of society fifty years ago, the child to-day occupies the center of the stage. Every period of his existence is being studied and the best intelligence in the world is busy in trying to secure for him conditions and opportunities which will render him an efficient, healthy, full grown member of society.

HOUSING AS A FACTOR IN HEALTH PROGRESS IN THE PAST FIFTY YEARS

LAWRENCE VEILLER, A. B.

Secretary, National Housing Association

FIFTY years ago the only community in the United States that was conscious that it had a housing problem was the city of New York, which then had a population of a little less then a million.

To-day there is no city in the entire country that is not aware that it has such a problem. Only, to-day, the conception of that problem is expressed in different terms.

Fifty years ago the housing problem was not only a health problem, but was so conceived by those conscious of its existence. To-day it still is largely a health problem, but at the moment it is not so conceived.

Owing to the widespread shortage of houses at the present time — a world-wide condition—the housing problem in the minds of most people to-day is solely the problem of supplying a sufficient *quantity* of houses in the shortest possible time.

But that is a shortsighted view to take of this great question. The problem in its essence is to-day the same as it was fifty years ago; and while it is an economic, a social and an industrial problem, it is also very largely a health problem.

The bad conditions of housing which prevailed fifty years ago were limited to a few cities and to a few spots in those cities. In such great centers of population as New York were slums chiefly to be found.

To-day the slum has spread all over the United States and its menace has increased a thousand-fold. No part of the country is free from this blight — East, West, North, South; in the great city and the small one; in the town, village and suburb — even on the prairies this evil is to be found.

The housing problem is indissolubly linked up with the public health movement; for it concerns itself with such questions as ventilation, sewage disposal, water supply, disposal of wastes, insect-borne disease, personal hygiene, the spread of communicable disease and even public health education.

To appreciate fully the changes which fifty years have wrought one must orientate himself back into the conditions of that time. It was only a few years before 1872 that the one great metropolitan center of the country, the city of New York, had been visited by serious epidemics of typhus, typhoid, cholera, smallpox and other communicable diseases.

So serious had the conditions in that city become that the year 1864 saw the formation of the famous Council of Hygiene from whose epoch-making work resulted the first health law in this country, namely, the New York Metropolitan Health Act of 1866. A year later saw the enactment of the first housing law in this country, the New York Tenement House Law of 1867.

It is a far cry from the conditions which prevailed in New York City in those days, as disclosed by the report of the Council of Hygiene, to the conditions of today.

While the function allotted to me has been to trace those changes which have taken place in the last half century only with reference to housing insofar as they have a bearing on health; and while others will undoubtedly set forth more authoritatively and more definitely than I can the great changes which have come about in all fields of the public health movement, yet it is impossible even to outline the marked advances in the field of housing that must be recorded, without at the same time commenting upon the general advance in knowledge of public health questions that has marked the period under review. Without such an understanding no true appreciation can be had of the great gulf which spreads between the conditions of then and now.

In attempting to determine and set forth the advances that have been made in the last half century in the field of housing in this country one is handicapped at the very outset of his task by the fact that it is not possible to make any general statement that holds good for the entire country. For naturally in a country as vast as ours, progress must necessarily be slower in some parts than in others. It is not strange that the greatest advances have been made in the great metropolitan centers and that to-day there are still many parts of the country, especially the more sparsely settled portions of it, where conditions at present are almost identical with those which prevailed fifty years ago in our great centers of population.

And so what one has to record is the general *trend* of advance, the tendency which has manifested itself in the great centers of population and is beginning now to slowly develop throughout the whole country.

VENTILATION

Probably there has been no greater advance in any phase of the public health movement than in the increased knowledge that has come of the true principles of ventilation and their application to the homes of the people.

In 1872 it was the practice to build houses, especially houses intended to be occupied by the working people of the large cities, in which there were many unventilated rooms — interior rooms — with neither light nor ventilation which secured their air from an adjoining room.

A few years later there came the first important change in this practice with the enactment in New York State of the Tenement House Law of 1879, under which law such interior unventilated rooms were outlawed in future construction.

Then as an improvement over this extraordinary condition and type of building came the so-called "airshaft," devised as a means of improvement over the interior unventilated room and in the belief that it would afford adequate ventilation to the rooms which opened upon it.

Twenty years of the airshaft, as it was developed in New York's tenements, proved it to be a greater evil even than the interior, unventilated room. It rightly was termed "a culture tube on a gigantic scale."

Twenty years ago the airshaft was outlawed and a revolution achieved in the ventilation of the dwellings of the poor. In place of narrow airshafts, closed at the bottom and without means of ventilation, there came into general existence, reinforced by the strong arm of the law, the recognition that rooms should be ventilated as much as possible either on the street or on a large backyard; and, failing this, that courts should be provided so arranged that there would be constant circulation of the air in them.

As has already been pointed out, it would be misleading to give the impression that these changes have become general throughout the whole United States. Unfortunately that is not the case; but many states and a number of cities have of recent years enacted laws requiring the ventilation of buildings in which people live to be along these lines. It is, as I have stated, a tendency which is quite discernible to every intelligent observer.

LIGHT

Fifty years ago there were no requirements of law in any city of the country which prevented the building of new dwellings containing completely dark, interior rooms as well as dark hallways.

It was the practice, we regret to say, in many communities, and especially in New York City — where even at that time land values were beginning to feel the effect of a constantly augmented immigration — to build new houses in which from one-half to two-thirds of the rooms in which the people were to live were totally dark, securing no light whatever, except such as might filter through the doorway of an adjoining room. The builders of that time enjoyed "self-determination" with a vengeance; for they could build as they pleased, subject to no restrictions of law, nor were there a sufficient number of people who had knowledge of the dangers of such practices, or who cared enough about the way in which the masses of the people lived, to organize public sentiment so as to prevent evils of this kind.

A few years after the beginning of the period under review, namely, in 1879, the airshaft, or lightshaft, as it was variously called, came into existence — a most inadequate method of attempting to provide light for the interior rooms of tenement houses. As the shafts were narrow and small they did not furnish adequate light even to the rooms on the top floor; and for the rooms on the lower stories of the four and five-story tenement houses which were being erected at that time they were indeed a hollow mockery.

To what extent the early living in these dark caves of dwellings was responsible for the spread and development of tuberculosis in our great cities it would be hard to say, but that it must have exercised such an influence can hardly be gainsaid.

Twenty years ago a revolution in the lighting of dwellings, equal to that above described in ventilation, came with the outlawing of the lightshaft and the substitution of the large court, which, while it did not admit sun*shine* into the rooms which opened upon it, at all times of the day, did provide light, so that from 1900, with the beginning of the new century, one may say that darkness became outlawed and the dark room a thing of the past.

At the same time, there came a greater recognition of the necessity of adequate open spaces of all kinds, not merely in interior courts, but at the rear of buildings as well.

More recently there is beginning to come throughout the whole country an appreciation that has never before been had of the great importance of sufficient open spaces. In most parts of the country it is not the custom to build houses in continuous rows, but generally the detached or semi-detached house, with open space on three or four sides of it, is the prevailing type. Unfortunately, in many cities, owing to unwise property subdivision by which lots have been made too narrow, it has not been possible to leave an adequate space between adjacent buildings, and the serious problem of light and ventilation which confronts most cities in the United States to-day is this problem of securing adequate distance between adjacent dwellings.

In many communities the very inadequate space of but 3 feet is often left between buildings, while in most communities seldom does one find more than 6 feet; whereas 20 feet between adjacent buildings, even when they are only two stories high, is the minimum which the best practice indicates should be left.   I am glad to say that an appreciation of the importance of these wider open spaces is spreading rapidly throughout the entire country, due to the educational work of such bodies as the National Housing Association, which, for the past ten years, has been campaigning on this subject.   The standards adopted by the Federal Government in its war housing operations marked a new step in advance in this direction.   Not only is this demand for adequate light becoming general throughout the whole country, but a newer and far more advanced standard is beginning to appear in the insistence on sun*shine*.   The city-planning movement, which has made great strides in recent years, is bringing to people's attention more and more forcibly every year the importance of the proper orientation of dwellings — of their being placed upon the property in such manner as to secure a maximum amount of sunshine in all rooms throughout the day.   New standards are distinctly visible.

DISPOSAL OF WASTES

Probably the greatest advance in sanitary science in the housing field that is to be recorded in the past half century is the great change which has come about with regard to the disposal of human wastes.

Fifty years ago the privy vault was practically not only the universal means but the only means of disposing of human excreta.

Then came the building up of the science of sanitary plumbing and of sewage disposal.   With the more general installation of sewers — which naturally were first found in the large cities — the privy vault was soon outlawed, and in its place came an evil almost as great, namely, the sewer-connected vault, known variously as the "school-sink" and the "catch-basin" privy.

With the single exception that this contrivance is free from the danger of soil contamination that exists with the ordinary vault, it marked little, if any, advance over the vault.

Fifteen years after the beginning of the period under review, New York City, the first in the country to take this step, enacted a law prohibiting the privy vault in all new construction, requiring in place of this evil the sanitary water-closet.

The great revolution in this field, however, came at the beginning of the present century with the Tenement House Act of 1901, when not only were modern sanitary water-closets required for all new construction, but the private closet, with its use limited solely to a single family and located inside of the apartment used by that family, became the required practice.

Not only did the law thus make this immeasurable advance with relation to tenement houses to be constructed from that time on, but at the same time, recognizing the serious consequences of the existing privy vaults which were found in large numbers even then, and with the new knowledge that had come of the relation between vaults and fly-borne disease, this new law outlawed all existing vaults; and property owners were required at very considerable expense to themselves to remove all such vaults within a limited time and replace them with modern, sanitary water-closets, placed, as a rule, inside the buildings.

The example thus set by the great city of New York has been slowly followed, but each year is being followed more and more by the other cities of the country.

While much progress has been made in this direction, the great task which confronts the health officers of the country to-day, and the work which is more urgent than almost any other phase of their activities is the removal of the hundreds of thousands of vaults which still exist in sewered communities thoughout all parts of the country. Less than 10 years ago an investigation made in 40 cities showed that in a city of 350,000 population there were then 60,000 individual privy vaults, and that 50,000 of these were located where sewers were available. In another city of 490,000 population it was disclosed that there were 27,000 privy vaults, of which 20,000 were located where sewers were available.

With the knowledge that has come of the part that insects play in spreading disease, the obligation to get rid of the privy vault has become more and more insistent. If we are to abolish typhoid, we must abolish our vaults. A study of the relation of typhoid fever to the presence or absence of sewage systems, made a few years ago by the New York State Health Department and embracing the records of twenty years, showed this conclusively. In the unsewered communities the typhoid death-rate had a 26 per cent excess over the rate in the sewered communities.

While conditions vary greatly in different parts of the country—and especially in the rural and semi-rural sections—yet great advances have been made, for to-day the standard, both of health and decency, is the private water-closet located inside the house, with one water-closet for each family.

In those rural sections where sewers have not yet been installed and where the privy vault is a temporary necessity, the standard is a fly-protected sanitary privy as distinguished from the old vault.

DISPOSAL OF OTHER WASTES

Not only in the disposal of human wastes has there been marked progress in the past fifty years, but in the disposal of all wastes. When one contrasts the conditions which prevail to-day in most of our cities with those that prevailed fifty years ago, one realizes how great a change has come about. Then, the streets of most cities, especially in the poorer quarters, were filthy and littered with rubbish and wastes of all kinds, with scattered heaps of garbage, and with pigs and cattle roaming freely through the thoroughfares.

While it is true that there are still some parts of the country in a similar condition to-day, yet the prevailing condition and the whole general trend is very far removed from such a state of affairs. In most communities the streets are kept clean and neat; the alleys, where alleys exist, unfortunately as a rule are not so well kept. In place of heaps of garbage and rubbish there is regular and prompt removal of these wastes; and to-day the metal-covered garbage can replaces the unpleasant piles of decaying materials which were to be found in most cities fifty years ago.

DRAINAGE

With the knowledge that has come of the true character of malaria and the means of infection through the anopheles mosquito, the drainage of the surface surrounding our houses has taken on a new significance. In place of the surface pools of water and slops that were so commonly found a half century ago, breeding mosquitoes, there is to-day in most parts of the country, certainly in the cities, a proper system of surface drainage.

PLUMBING

Practically the whole science of modern sanitary plumbing has been developed in the past fifty years. Developed primarily as a health necessity, it is interesting and significant to find that the best authorities today are unwilling to associate plumbing with health work. We no longer believe, as we did fifty years ago, that diphtheria is caused by sewer gas. While it may not be possible to establish any direct causal relation between bad plumbing and disease, it is unquestionably true that modern sanitary plumbing makes greatly for better living conditions.

ROOM-OVERCROWDING

This is the one phase of housing in which we have made the least progress in the last half century. Strangely enough, it is the one phase of housing where a direct causal relation between housing and disease has been established to the satisfaction of the authorities, for room-overcrowding is a most potent factor in the spreading of communicable disease.

In respect to this subject, however, we stand where we did fifty years ago. A few laws have been enacted, but they have seldom, if ever, been enforced. Today, owing to the great shortage of houses—which is world-wide—and to the high rents which have resulted from this shortage, there has been a doubling up of families, a contraction of living accommodations, with probably the worst room-overcrowding resulting therefrom that the world has ever known. It behooves the health authorities of the country to give most earnest attention to this serious situation. It is one that is fraught with menace.

LAND-OVERCROWDING

Congestion or land-overcrowding was an almost unknown term fifty years ago, but with the constant trend of the population from the country districts to the cities and the rapidly increasing city population, land-overcrowding has become a more or less serious problem in all of our large cities.

Fortunately a new consciousness of the dangers of such congested conditions pervades the country. Through zoning laws and housing laws the remedies for this situation are beginning to be applied, by limiting the height and area of buildings, and thus the number people living on a given area of land.

WATER SUPPLY

The substitution of a central water-supply, whose purity is insured by vigilant inspection, filtration and chlorination, for the individual surface well and yard pump, has become almost complete in the cities, and is being extended into the towns and villages over wider and wider areas.

With the elimination of the individual well and the abolition of the vault, typhoid will soon be relegated to the limbo of lost diseases.

GENERAL CLEANLINESS

General cleanliness of the home and of the person has added to personal hygiene while the providing of an ample supply of pure water in the home throughout our large cities has done much to induce personal cleanliness and stimulate the bathing habit. With the new knowledge that has come since the War of the spread of typhus fever through the body louse, the increase in habits of personal cleanliness becomes an important factor in combatting the spread of this disease, which is constantly seeking a foothold here from the other side of the ocean. The conditions which exist to-day in this respect are in striking contrast to the conditions which generally prevailed a half century ago.

THE HEALTH OFFICERS' EQUIPMENT

This record would be singularly incomplete if it left out of consideration the better equipment of the health officers throughout the country in their fight against bad housing and insanitary conditions generally. It is no exaggeration to say that we are at the dawn of a new era, when periodic sanitary inspection will be substituted for inspection solely on complaint.

There are already signs quite manifest that the health officer of the future instead of sitting down and waiting for trouble to come to him will be out looking for trouble. An ounce of prevention is worth many pounds of cure in the public health movement. The pioneer steps taken by New York City, Detroit and Chicago in adopting periodic sanitary inspection as the basic condition of their sanitary work is merely a precursor of what is to come in this direction throughout the country generally.

And, finally, we must not fail to record the changed viewpoint that exists to-day with regard to the important influence of environment — an influence hardly thought of, and certainly not discussed, in 1872. At that time, not merely was tuberculosis considered a hereditary disease, but nearly everything else. To-day there is a totally new attitude and atmosphere with regard to the important part which environment plays in the development of the human race, and with that changed viewpoint has come new knowledge.

Great as the advances have been in the field of housing and health in the last half century, the fifty years to come will see even greater advances.

WHAT FIFTY YEARS HAVE DONE FOR VENTILATION

GEORGE T. PALMER, D. P. H.

*Epidemiologist, Detroit Department of Health. Formerly Chief of Investigating Staff,
New York State Commission on Ventilation*

"VITIATED air produces deformity, imbecility and idiocy." Thus
wrote an American physician in 1850. And that is not all that
vitiated air was charged with. It encourages "pusillanimity and
cowardice, vice, and intemperance in the use of intoxicating drinks." It
"produces inaptitude for study and, therefore, ignorance."

These contentions sound a bit exaggerated. Surely the most
rabid open-air enthusiasts, even those intrepid individuals who break
the ice for a stimulating dip in midwinter, would hardly dare to be so
dogmatic to-day.

In fifty years' time we have at least learned to be analytical, to
separate a problem into its elements, to consider a number of possibilities before drawing conclusions. This has been made possible by
an advancing knowledge of physics, chemistry, physiology, and soci-
ology. Bad ventilation is detrimental to health. This has been
proved. That ventilation is at the base of all our social shortcomings
is a stupendous exaggeration. It is not only untrue, but it is unnecessary to charge so many evils to bad ventilation. There are reasons
scientifically sound for demanding good ventilation on the grounds of
comfort, health, and efficiency without going further.

Perhaps the most outstanding change in ventilation since 1870 has
been the substitution of experimentation for guesswork. It is for this
reason that we are vastly nearer the true causes of bad ventilation to-
day, and we are in consequence in a better position to prescribe
effective remedies for bad ventilation.

CONCEPTIONS OF VENTILATION HAVE CHANGED

Ventilation, as we understand it to-day, has outgrown its etymological swaddling clothes. Literally, ventilation means "to air", or by fanning or blowing "to replace foul air with pure air." This definition is somewhat narrow and restricted now because in its broad meaning ventilation involves certain physical characteristics of air, such as temperature, humidity and movement, factors which the words "foulness" and "purity" do not suggest. Broadly, *ventilation is the adjustment of the indoor air environment to meet the requirements of comfort, health and efficiency.*

Our conceptions of the causes of bad ventilation have, it is true, changed in fifty years, but unchanged still is the belief in the necessity for ventilation. To-day in many offices, schools, factories and theaters we can experience that sensation of stuffiness, oppression, discomfort, uneasiness, which are the products of poor ventilation. These same uncomfortable feelings were well known in the 70's. They were known and described long before that time. All mankind is and has been conscious of the fact that you cannot crowd human beings into an enclosure and expect them to remain in comfort unless some provision is made for an interchange of, or an alteration in, the air.

THE REASONS FOR VENTILATING

Human beings give off heat, moisture and odor. Through respiration they convert oxygen into carbon dioxide. Our ordinary habitations are not air tight, and there is constantly taking place an interchange of air between the inside and outside, through walls and through cracks around doors and windows. This natural interchange of air is usually sufficient to maintain comfort when there is ample space and there are few people. As the ratio of people to space is increased the natural interchange of air becomes increasingly less effective in keeping down the accumulation of heat, moisture and odor. The crowding may proceed much further, however, before oxygen is diminished or carbon dioxide is increased to the point of discomfort or danger. In short the body's ability to withstand alterations in the chemical substances, oxygen and carbon dioxide, is vastly greater than its ability to withstand changes in the physical characteristics of the atmosphere. Furthermore, the natural diffusion of the chemical constituents is much more rapid than the diffusion of heat and odor.

The internal body temperature in health is approximately constant, being maintained at all seasons of the year within one or two degrees either side of 98° Fahrenheit. Although man can adjust himself to a wide range of external air temperature, there is an optimum in the neighborhood of 65° F. This is attested by the history of civilization, for the greatest advances have been made in the temperate zones of the earth.

In winter, man secures comfort by wearing heavier clothing, by supplying buildings with heat and conserving that heat by keeping windows and doors closed. In summer artificial heat is cut off, doors and windows are opened, and lighter clothing is donned. Practically, human comfort depends more on maintaining a proper temperature balance between body and surrounding air than upon any other factor in the atmosphere. The ventilation requirement of greatest importance, both winter and summer, is, thus, a control of temperature within a short range of the optimum. This is a twentieth century conception of ventilation needs. As we shall show, the conception of ventilation was quite different in 1870. As our understanding of the subject has changed, so have the methods used to secure ventilation.

The Carbon Dioxide Bogy

It is difficult to trace chronologically the theories respecting the underlying badness in used or confined air. The pendulum has swung back and forth. Before the discoveries of oxygen and carbon dioxide as components of air the mysterious poison theory was uppermost. When the physiology of respiration — the conversion of a portion of oxygen into carbon dioxide in the lungs — came to be understood, leading scientific thought seized upon carbon dioxide as the culprit. Knowing that oxygen was essential to life and that an animal would soon die from suffocation in an air-tight box, it was assumed that the diminution of oxygen and the increase in carbon dioxide in the ordinary room was also harmful. This was the situation in the 70's, and as it is our purpose to trace the ventilation problem during the lifetime of the American Public Health Association, it is not to the point to go back of this date.

The whole thought of ventilation in the 70's was to prevent people from being poisoned by their own exhalations. A lay writer, John Brown, expressed the popular sentiment of the time in the following sentence: "Everybody knows that carbonic acid gas is fatal, but everybody does not realize how much we suffer from the moderate doses of it which we are constantly inhaling."

This sentiment prevailed to a widespread degree through the 80's and 90's and in fact reveals itself in the expressions of some even at the present day. It is strange how persistently belief in the harmful nature of carbon dioxide has remained in lay and scientific thought. It is like the memory of a long-lost friend that will not down. The strangeness of this persistence is referred to because as far back as 1842, Leblanc showed that an animal can breathe an atmosphere containing 30 per cent of carbon dioxide for three quarters of an hour, so long as the percentage of oxygen was kept around 70, and then recover on removal to the normal atmosphere. Furthermore, he showed that the increase in carbon dioxide which takes place in theaters and crowded places is surprisingly slight relatively, and that the reduction of oxygen is quite insignificant.

In 1857, Claude Bernard performed a variety of experiments with animals, all tending to show that the increase of carbon dioxide in commonly occupied places was far below a lethal or even an irritating limit. In 1863, Von Pettenkofer proclaimed the harmlessness of carbon dioxide as it occurred in the ordinary occupied room. He did not believe that rebreathed air was a poison in the ordinary sense of the term, but he did believe that vitiated air increased susceptibility to disease. Von Pettenkofer unwittingly fastened odium upon carbon dioxide by proposing the carbon dioxide test as an indication of the amount of other impurities in the atmosphere.

It is probably because the CO_2 test has become so universally used in ventilation studies that a belief in the harmfulness of the gas itself still persists.

ORGANIC EFFLUVIAL POISON

Carbon dioxide slowly but surely lost its adherents during the 80's. Perhaps experience had proved that its harmfulness in small quantities was unfounded. Crowded rooms still caused discomfort, and some reason for the annoyance had to be advanced. Nothing was known about "organic effluvia," and it was consequently elevated to the throne of iniquity. It was spendidly fitted for the part. It possessed an element of mystery that was tremendously satisfying. Greenleaf, a civil engineer, wrote in 1885, as follows: "Now the best opinion is in favor of the view that the vitiating of air by human beings, so far as it is made unfit for use, is due chiefly to the organic matter given off."

Griscom had hinted at this in 1850: "On the whole, it would appear that sulphuret of ammonia is the morbific agent exciting typhus fever, sulphuretted hydrogen being the pestilential virus producing yellow fever and the bilious remittents and agues of tropical climates." Griscom refers to no less an authority than Liebig as having found ammonia in the atmosphere, and he "has well-nigh established the identity of malaria with sulphuretted hydrogen."

The organic poison theory of bad air found a ready champion in Brown-Sequard and d'Arsonval, who reported, in 1887, that expired air from healthy men and dogs had the power of producing toxic phenomena. They injected the washings from the trachea and condensed moisture from the breath into animals, and death ensued in from a few days to several weeks. They were convinced of the presence in the expired breath of a volatile poison in the nature of an organic alkaloid.

They performed also another experiment which has had great weight in inducing people to believe in the dangers of vitiated air. They confined rabbits in a series of tight metallic boxes connected by rubber tubing through which a constant supply of air was drawn. The animal in the fourth cage breathed the air passing through the other three cages. The third animal breathed the air of the first two, the second animal the air from the first, and the first animal received air directly from outside. In a few hours the animal in the fourth cage died. Some time later the animal in the third cage died. The first two animals usually remained alive. Inasmuch as the air in the last cage rarely showed by analysis more than from 3 to 6 per cent of CO_2, they concluded that death was caused by a volatile poison. This belief was supported by the fact that when the air from the third cage was passed through sulphuric acid before entering the fourth cage, the fourth animal remained alive, whereas the third animal died. The acid, they said, absorbed the poison and thus protected the fourth animal.

Brown-Sequard and his colleague succeeded in stimulating a great amount of experimentation, the results of which largely failed to confirm their findings. For instance, Haldane and Smith, in 1892, confined a person in a small chamber until the vitiation was from ten to twenty times as great as in the most crowded and worst ventilated building, and yet there was no perceptible odor or sense of oppression.

Billings, Mitchell and Bergey repeated Brown-Sequard's work and were unable to secure any evidence which pointed to the presence of a volatile poison in the expired breath. For instance, six rabbits were kept in a series of bell jars for forty-two days, the proportion of CO_2 in the last two jars much of the time being from 4 to 7 per cent, and of oxygen from 12 to 16 per cent. *None of the animals died or were seriously ill.* "*Those in the first three and in the fifth jar gained in weight, those in the fourth and sixth lost slightly in weight.*" They concluded that death occurred in the latter jars of the series when the CO_2 increased to 12 or 14 per cent and oxygen was diminished to 4 or 6 per cent. Death did not occur when the CO_2 remained less than 10 per cent unless the oxygen was reduced to below 7 per cent of the mixture. They believed the sulphuric acid did nothing more than to interpose a resistance in the circuit so that leakage of air took place around the connections to the last jar, thus reducing the CO_2 content and increasing the proportion of oxygen.

The idea that an organic poison actually exists in the exhaled breath was not by any means dispelled in 1895. In fact, as late as 1911, Rosenau and Amos believed that they could demonstrate this fact by producing anaphylaxis in animals following the injection of small quantities of condensed matter from the breath of other animals, to whose breath the animals under experiment had previously been exposed for some time. Subsequent work along this line independently by Leonard Hill, Weismann and Lucas have failed to substantiate Rosenau's claims.

TEMPERATURE AND MOISTURE GAIN A HEARING IN 1895

While there is occasional reference prior to 1880 to high temperatures and moisture as being undesirable and discomforting, the references are given half-heartedly. Heat and moisture were merely looked upon as accentuating the poisonous effects of organic matter and carbon dioxide. They were not given primary weight of themselves. In 1883, Hermans was bold enough to suggest that chemical impurities were insignificant as causes of discomfort in occupied rooms, and that bad ventilation was in reality due to excessive temperature and moisture. Like so many pioneers, Herman's voice carried little weight at the time. It was not until 1895 that the dawn of a new conception of ventilation appeared. Evidence of this is found in the refreshingly clear statements of Billings, Mitchell and Bergey. After a review of the experimental work up to that time and a repetition of much of this work under their direction they came forward with the statement that it is *"very improbable that the minute quantity of organic matter contained in the air expired from human lungs has any deleterious influence upon men who inhale it in ordinary rooms, and, hence, it is probably unnecessary to take this factor into account in providing for the ventilation of such rooms."*

We cannot forbear quoting further from these authors, for their pronouncements in 1895 are so closely in agreement with our understanding of the situation to-day after twenty-five years of further experimentation:

The discomfort produced by crowded, ill-ventilated rooms in persons not accustomed to them is not due to the excess of carbonic acid, nor to bacteria, nor, in most cases, to dusts of any kind. The two great causes of such discomfort, though not the only ones, are excessive temperatures and unpleasant odors. Such rooms as those referred to are generally overheated, the bodies of the occupants, and, at night, the usual means of illumination, contributing to this result.

They conclude from their researches that some of the theories of ventilation prior to this time were either without foundation or were doubtful, and that the problem of securing comfort and health in inhabited rooms was one of preventing or disposing of various dusts, of regulating temperatures and moisture, and of preventing the entrance of poisonous gases such as carbon monoxide "rather than upon simply diluting the air to a certain standard of proportion of carbonic acid present."

We have dwelt at length on the theories of ventilation because of their importance, and we shall return to this question later on. The reader must appreciate the fact that so long as people were worried to death over a mysterious poison in the air of a crowded room, and over a distressingly slight excess in carbon dioxide over that in outside air, they could not think of ventilation except in terms of flushing rooms with air so as to keep down the concentration of these supposedly evil substances. They saw poison and suffocating gas and their remedy for these supposed conditions was the proper one. They failed to secure universal comfort because in spite of ample air dilution they made no special effort to keep rooms cool.

THE SERVICE PERFORMED BY STEAM HEAT AND THE MECHANICAL BLOWER

Because the word "fail" has been used in the paragraph above, it must not be taken for granted that progress in ventilation was lacking from the 70's to the 90's. On the contrary, there were well-defined advances during this period. In the 50's and 60's steam radiators, both direct and indirect, made their appearance, and these devices, taken in conjunction with the blower fans, made possible voluminous flushing and aeration with tempered air, which had not been satisfactorily worked out prior to this time.

To be sure, the House of Commons in England was ventilated by a crude centrifugal fan back in the eighteenth century, and later, in 1846, the United States Custom House in Boston installed a steam-driven fan. But this was in the perplexing days of trial. Prior to 1870 fans were confined largely to industrial plants to remove dusts and gases. It was after 1870 that mechanical ventilation began to find its way into school buildings and larger places of assembly. It performed a distinct service, because air flushing was an improvement over conditions that had existed, and temperature could be controlled within narrower limits, School buildings, for instance, formerly depended on natural draft or warm air furnaces. Ducts were provided for supply and exhaust, but they were small and poorly located. In New York City to-day one can find old schools with exhaust registers one or two feet square placed in an out-of-the-way corner, the exhaust ducts frequently being in or near the cold-exposed wall with a mighty slim chance of air leaving the room through such a portal. The responsibility for this error has been laid at the door of the architect, it being charged that he was more interested in the beauty of arrangement than in the utility of the ventilating equipment. Perhaps the architect was at fault, although he may have an alibi. Perhaps the school commissioners insisted on putting those unsightly registers in an inconspicuous place. They succeeded, at least. Regardless of who was at fault, ventilation did not have a ghost of a show with such treatment.

The power fan did force some air through the rooms, and a badly located register could not altogether prevent this. At times this airflow cooled the densely populated rooms, but as a rule room temperatures still fluctuated widely and overheating was all too common.

Thus, while positive air-flow helped to keep down carbon dioxide and to lower temperatures, it did not insure cool rooms at all times, the cooling being purely incidental. Nor did air-flushing keep down odor. As Billings pointed out in 1893, the smell of organic matter may not be perceptible when the CO_2 content due to respiration amounts to an excess of 5 parts per 10,000; and, again, odor may be very decided when the CO_2 does not exceed 3 parts. It depends on the temperature and moisture and the amount of diffusion going on, and odors do not diffuse as rapidly as CO_2.

STANDARDS OF AIR-FLOW

Again do we feel the urge of apologizing for our rather free criticism of the shortcomings of ventilation in the period of 1870 to 1900.

As has been said, progress was measurable during this period, and against the background of the fifty preceding years it was a very marked advance. The air-flow standard of 30 cubic feet per minute per person was well established at this time. Back in 1824, Tredgold, an English engineer, had the temerity to propose that a certain amount of air change was necessary, and he very modestly suggested a standard of 4 cubic feet per minute per person. In 1835, Dr. Reid, who was identified with the ventilation of the House of Commons, looked upon 10 cubic feet of air as essential. In 1857, the Barrack Commissioners of England fixed upon 20 cubic feet as the proper amount. Morin, in 1873, regarded 8 feet cubic as necessary in schools for children under 15, and 14 cubic feet for children over 15. For theatres he recommended 25 cubic feet, and the same for army barracks at night.

It remained for De Chaumont, in 1875, to interpret good ventilation as demanding less than two parts of CO_2 per 10,000 above the normal. To maintain this level of 6 parts CO_2 requires 50 cubic feet per minute per person. This was the standard adopted by Dr. Parkes and many English writers. Billings looked upon 30 cubic feet as a minimum, but with provisions for increasing this to 60 should the occasion demand.

The standard of 30 cubic feet per minute per person for schools met general acceptance in this country and is incorporated in the statutes of a number of states to-day.

The period from 1870 to 1890 thus may be credited with giving us our present-day standards of air-flow, which are widely used by engineers. While superior to preceding standards, they have led us astray by focusing so much attention on air volume as to obscure the important matter of temperature, and the desirable feature of fluctuation in air-flow.

TWENTIETH CENTURY CONTRIBUTIONS TO VENTILATION

The last twenty years have been characterized mainly by an increasing respect shown to the thermal factors of the atmosphere with a corresponding diminishing importance attached to the chemical constituents.

That the badness of bad air is due more frequently to overheating and excessive moisture than to any other cause was brought out in most convincing fashion in 1905, by Flügge and his pupils, Heymann, Paul and Ercklentz. They placed normal people in a cabinet of 3 cubic meters' capacity. In four hours' time the CO_2 had risen to 1.0 and 1. 5. per cent (100 and 150 parts per 10,000 as compared with 4 parts in outdoor air.) No illness or discomfort was felt so long as the temperature and humidity were kept down. When the temperature was allowed to rise, discomfort was felt. At a temperature of 75 degrees and 89 per cent relative humidity, and a CO_2 content of 1.2 per cent, the subjects felt very uncomfortable. Breathing fresh air from outside gave little, if any, relief. A person on the outside experienced no discomfort on breathing the air of the chamber through a tube. A person entering the chamber experienced immediate discomfort. When a fan was set in motion within the chamber, stirring up the air, there was immediate relief, even with no fresh air from outside. The layer of warm, moist air next to the skin was set free and distributed more thoroughly over the entire chamber.

The interpretation of these experiments is that it is not the chemical constitutents of used air which cause unpleasantness to those in the room. It is wholly the increasing heat and moisture which are responsible for discomfort.

This work has been repeated a number of times with the same results. Leonard Hill and his English colleagues, Flack, McIntosh, Rowlands and Walker, in 1913, published their account of a repetition of Paul's work with complete confirmation.

The New York State Commission on Ventilation found substantially the same results in 1914 and 1915, and their work was on a larger scale and covered longer periods of time. Instead of hours, subjects were kept under varying atmospheric conditions for the entire day, day after day, and for as much as six successive weeks. The Commission found that overheating, even slight overheating, 75°F, increases discomfort and brings on premature fatigue. It increases body temperature and the heart rate. When working on the piecework basis, a bonus being paid for quantity of work done in addition to a flat wage, subjects did 13 per cent less work at 75°F, than at 68°F. *It mattered not whether the chamber was bathed in fresh outside air (45 cubic feet per person per minute) or whether it was sealed so tightly that the CO_2 rose to 30, 50 and even 130 parts per 10,000. So long as the room temperature was kept down to 68°F., the subjects did just as much work and were quite contented.* But if the temperature rose to 75°F., even though the humidity did not exceed 50 per cent, work slackened, perspiration began and discomfort arose. The only indication of any unfavorable effect of stale air —that is air undiluted with fresh air — was in the slightly lessened food consumption, and this was most noticeable in the first or second week, largely, if not entirely, disappearing in the following weeks.

The above are the contributions of the laboratory men —physician, physiologist, chemist and physicist. The practical ventilating engineer, architect and layman may look askance at these experiments on a few people in small rooms, suspecting that the same laws will not hold true with many people in large rooms. This question has often been propounded: Even if these short-time experiments prove that air vitiated by the products of human exhalations is not harmful, is it not possible that a long-continued stay under these conditions, even though the air is cool, will eventually affect health? The answer to this is that the best of experimental evidence shows that the chemical constituents of vitiated air of ordinary occupied rooms are innocuous to health, and until evidence is produced to the contrary it is entirely logical and scientific and a matter of common sense to abide by these findings.

How the Newer Experimental Evidence Has Affected Ventilation Practice

Ventilation has inevitably been closely associated with heating. In the days before the mechanical blower and the steam radiator, buildings were heated by stoves and furnaces. The stove heated the single room. The furnace was an elaboration of the stove with the addition of a jacket through which air passed and then ascended through ducts to a number of rooms. The temperature of the air had to be high, that is above 100° Fahrenheit, to do its work. It was found that the distribution of this heated air was seriously interfered with by outside winds. Furthermore, the great heat of the air caused an annoying sensation of dryness to the occupants.

The steam and hot-water radiator provided a convenient means of direct heating. This solved the heating question for the time being but left the matter of ventilation to be dealt with independently. Air ducts were then added, and in the exhaust ducts it was customary to place steam-pipes or burning gas jets to accentuate upward air currents. These ducts were usually too small in area to be effective, and consumed a great deal of fuel.

The next step was the introduction of the steam-driven fan which forced air over heated coils or radiators. This method was used to ventilate, and it was also depended upon to do the entire heating. This again introduced the same objections associated with the hot-air furnace.

A modification of this plan was the placing of direct radiation within the room to supply heat, and the use of blowers and indirect heating coils to furnish tempered air for ventilation. This is the arrangement most common to-day.

The introduction to rooms of large volumes of air in order to maintain the standard of 30 cubic feet per minute per person necessitated the use of more spacious ducts, for otherwise the velocity of the entering air was so great as to cause annoying draughts. Larger exhaust ducts naturally followed.

Improvement took place in air distribution, which involved more careful placement of inlet and exhaust registers. Engineering details likewise advanced as the use of this equipment became more general. The steam-driven fan gave way in many instances to the electrically driven fan, and direct connected motors replaced the belt connections between motor and fan. Automatic temperature control replaced manual control, and to-day the thermostat is an essential part of indirect heating and is quite common in connection with direct heating.

We can see to-day many efforts to effect improvement in air distribution. The exhaust fan was added to assist the plenum fan in keeping the flow of air confined to the channels provided, and also to assist in the proportioning of this flow over the building.

Efforts have been made to maintain air circulation wholly by exhaust fans, the plenum fans being omitted and air being admitted to each room through apertures in the outer wall, the air temperature being raised by contact with the direct radiation. The passage of cold air over the radiators resulted frequently in frozen pipes, particularly when steam pressure was low. Furthermore, a strong suction from the exhaust duct at times drew air from open doorways or other apertures, and caused short-circuiting with consequent reduction in the aeration of the room as a whole.

INDIVIDUAL ROOM DUCTS FOR TEMPERATURE ADJUSTMENT

When the sun is shining the rooms in its path are warmed more than rooms on the shaded sides of a building. Consider the effect of this when the temperature of the indirect air supply is the same for all rooms. Some rooms become overheated, and to correct this condition the temperature of the air supply to the sun-exposed rooms should be reduced. The practice most commonly used now is to have a separate cold air supply controlled by dampers operated by thermostats in each room. A room that is too warm will have its warm air supply cut down by the damper, and some cold air will be admitted to lower the temperature. This involves individual ducts to each room from the hot and cold air-chamber in place of the single trunk duct leading up to a certain section of a building, with branching ducts to each room.

HUMIDIFICATION

The use of humidified air was ushered in just prior to the twentieth century, and was prompted by both hygienic and economic considerations. There are many industrial processes, such as weaving, which require a relatively high moisture content in the rooms. Then, also, mechanical ventilation, with its large volumes of air, produced so much evaporation from the bodies of occupants as to cause annoying sensations of dryness. When cold outdoor air is heated to 60 or 70 degrees, the relative humidity changes from the 70's and 80's to 20 and 30 per cent.

The heating of air reduces its relative humidity. When air is saturated with moisture (100 per cent relative humidity) a cubic foot contains, at 30° F., 1.94 grains of water, at 70° F., 7.98 grains. Thus when outdoor air at 30° and 80 per cent relative humidity is taken into a building and heated to 70° the resulting *relative* humidity is only 19 per cent. *The actual* quantity of water (absolute humidity) present is the same, but at 30° this amount represents 80 per cent of all the moisture that the air could contain, whereas at 70° this same amount represents only 19 per cent of what the air could contain. Warm air at low relative humidity tends to extract moisture from the surroundings. It was to correct this condition that humidifying pans and steam jets were added to ventilating equipment. These have been superseded largely by air-washers which not only add moisture to the air but also remove dust. Many installations to-day include air-washers as an integral part of the ventilation equipment. This involves also some means of automatic humidity control.

CHANGES IN HEATING PRACTICE

In 1870, the stove and hot-air furnace were most widely used for heating and ventilating. Hot-water heating was being advocated for houses, and steam was confined mostly to factories. Gravity ventilation in schools with supply ducts and heat acceleration in the exhaust ducts were not uncommon, but most schools had no provision whatever for ventilation. Mechanical ventilation was unknown in school buildings.

Thirty years later conditions had changed. We have an interesting picture of school ventilation in 1899 from the report of Mr. John Gormley. The Board of Education of the city of Philadelphia then had supervision over 447 schools.

13 were heated by direct steam radiation.

38 were heated by direct and indirect steam radiation.

152 were heated by hot-air furnaces.

14 were heated and ventilated by blowers and steam coils.

4 were heated and ventilated by batteries of hot-air furnaces, through which blowers forced air into the rooms,

the blowers being operated by gas engines.

None were heated by hot water.

Many of the remaining were heated by stoves or by combinations of stoves and furnaces.

In schools heated by hot-air furnaces and blowers driven by gas engines there was much complaint of the smell of hot oils, gas and noisy machinery. There was much vibration in the rooms above the machinery. Evaporating pans were provided for humidification, but were rarely used.

In 1921, the stove-heated school building has disappeared, at least in the larger cities. Furnace heat in large schools is a rarity. Gravity ventilation with direct heat and the various mechanical systems — plenum, combined plenum and exhaust, and exhaust alone with direct-indirect heat — are in most common use.

RECIRCULATION

As may be appreciated from the foregoing, the development of ventilation has proceeded from the simple to the complex. Each year has witnessed new and more elaborate equipment, and along with this advance has gone mounting cost. To offset the increasing expense there has been proposed a recirculation of the air within the building. Obviously much fuel will be saved if, instead of cold air from the outside, the warm air drawn from the building can be sent back through the supply ducts. Presumably this proposal would have been hooted with scorn in the days when carbon dixoide and organic effluvia reigned in their poisonous glory. However, Walter Snow urged recirculation of factory air as far back as 1891. Where the cubic space is great, this is an entirely feasible plan, for natural leakage through walls and around doors and windows is sufficient to prevent any unusual accumulation of odorous material in the air. Recirculation has worked out with apparent success and appreciable saving in fuel in the gymnasium of the Young Men's Christian Association Training School in Springfield, Massachusetts. This method has much to commend it in places where the air space is ample and the vitiating factors — from human beings, illuminating gases and industrial processes — are relatively slight.

The best example which has come to our attention concerning this practice in a school building was described by Professor Larson in 1916. The Wisconsin High School, at Madison, was ventilated with apparent success by utilizing only the air which was returned from the rooms and none from outside. The air supply was cut down to about 15 cubic feet per person per minute. Room temperature ran from 65° F. to 67° F., and relative humidity around 60 per cent. All air was passed through a washer before readmission to the rooms. The velocity of air entering the rooms was around 600 feet per minute, or double that in usual practice. Carbon dioxide ran as high as 20 parts per 10,000 and averaged above 10. By this method there was a saving in fuel of from 40 to 50 per cent. Larson makes this commentary: "Ventilation by recirculation is both efficient and economical. At the end of a year's run the teachers are almost unanimous in their praise of the system."

The point to be borne in mind in connection with this work is that this building was occupied only to about 75 per cent of its capacity, and the cubic feet of space per student was more than 350, as compared with a standard of 200 cubic feet in grade schools.

Thus, with buildings having a large ratio of air space per occupant, and with occupants moving about at frequent intervals during the day, recirculation offers an attractive method of ventilation. For crowded rooms or buildings it has disadvantages. Thus, the New York State Commission on Ventilation found that recirculating the air of a single class-room was associated with physical discomfort and odor. Some outside air had to be admitted to reduce odor. Air-washing intensified odor, and recirculation was more successful with the air-washer shut down. Ozone was used to reduce odor, but this likewise aggravated rather than helped the situation. The combination of ozone with the room odor was worse than the room odor by itself. Odor was less noticeable with humidities around 40 per cent or below than with higher humidities.

The Newer Ventilation Standards

The primary purpose of ventilation in 1870 was to remove carbon dioxide and organic effluvia. This view had not altered greatly in 1891, for Leicester Allen, a mechanical engineer, wrote as follows:

"The end and purpose of ventilation is, therefore, to remove from inclosed spaces these emanations (referring to organic matter given off from human bodies, and also carbon dioxide) together with any other poisons which may have become added to them either from leaks in gas pipes or fixtures, from soil pipes, from defects in water closets or any other source."

The carbon dioxide content was the measure of ventilation. Allen states that, "When by the presence of people in an enclosed space the percentage rises from 6 to 7 parts (of CO_2) in 10,000, the ventilation is bad. When the proportion is less than this the ventilation is good."

The change in our conceptions of ventilation since the nineteenth century may be judged from Winslow's definition of good ventilation as recorded in Park's *Public Health and Hygiene*, published in 1920.

1. "The air should be cool but not too cold."
2. "The air should be in gentle, but not excessive, motion, and its temperature should fluctuate slightly from moment to moment."
3. "The air should be free from offensive body odors."
4. "The air should be free from poisonous and offensive fumes and large amounts of dust."

Notice, if you will, the order of these requirements. Observe the omission of the CO_2 standard, and the air-supply standard of 30 cubic feet per minute per person. Take note of the avoidance of set values in the definitions. The physical and cutaneous factors — temperature and air movement — take precedence over the chemical and respiratory elements. There is a suggestion of variability in temperature and air motion as a desirable condition as opposed to uniformity in these conditions.

From the standpoint of the engineer who is called upon to design ventilating equipment, this definition will be criticized as too general.

The engineer needs something more specific. What temperature? How much air supply? What limits of fluctuation in temperature and air movement?

Winslow suggests a temperature between 65° F. and 68° F. in the office and schoolroom and even lower in the factory and open-air school where physical work is performed or heavier clothing is worn.

No mention is made of the degrees of fluctuating air movement. Further experience must determine this figure in specific terms. The engineer may, however, act upon the theory that variability is wanted rather than uniformity, and in planning his fan equipment this point must be borne in mind.

As to air volume and rate of change, there is no dogmatic assertion. This is a matter that must be worked out for specific purposes. In commenting on this point Winslow states:

> The fact is that while 30 cubic feet per minute may be set as a rough standard often desirable to attain, it may be insufficient in certain cases and in many other cases may be an unnecessarily high figure. Hygienists must insist on standards of air conditions actually maintained rather than on any arbitrary mechanical standards assumed to be capable of maintaining them. Any system which does not guard against overheating is inadequate, however large a volume of air may be forced into a room.

As to humidity, Winslow agrees that high temperatures combined with high humidities are particularly harmful. He does not lay stress on the hygienic influence of humidity at lower temperatures.

Deficiencies in Existing Laws and Enactments on Ventilation

How do existing statutes and regulations conform to this definition?

They differ primarily in the air-supply standard. The New York state law passed in 1904 recites that the "Commissioner of Education shall not approve any plans for the erection of any school building in third-class cities or incorporated villages or school districts, the cost of which building or addition exceeds $500, unless provision is made therein for assuring at least 30 cubic feet of pure air every minute per pupil, and the facilities for exhausting the foul or vitiated air therein shall be positive and independent of atmospheric changes."

The Pennsylvania law enacted in 1905 requires that school-houses "shall provide for an approved system of indirect heating and ventilation by means of which each classroom shall be supplied with fresh air at the rate of not less than 30 cubic feet per minute for each pupil and warmed to maintain an average temperature of 70° F. during the coldest weather."

In 1914, the American Society of Heating and Ventilating Engineers promulgated a set of minimum ventilation requirements for public and semi-public buildings, which were recommended as model compulsory heating and ventilating laws. Those which applied to schools specified that: "A positive supply of outdoor air shall, while school is in session, be provided the following rooms, and the quantity of this positive supply shall be equal to, or in excess of, the following minimum requirement per occupant per hour."

The standard for classrooms, study and recitation rooms was given as 1,800 cubic feet, or 30 cubic feet per minute per person. Gravity indirect heating and ventilating systems are accepted for small schools not exceeding 8 classrooms, in localities where it is impossible to secure proper motive power, provided such gravity systems are capable of supplying at least 30 cubic feet of air per minute for each pupil.

San Francisco has a section in the building law which requires "30 cubic feet of pure air per minute for each occupant" of all buildings designed to be used in whole or part, as public buildings, public or private institutions, schoolhouses, churches, public places of assemblage or places of public resort, including theatres and audience halls, factories, workshops and mercantile establishments.

The Sanitary Code of Chicago, adopted in 1911, is very comprehensive and specific in the matter of ventilation. Temperature exceeding 68° F. or 70° F. is prohibited in certain types of occupied buildings during the heating season. In street-cars, elevated and railway trains a range from 50° F. to 75° F. is permitted. There is nothing said about the fluctuation in air-flow. There is a provision requiring the removal, so far as practicable, of all noxious or poisonous fumes or gases or dusts arising in connection with a manufacturing process.

The Chicago Code specifies floor and cubic space requirements for different types of buildings, as well as quantities of air to be passed through them.   Air-flow requirements vary from about 1,000 to 2,000 cubic feet per hour per person.   A maximum CO_2 standard of from 10 to 12 parts per 10,000 is specified.

There is also included a section requiring that the relative humidity of certain enclosures shall not be less than 40 or 45 per cent and not more than 80 to 85 per cent.   The lower limit of humidity would seem to be unjustified from existing experimental evidence.

The intent of the above laws and regulations is to provide good ventilation.   A criticism that may be leveled against them is that they are too specific in the matter of air-flow.   There is not sufficient justification for demanding a continuous air-flow in the proportion of 30 cubic feet per minute per person for so varied a group of buildings.

For instance, it is entirely feasible to maintain good ventilation in such places as schoolrooms, when equipped with:

    a.   Direct radiation.
    b.   Window deflectors.
    c.   Spacious gravity exhaust-ducts on the inside wall.
    d.   Readily adjustable windows.
    e.   Readily adjustable temperature control, automatic or hand.

This type of ventilation shows from the experience of the New York State Commission on Ventilation great promise in providing cool atmospheres, with fluctuating air movement, free from offensive odors and large amounts of dust.   And yet under the above rules and regulations this method is completely ruled out because of the positive air-flow requirements of 30 cubic feet per minute which can be produced only by mechanical means.   Recirculation likewise is rendered impossible by many of these laws and regulations.

Notwithstanding the inconsistencies as pointed out above, there is a uniformity of opinion on certain fundamental ventilation requirements, which we may group as follows:

    1.   Except in rooms occupied by a few persons only, ventilation solely by means of windows located on one wall of a building is

unsatisfactory. Consequently a schoolroom with window exposure on one side only, and without exhaust-ducts, cannot be ventilated in a satisfactory manner.

2. Assembly rooms, audience halls, theatres, court-rooms and other places where people congregate in such large numbers that the floor space per person is not more than 10 square feet cannot be satisfactorily ventilated during the heating season except by means of mechanically propelled air.

3. During the summer time moving picture theatres and other places where people congregate to a similar extent demand mechanically propelled air for comfort. This may be accomplished by numerous circulating fans distributed at various points or by blower fans sending cool air through the enclosure, or by a combination of the two. The cooling of the air is done in various ways—by means of an air-washer, ice or brine coils.

As to the ventilation of schoolrooms there exists a divided opinion. As already stated, the work of the New York Commission indicates certain undeveloped and hitherto unrecognized advantages of window ventilation with gravity exhaust. There is no question that the statutes regarding air-flow for this type of room should be altered so as to permit the use of window ventilation.

Perhaps the most unsettled question at the present time is that of humidity. In rooms which are not overheated is humidification necessary for health and comfort? There is much to be said pro and con. The fact remains that we still have much to learn on this point. High humidity with high temperature is detrimental to health. Whether low humidity with temperatures below 70° F. is objectionable is a matter still awaiting convincing evidence.

The study of the sanitary insignificance of bacteria is a new development dating from 1870. While within the period from 1880 to 1910 there was considerable perturbation over the danger of bacteria floating about in the air, as evidenced by our past efforts at gaseous fumigation, their significance from a ventilation standpoint is almost nil, a possible exception being in hospitals and operating rooms, and certain industrial processes, such as the handling of hides and furs which may contain anthrax spores. There are other ways far more effective than ventilation for limiting the spread of infectious disease.

Dust is a factor to be reckoned with in industrial establishments and in mines. It may be annoying in other buildings but its significance below the limits of sensibility is slight. The suppression of dust in school, theatre and mercantile establishments is largely a matter of floor cleanliness or location of air intake, rather than of air flushing.

MEETING THE PRESENT DAY VENTILATION NEEDS

Aside from the special ventilation problems of industry involving dust and fume removal, the greatest need to-day in homes, offices, schools, barracks, prisons and hospitals is for facilities for maintaining a proper temperature range. This means easily adjustable windows, window deflectors, direct radiation, ready control of heating unit, either automatically or by hand, and where it is impossible to secure cross ventilation by windows there should be provision for exhaust ducts with dampers near the interior of the room. It must be the aim of the engineer and the architect to provide people with the means to keep comfortably cool. We have had enough of the overheated radiator which cannot be turned off, the traversing of an occupied room by uninsulated steam pipes whose heat it is impracticable to cut off, the window which will not budge. More attention must be paid to these details in order to improve indoor air comfort in the less crowded enclosures.

In schools which are mechanically ventilated, we must discard the 30-cubic-feet standard and also give up the idea that it is necessary to send air to every point in the room. The extremists, in 1870, wished to flush a room as a body of policemen would clear a hall, pushing all before them. This was ventilation by displacement. We now ventilate by dilution. It would seem that still better results could be accomplished in schools and auditoriums by substituting surface skimming in place of flushing. We must also substitute the intermittent or ejector type of air-flow for the monotonous uniformity which now characterizes mechanical ventilation. This will mean changing the inlet register from its accustomed place on the inner wall to the space between the direct radiation and the outer wall. The course of air-flow will be upward across the upper levels of the rooms and down the inner wall to the outlet. Windows may then be opened with impunity, the mechanical air-flow creating an aspirating effect which will draw in the cold outside air and send it over the room. By this means we shall harmonize the conflicting interests of the teacher who wants the window open and the janitor who wants it kept closed.

The occupants of the room, it is true, will not be uniformly perflated. At times they will sit in an atmosphere higher in CO_2 than under the old arrangement, but they will not sit in direct draughts of unvarying air currents, and consequently they can stand lower temperature. It is almost impossible in many fan-ventilated schoolrooms to secure comfort at 68° F. temperature, because of the appreciable air-flow through the room, which cools by convection and evaporation. Seventy, and even 72° degrees, are more comfortable. Direct the circulating air over the upper portions of the room and temperatures of 68°F. and even 65°F. are not uncomfortable. Dryness will not be noticed with overhead air circulation. Air from the windows will aid in giving a pulsating or fluctuating motion to the mechanically propelled air stream, which will be both pleasant and stimulating.

The adoption of this general plan for the ventilation of a theatre has been recently described by Samuel R. Lewis. Its adaption to auditoriums and rooms similar to the ordinary schoolroom holds out great promise.

Another weakness of present-day ventilation is the great and unnecessary waste of fuel. There is no reason, other than the 30 cubic feet of pure air standard, which militates against the use of recirculated air for many types of enclosures with ample space provisions, such as gymnasiums, churches, large assembly halls sparsely occupied, stores and factories. The same air might just as well be recirculated with a consequent saving in fuel. The natural dilution that takes place will meet all hygienic requirements so long as the temperature is kept down below 70°F., and if this is done humidification will in most cases be unnecessary. Odors are less pronounced in a dry atmosphere than in one of high relative humidity.   In short, let us be free to apply the remedy that will insure maximum comfort, health and efficiency to each specific case, without being prevented from so doing by well intentioned but overzealous requirements of air-flow.

The deficiency of ventilation in warm weather is being overcome by the increasing use of the disc fan for evaporative cooling and the use of the air-washer in theatres for lowering temperature by vaporization.   This is a distinct advance of recent date in ventilation practice.

One further unsolved problem of the present day is the ventilation of railway coaches, parlor cars and sleepers during winter weather.   This is almost wholly a matter of temperature control. There has been a signal failure in providing passengers with air comfort while traveling, and the journey without most uncomfortable overheating day and night, or else extreme underheating, is a rare one. It is to be hoped that railroads will some day cater to their patrons to the extent of allowing them to be cool if they so wish.   Screened, openable apertures in the side of the cars, accessible from the berths, would do wonders in placating the traveling public.   As it is, a passenger must lie like a prisoner in a sweltering and suffocating berth powerless to alleviate his discomfort.

THE CONTRIBUTIONS OF VENTILATION TO BETTER HEALTH

Have advancements in ventilation contributed anything to human happiness, health and longevity in the last fifty years?

Most decidedly, yes!

The unnecessarily hot, damp factory which fatigued operatives prematurely and reduced resistance to colds and pneumonia has largely disappeared in this time.   Some form of ventilation is now looked upon as an integral part of many types of buildings.   It was purely an incidental factor fifty years ago.

The dust and fume exhaust system has without question contributed to our declining tuberculosis rate.

To-day the open window by day, and more particularly at night, is known and utilized by many more than formerly.   The lack of ventilation in living quarters is responsible to-day for much of the tuberculosis in the land of our good friend and ally, the French Republic. The American doughboy who sojourned overseas can tell you that good ventilation is an adjunct to health.

Air comfort prevails in theatres, in assembly halls and in schools in an increasing measure each year, and pneumonia is losing its victims with each advance. Good ventilation, as defined in the terms of 1921, is a big factor in the war on respiratory disease. As Dr. S. Josephine Baker has shown, cool rooms with fluctuating temperature and air-flow specifically proved their value in reducing colds and respiratory affections among New York City school children in 1916 and 1917.

The mechanical blower and the steam radiator have been a godsend to the factory operative and the girl at the department store counter. Even though located a long distance from the open window, these workers in our immense twentieth century buildings may be supplied with cool, revivifying air. There is no longer any excuse for adding high temperature fatigue to the normal fatigue of physical exertion.

To permit ventilation to aid still further in the cause of human welfare, there remains only the reframing of our laws, rules and regulations in the light of recent experience, so that ventilation essentials will be insisted upon, and non-essentials be relegated to their proper subordinate position.

Just so soon as the hygienist incorporates in clear and understandable phraseology the health, comfort and efficiency demands of ventilation, attributing to each element its proper weight and no more, and so soon as the weight of an enlightened public opinion transforms these requirements into legal enactments, we can depend upon those who build our enclosures—the engineer and the architect — to provide for us the condition desired.

HISTORY OF INDUSTRIAL HYGIENE AND ITS EFFECTS ON PUBLIC HEALTH

GEORGE MARTIN KOBER, M. D., LL. D.*

Professor of Hygiene and Preventive Medicine, Georgetown University Medical School, Washington, D. C.

INTRODUCTION

Edgar L. Collis, in his retrospect of prehistoric industry, writes:

Industry may be considered as an outward and visible sign of the progress of the human intelligence, and the mile stones along the road — the stone age, the bronze age, the iron age, the machinery age — gather additional interest when considered as stages in the evolution of mind. . . . . The statement may be made that the intelligence of a race is measured by its industry, and that the primary *raison d'être* of industry is safety and health. In other words, industry is the means human intelligence employs to insure the existence of the race.

It is not surprising, therefore, that the anthropologist should find evidences among the "shell mounds and flint heaps" of prehistoric man that there were in reality factories for the manufacture of implements which were used for weapons of offense or defense, and that some of the best preserved remains of prehistoric man in addition to flint also reveal the presence of bronze arrow-heads. Industry, however, did not originate solely for offensive and defensive purposes, but also to improve living conditions in the life of the race struggling for existence. Buecher, cited by Price, has classified the methods of industrial production as follows: domestic production, handicraft production, and the modern factory system.

Domestic production is production in and for the house from raw materials furnished by the household itself. In its purest form it presupposes the absence of exchange and the ability of each household to satisfy by its own labor the wants of its members. All that the house-

---

*The compiler expresses his indebtedness to Mr. Felix Neuman and Sergeant M. Katz of the Library of the Surgeon General's office and to the Rev. Francis Tondorf of Georgetown University for valuable assistance.

It is a matter of regret that lack of space compels the omission of a complete list of biographical references.

hold has it owes to its own labor, and it is scarcely possible to separate the operations of the household from those of production.

Handicraft production, also known as custom production, is carried on within or outside of the house, usually by free workers. The handicraft man always works for the consumer of his production; the region of the sale is local — that is, the town and its immediate neighborhood.

The modern factory system supplies the economic wants of persons, communities and nations by wholesale production and the aid of machinery and motive power in specially constructed plants operated by industrial wage-earners.

It is very evident that at no time did one method of production exist to the exclusion of the other, and that there was a tendency, even in ancient times, toward a "localization of human industries." Lehmann tells us that the father of Demosthenes had a knife-factory employing 30 slave-workers, and that Lysias operated an armor-shield factory with 120 slave-workers. The Romans during their occupation of Britain, according to Cooke-Taylor, cited by Collis, established a manufactory of woolen clothing for their troops, also a manufactory of pottery, and at least one military iron-forge, or *fabrica;* but on their departure all was swept away, and for 900 years no great centers of industry and no factories existed. Now and again sprang up a very few notable and apparently temporary exceptions, such as the great clothier, "Jack of Newberry," who is said to have employed over 1,000 persons in the reign of Henry VII, but before the eighteenth century, industry as we know it did not exist in England. The only factories were the parish water-mills or windmills where corn was ground between stones brought from near Paris or Andernach on the Rhine. Only here and there was there any local industry in the thirteenth century.

Manufacturers of cloth are noted — scarlet at Lincoln; blankets at Bligh; burnet at Beverly; russet at Colchester (eight weavers are enumerated at this town in the rolls of Parliament under the year 1301); produce of linen fabrics at Shaftesbury, Lewis and Aylesham, of cord at Warwick and Bridgeport, the latter being cited also for its hempen fabrics; of fine bread at Wycombe, Hungerford and St. Albans; of knives at Maxstead; of needles at Wilton and razors at Leicester.

Space will not permit tracing the rise and growth of domestic and handicraft industrial production and its influence upon the health of the operatives, which doubtless was very important, the workshops of the mediaeval towns and cities being extremely primitive in character.

There is evidence to show that the factory system began in Italy in the fifteenth and sixteenth centuries with the manufacture of silk and woolen goods. In France, from the middle of the sixteenth century, the cloth, carpet, arms and porcelain industries grew rapidly. Similar progress was also made in England, Holland and Germany. According to Stieda, there was a large sugar refinery at Augsburg in 1573, a gold and silver works at Nuremberg in 1592, a soap factory in Augsburg in 1593, a blue-dye factory at Annaberg in 1649, and a woolen cloth factory, with 50 weavers and 300 spinners, at Halle in 1686. Some years later a wool and silk factory, with 500 workers, was established in Magdeburg. In 1710 a porcelain factory was established in Meissen, and another one in 1718 in Berlin. In 1764 a linen factory, with 800 workers, was founded in Tournai, Belgium. Prior to 1801 Germany had about 20 factories, each employing between 100 and 500 persons.

The modern factory system started in England in the latter part of the eighteenth century. Up to the beginning of that century, England was largely devoted to agriculture and sheep culture, and it is quite natural that the first mechanical industries should have been devoted to the production of material for clothing. The spinning-jenny, invented and perfected by High Kay and Hargreaves in 1767, supplemented by Arkwright's spinning machine in 1771 and Cartwright's power loom, patented in 1785, laid the foundation for the textile industry on a large scale. With the invention of the steam-engine by Watt and its practical application to factories in 1785, a tremendous growth in the mechanical and manufacturing industries occurred. This is shown by the fact that the importations of raw cotton into England increased from 5,000,000 pounds in 1775 to 273,249,653 in 1831 and 775,469,008 pounds in 1849, and also by an unusual demand for labor, especially apprentices and child labor to feed the machines. England in 1810 already operated 5,000 steam-engines, against 200 in France, while Germany introduced its first steam-engine as late as 1841.

With the development of the modern factory system of increased production came also a concentration of the population in certain manufacturing districts, as shown by an increase of the population in the Lancashire district from 166,200 in 1700 to 1,336,854 in 1831. But most important of all, occupational diseases and accidents came to be more and more seriously regarded. It soon became apparent, in countries like England, France, Germany and Italy, that death was exacting a very heavy toll in many of the industries. Indeed, the workmen in these countries began to believe that steam and speed had not improved their lot in life, branding their condition as one of slavery, and their factories and workshops as "slaughter-houses."

This was not an unreasonable conclusion, when it is recalled that in 1833 in factory towns like Manchester, "the youthful population was physically worn out before manhood," and that the average age of the laboring classes was only 22 years as compared with 44 years among the upper classes. Even later there was a period when, with a general death-rate for the whole of England of 22 per 1,000, the death-rate in the laboring districts was 36 out of every 1,000 per annum.

EPIDEMICS IN INDUSTRY

Collis, in his chapter on "Industry and Epidemic Diseases," brings out a number of interesting facts and shows very clearly that the typhus fever epidemics in Great Britain in the late eighteenth and early nineteenth centuries were generally influenced by a combination of want, overcrowding and other economic circumstancs. He refers to Tiverton, which in the first half of the eighteenth century was a fairly prosperous town with 8,000 inhabitants mainly engaged in weaving. In 1720 business began to slacken, and affairs became worse after a fire in 1735. Then followed a hard winter in 1739–40, which reduced the inhabitants to acute distress. In 1741 spotted fever was epidemic, and one in every twelve of the inhabitants died. At the close of the century Tiverton was less populous than at the beginning.

Whether history will repeat itself is a matter of speculation, but in the light of recent experience no one can deny that the aggregation of human beings in the industries, as in the army and navy, has favored contact infection, and the epidemic extension of influenza, pneumonia, septic sore throat, and other communicable diseases. It is also generally recognized even now that abject want and other economic conditions play an important rôle in the spread of typhus fever.

PROGRESS OF INDUSTRIAL HYGIENE IN THE UNITED STATES

As in Europe, so in this country, the mechanical industries had their origin in the textile industry. According to Wright, cited by Price, the first spinning-jenny in this country was exhibited in Phila-delphia in 1775. The first cotton factory to apply Arkwright's inven-tion was started with three cards and 72 spindles in Rhode Island in 1700, by Samuel Slater of England. It is reported, however, by a writer in the *American Museum* for July, 1790, that a man in South Carolina completed and had in operation on the Santee, ginning, card-ing and other machines driven by water and also spinning-machines with 84 spindles each. Waltham, Massachusetts, has the credit of having set up the first power loom in 1814, and of having established for the first time in history a factory in which all the processes involved in the manufacture of goods from the raw material to the finished product were carried on in one establishment.

The wonderful progress in the cotton textile industry in the United States is shown by the increase of spindles from 4,500 in 1805 to 1,246,703 in 1831. The following table shows the growth of the factory system as illustrated by the cotton industry in Great Britain and the United States:

	Year	No. Mills	No. Spindles.	No. Looms	No. Employees
Great Britain	1838	1151	9,333,000	100,000	237,000
	1878	2671	39,527,920	514,911	482,903
United States	1831	801	1,246,703	33,433	57,466
	1880	756	10,653,435	225,759	172,544
	1899	1055	19,008,352	450,682	302,861
	1914	1328	30,815 731	672,734	393,404

According to the Department of Commerce, the number of cotton bales (500 pounds to each bale) exported from the United States increased from 1,987,708 bales in 1870 to 10,681,382 bales in 1912, and fell to 9,256,028 in 1914.

CHILD LABOR IN THE UNITED STATES

Both in England and in this country the application of machinery resulted in the exploitation of child labor. It cannot be claimed, however, that we followed the example of England to the extent of trafficking with the poor-law officials in a form not greatly different from the methods of ancient slave-dealers. It is reported by Price that the first cotton mill established in 1770 in Rhode Island began work with four spinners and carders, but five children were soon added whose ages ranged from seven to twelve years, and in 1831 the number of children engaged in the cotton mills of that state was about one half of the total number of employees. According to Miss S. S. Whittelsey's "Essay on Massachusetts Labor Legislation," the subject of child labor received attention in 1836. The act provided for at least three months schooling during the working year for every child employed under the age of fifteen, and, as amended in 1842, for a ten-hour working day for children under fourteen years. In 1842 similar legislation was enacted in Connecticut.

According to Price, as early as 1827 a bill was introduced in the House of the Pennsylvania Legislature which provided that no minor between twelve and thirteen should be employed in the manufacture of cotton or wool unless producing a certificate from a schoolmaster or two citizens stating that the minor in question could read and write English and German or some other modern language, or unless the manufacturer should provide for instruction of said minor. The bill passed the House but failed in the Senate, and nothing more was done until 1837 when the Senate appointed a committee to investigate child labor. This committee found that one fifth of the entire number of workers in the cotton mills in the state were under twelve years of age, and that the time spent at work ranged from eleven to fourteen hours a day, with an average working week of seventy-two hours. The committee also reported that only one third of the cotton-mill workers under eighteen years could read or write. In spite of this deplorable condition no action was taken until 1848 when a bill was passed which forbade the employment of minors in any cotton, woolen, silk or flax factory. The bill provided a legal working day of ten hours in all such factories, with a proviso that minors above the age of fourteen might be employed more than ten hours by special contract with parents and guardians. In 1849 the minimum age was raised to thirteen years, and the law was extended also to the paper and bagging industries.

In New York the first school law was enacted in 1852, and it was not until 1874 that the law was framed making compulsory fourteen weeks of schooling each year. In 1886 the first factory law to regulate the employment of women and children in manufacturing establishments was enacted, and Illinois followed soon with a similar law. Since then commendable advance has been made. The compilation of labor laws by the Department of Labor in 1892 shows that thirty-four states had laws relating to the employment of children and females. Forty-three of the forty-five states in the Union in 1892 also had laws relating to minors who could be bound out as apprentices. Most of the laws required that the apprentice be given an education, good and wholesome provisions, and all necessary clothing, washing, lodging and medical attention, and also that he be taught the trade to which he was indentured.

NATIONAL COMMITTEE ON CHILD LABOR

In 1906 by an act of Congress (Section 2, United States Statutes, Number 1180) the National Committee on Child Labor was incorporated. The objects of this corporation are to promote the welfare of society with respect to the employment of children in gainful occupations; to investigate and report the facts concerning child labor; to raise the standard of parental responsibility with respect to the employment of children; to assist in protecting children, by suitable legislation, against premature or otherwise injurious employment, thus to aid in securing for them an opportunity for elementary education and physical development sufficient for the demands of citizen-ship and the requirements of industrial efficiency; to aid in promoting the enforcement of laws relating to child labor; to coördinate, unify and supplement the work of state or local child labor committees, and encourage the formation of such committees when not existing. This Committee deserves special credit for what has been accomplished in the way of child-labor legislation in this country.

FEDERAL LABOR LEGISLATION

The fundamental legal requirements relating to occupational diseases and accident and industrial hygiene are found in the statutes of the state and of the federal government, as interpreted in case of disputes by courts. These statutes rest upon the "police power" of the government; that is, the exercise of public authority to secure the public welfare by restraint and compulsion. Federal labor legis-lation began rather late in the history of the United States, and this because all such legislation was entrusted under the Constitution to the police powers of the various states. It was only after the govern-ment directed the affairs in interstate commerce and increased the number of civilian employees that federal legislation became more necessary. The following is a chronological list of federal enactments:

1875. The first federal statute relating to labor which the writer found was an Act of March 3, 1875, in Section 2 of which the involuntary transportation of any subject of China, Japan or any other oriental country is prohibited. The same Act also requires preference to be given to all domestic materials and labor for public works.

1882. The Act of May 6, 1882, as amended July 4, 1884, suspends the coming of Chinese labor to the United States and the Act of September 13, 1888 prohibits immigration of Chinese labor. Section 7 of the Act of May 4, 1882, grants the privilege to any keeper or member of a crew of a life-saving or life-boat station disabled by reason of any wound or injury received or disease contracted in the line of duty and which unfits him for the performance of his work, of being continued upon the rolls of the service and entitled to receive his full pay during the continuance of such dis-ability, the period of one year, applicable to this regulation, not to be extended unless upon recommendation of the general superintendent.

Section 4418 of the Act, as amended by the Act of March 3, 1905, requires inspec-tion of the boilers and appurtenances in all steam vessels before the same shall be used and once at least every year thereafter.

1885. By a resolution of January 6, 1885, the employees of the Navy Yard, Government Printing Office, Bureau of Engraving and Printing and all other per diem employees of the government shall be allowed the following holidays: the first day of

January, the twenty-second of February, the fourth of July, the twenty-fifth of December, and such days as may be designated by the President as days for national thanksgiving, receiving on these days the same pay as on other days.

1886. The Act of June 29, 1886, deals with labor organizations, and particularly with the incorporation of national trade unions.

1887. By a resolution of February 23, 1887, all per diem employees of the government on duty in Washington or elsewhere in the United States shall be allowed as holidays each year the day which is celebrated as Memorial or Decoration Day and the Fourth of July, and shall receive on these days the same pay as on other days.

1888. The Act of May 24, 1888, prescribes eight hours as a day's labor for letter carriers. By an act of June, 1900, the hours shall not exceed 48 during the six working days of each week, such number of hours, not exceeding eight, to be spent on Sunday as may be required by the needs of the service.

1890. Section 4509 of the Act of August 19, 1890, provides that to be apprenticed for sea service a boy must have the consent of his parents or guardians, and must be not less than 12 years of age, and of sufficient health and strength.

1890–91. Chapter 564 refers to an act relating to coal-mines, covering, among other subjects, inspections, defective conditions, ventilation, sprinkling, shot fire, escape shafts, furnace shafts, safety cages, and accidents. Employment of children under the age of 12 is prohibited in the underground workings of mines.

1892. The Act of August 1, 1892, as amended by Chapter 106, Act of 1912–1913, in Section 3738, declared that "eight hours shall constitute a day's work for all laborers, workmen and mechanics who may be employed by or on behalf of the Government of the United States."

1893. The Act of March 2, 1893, deals with safety appliances on railroads.

1895. The Act of January 12, 1895, as amended by the Act of August 24, 1912, fixes the limits of wages, holidays, and night work of certain federal employees.

1897. The Act of January 18, 1897, refers to inspection of boats propelled by gas, etc., also to tug and freight boats, and the inspection of boilers.

1897. The Act of March, 1897, refers to inspection of steam boilers on foreign vessels.

1899. By an Act of March 1, 1899, to railway postal clerks whose duties require them to work 6 days or more per week, 52 weeks a year, an annual vacation of 15 days with pay may be granted by the Postmaster General. Section 4153 of the same Act requires not less than 73 cubic feet and not less than 12 superficial feet for each seaman or apprentice lodged on vessels.

1901. Section 1990 of the United States Statutes compiled in 1901 abolished peonage. Section 2158 prohibits engaging in coolie labor. Section 4801 deals with hospital relief for sick and disabled seamen, and Section 5344 with negligence of employees on steamboats, causing death. Section 4569 requires every vessel of 75 tons or upwards to be supplied with a medicine chest, and Section 4572 makes provision for clothing and fuel on vessels. Section 4611 prohibits flogging and all other forms of corporal punishment on board of any vessel.

1902–3. Chapter 976 deals with the application of the law of 1893 regarding safety appliances on railroads.

1906–7. Section 2, Chapter 1180 of the Acts of 1906 provides for the incorporation of a National Committee on Child Labor.

Chapter 2558 creates a foundation for the promotion of industrial peace.

Chapter 2939 regulates the hours of labor of employees on railroads.

1908. Chapter 149 of the Acts of 1907–1908 deals with liability of railroad companies for injuries to employees in interstate commerce.

Chapters 200 and 225 deal with inspection and test of railroad safety appliances.

1908. On May 30, 1908, the Federal Government enacted a limited compensation law for the civilian employees of the United States applicable only to certain hazardous employments.

1909. Chapter 240 of the Acts of 1909–1910 creates a Federal Bureau of Mines in the Department of the Interior.

1910. Chapter 103 of the Acts of 1910–1911 relates to inspection of locomotive boilers.

1911–12. Section 1, Chapter 355 of the Acts of 1911–1912 relates to plate printers, rates of wages and power presses in the Bureau of Printing and Engraving of the United States Treasury Department. Chapter 389 of the Acts of 1911–1912 relates to the construction of sound and sanitary postal railway cars, and to the provision in these cars of sanitary drinking-water containers and toilet facilities.

1912. By an Act of Congress, approved April 9, 1912, the use of poisonous white phosphorus matches was abolished in our country by the establishment of a prohibitive tax of 2 cents per 100 matches. The creation of the Children's Bureau by an Act approved the same day was a significant and prophetic action. By an Act approved August 23, 1912, Congress authorized the appointment of a temporary commission on industrial relations, one of whose duties is to inquire into matters relating to the health of employees. This commission made several important reports.

1912–13. The Act of August 1, 1892, as amended by Chapter 106, Acts of 1912–13, provides in Section 3738 that eight hours shall complete a day's work for all laborers, workmen and mechanics who may be employed by or on behalf of the Government of the United States.

1916. On September 7, 1916, Congress enacted a model workmen's compensation law for the civilian employees of the United States, and in 1919 Congress extended this law to likewise protect the public employees of the District of Columbia.

STATE LABOR LEGISLATION

Because of the multiplicity of commonwealths in the United States and the lack of uniformity in the laws, it is quite difficult to offer anything like a complete historical review of all the laws of the states relating to the protection of wage earners in factories, workshops, and mines.

The first compilation of labor laws enacted in the United States was published by the United States Commissioner of Labor in 1892. The volume covers 603 pages and includes all legislation in force at the close of the year 1890. A revision of this compilation with additions was published in 1896. This volume of 1,383 pages includes all legislation up to the beginning of that year. The third compilation, covering 1,413 pages, appeared in 1904. The fourth compilation, covering 1,562 pages, was published in 1907. The fifth compilation, covering 2,473 pages, appeared in 1915, and includes all legislation up to the beginning of 1914, together with orders of the State Industrial Commissions of New York and Wisconsin, which under the laws of these states have the force of laws.

It is interesting to note that the laws enacted prior to 1890 deal largely with the protection of children and female employees, apprentices, and the right of action for injuries in nearly all of the states. The eight-hour labor laws as applied to roads and public works existed in thirty-three states. Thirty-four states had legislation on female labor. Of these, sixteen states regulated the hours of work for women, and nineteen required seats for women in certain occupations.

Only 14 of the states had made provisions for inspection of factories and workshops, and 22 states for inspection of mines. Fourteen of the states had provisions for reporting accidents in factories, and 22 states had statutes for the prevention of accidents in mines. Thirteen states required fire-escapes and doors swinging outwards; 23 states required inspection of steam boilers; 21 states had statutes relating to the health of employees, among these being statutes regarding ventilation and sanitation of workshops in general. (See Table I.) Thirteen states had laws requiring guarding of machinery. Three states, New Jersey, New York and Ohio, had laws requiring guards for vats containing molten metal or other hot liquids.

The following states had laws prior to 1890 on safety apparatus for mineshafts: California, Colorado, Illinois, Indiana, Iowa, Kansas, Kentucky, Missouri, Montana, Nevada, Ohio, Pennsylvania, Washington, West Virginia and Wyoming.

Michigan and New York had laws on safety appliances on railroads.

Seven states — Massachusetts, New Jersey, New York, Connecticut, Pennsylvania, Michigan and Missouri — had laws prohibiting "oiling of machinery in motion by women and children."

The following states had laws guarding elevators and hoistway openings: Massachusetts, New Jersey, Ohio, New York, Connecticut, Pennsylvania, Rhode Island, Michigan, Missouri, and Minnesota.

Massachusetts and New York were the only two states having laws on the use of explosives and inflammable material.

The following states had laws relating to ventilation of factories and workshops: Massachusetts, New Jersey, Ohio, New York, Connecticut, Pennsylvania, Rhode Island, Missouri.

Only two states, New Jersey and Ohio, had statutes on the subject of heating and lighting.

New York, New Jersey and Michigan were the only states requiring "limewashing or painting of walls of workshops."

Only five states — Massachusetts, New Jersey, New York, Pennsylvania and Illinois — had legislation to regulate the "sweating system."

Massachusetts was the only state requiring approval of plans for factories.

In 1908 and 1909 legislative attention was given largely to the subject of employer's liability, the common law defenses having been abrogated or modified in a number of states. Fifty-four laws were enacted in 32 states affecting the employment of women and children.

In 1910 the subject of workmen's compensation began to claim the attention of legislatures, and a number of industrial commissions were created. Retirement and pension funds also received attention in two states.

In 1911 the workmen's compensation acts continued to occupy the center of the legislative stage in 10 states, and occupational diseases also received attention in some of the states. The first American law for the compulsory reporting of these diseases was drafted by the Association for Labor Legislation and was enacted in California in March, 1911. These two subjects also held places of increasing importance from 1912 to 1914. Accident prevention and accident reporting, and female and child labor received attention in a number of states, and the conditions affecting employees in mines and on railroads also resulted in additional legislation.

In 1913 the subject of minimum wages and of support for mothers and dependent children was a prominent topic in remedial legislation.

After these preliminary remarks a clearer insight into the development of factory legislation may be given by sketching briefly the legislation of Massachusetts — the first state in the Union to recognize the fact that sanitary inspection of factories is essentially a public health matter.

FACTORY LEGISLATION

The bill passed by Massachusetts in 1852 regarding the safety of steam machines was the first legislation of this nature enacted by any state. An Act of 1870 also required supervision of steam-boilers. The enforcement of the child labor law had been assigned to the local school authorities and truant officers. In 1866 a single deputy detailed by the police department was entrusted to enforce this law, and only in 1877 was the right of entry into factories granted to the inspector. In the same year this state enacted a law setting forth certain requirements for the removal of dust. In 1879 the Governor was empowered to appoint two or more members of the district police to act as inspectors of factories and public buildings. The duties of these inspectors were (1) the enforcement of laws regulating the hours of labor in manufacturing establishments; (2) the enforcement of laws relating to the employment of children, and (3) inspection of factories and public buildings.

One of the inspectors, Rufus R. Wade, in his report made as Chief of District Police for 1879 (page 8), cited by Price, states:

In the matter of providing for speedy and safe egress in case of fire or panic, a large number of manufacturing establishments were found deficient. The horrors of Holyoke and Granite Mill at Fall River and other disasters that have occurred by reason of neglect to provide safe means of egress in case of fire or panic should not, through negligence or thoughtlessness of manufacturers or owners of buildings, be repeated.

The report also points out that the laws providing for education of child workers were not enforced, and that children were below the legal age, the youngest being nine years old. The board asked for two additional assistants, and, because of the magnitude and importance of the problem, recommended that the inspection of factories be made a distinct branch of the police service. The Governor in his message in 1880 approved the recommendation, but it was not put into effect until 1888.

In the meantime an act had been passed on March 24, 1887, to secure proper sanitary provisions in factories and workshops; another, on April 14, to secure proper ventilation and proper meal hours. On March 10, 1890, the law relating to accidents was amended and made more drastic.

In 1891 the corps of inspectors was increased to 26, two women inspectors being added. In 1893 a separate boiler inspection division with ten inspectors was created. In 1905 a reorganization of factory inspection was made, by which a number of state health inspectors were appointed, who took over a considerable part of the functions of factory inspectors. In the same year the State Board of Health submitted a brief but excellent report on the conditions affecting the health and safety of employees in factories and other establishments in Massachusetts. This report was supplemented in 1907 by a more extensive report and included a collection of ninety photographs. The photographs, based upon a study of dusty trades in Massachusetts made by Dr. William C. Hanson, together with charts and a collection of dust and other materials, demonstrated in a most effective manner that many of the insanitary surroundings and injurious factors in the leading industries are due to neglect of perfect ventilation, and hence are to a great extent avoidable. This was in fact the first exhibit in America relating to occupational diseases and industrial hygiene.

The report contained many excellent comments, as, for example:

> In the boot and shoe industry, the inspectors found four conditions which can be and ought to be remedied, viz.: Poor ventilation, inadequate removal of dust from machines, the conditions of water-closets, and spit upon the floors.
>
> In the majority of the factories visited the ventilation was very poor, and in many of them distinctly bad. Of the rooms not especially dusty, 102 were very badly ventilated and 26 were overcrowded. Of 84 of the many dusty rooms reported, 40 were also overcrowded; 35 were dark, 21 overheated, and 18 overcrowded, dark and overheated. In more than one-third of the factories inspected, most of the water-closets were dark and dirty, to very dirty. In 50 establishments no spitting on floors was noticed; in 173 there was some; in 115 considerable, and in 35 much.
>
> In 85 factories, or 23 per cent of those visited, a considerable proportion of the employees were noticeably pale and unhealthy.
>
> In the emery and corundum, sand-paper, and all other industries more attention should be given to keeping the dust away from the mouths and nostrils of the workmen. In the rag industry and cutting rooms of some paper mills very objectionable amounts of dust were found and some pale and sickly-appearing operatives, but there are mills using the same kind of stock, where the dust is kept away from the employees in a satisfactory manner, and much improvement is practicable in the former class.

In discussing the provisions of the Massachusetts law regarding the cleanliness of factories, the report points out that

> What is clean in an axe-grinding factory would not be so in a silk mill, but the law makes no distinction, and the judgment of the officer cannot be received as law. . . . The Board considers it impossible to specify in any law a standard of cleanliness applicable to all industries, and advises that the officer should be authorized to hold all factories in any industry up to the standard of cleanliness which he finds maintained in factories in the same industry and using the same grade of stock which are the cleanest. The same method is recommended for the enforcement of standards in other directions, subject to an appeal to the State Board of Health.

The writer feels that the pioneer work and methods pursued by the State Board of Health of Massachusetts have been of inestimable value not only to that commonwealth, but also to the country at large. The same agency which investigated the dangers of occupations was seeking also to control the evils which arise in the home and community life of the worker. The state inspectors of health were in constant communication with local physicians who could give information concerning not only merely communicable diseases, but also occupational diseases, as is brought out in a paper by Dr. William

C. Hanson.* The principles upon which the board was proceeding may be found in a paper by Dr. H. Linenthal,† one of the inspectors.

By a law enacted June 10, 1912, in spite of the good work done under the State Board of Health, the duties of the Board were transferred to a "Board of Labor and Industries," composed of one employer, one laborer, one physician and one woman. This Board was empowered to appoint a commissioner of labor whom it might remove at any time; to investigate conditions and to hold hearings; to seek expert advice and prosecute violators of the law, and to appoint industrial health inspectors and assistants, such persons not being legally required to have a medical training.

Considerable space has been devoted to the state of Massachusetts because it has led all other states in labor legislation, except in the enactment of the law relating to the reporting of occupational diseases.

Factory Inspection. There was no legislation in the United States for factory inspection prior to May 11, 1877, when Massachusetts led the way, followed, in 1883, by New Jersey and Wisconsin, Ohio in 1884, New York in 1886, Connecticut, Minnesota and Maine in 1887, Pennsylvania in 1889, Missouri and Tennessee in 1891, Illinois and Michigan in 1893, and Rhode Island in 1894.

The inspection service in 11 of these states included the enforcement of the laws relating to child and female labor. In Massachusetts, New Jersey, Ohio, Connecticut, Rhode Island, Maine, and Minnesota, the inspection covered seats for female employees.

In nine states the inspection law covered fire protection in the way of fire-escapes and ready egress by outward-swinging doors. In 10 states inspection applied also to the guarding of machinery. In the following states, which had laws providing for the removal of dust and objectionable gases by exhaust fans, the inspection covered this point, viz. — Massachusetts, New Jersey, New York, Connecticut, Michigan, Missouri and Minnesota. Michigan, by Act 136 of 1887, and New York, in 1890, required blowers to be provided for emery wheels in factories.

In 1908 the writer was able to report 12 additional states — California, Illinois, Indiana, Iowa, Maryland, Ohio, Oregon, Pennsylvania, Mississippi, South Dakota, Washington and Wisconsin — making 17 states which required mechanical devices for the removal of injurious dust and gases. Of these states quite a number laid down specific rules concerning the construction of work-benches and hoods. The latter

---

*Wm. C. Hanson, M. D., Fifteenth International Congress of Hygiene and Demography, 1913, vol. III, p. 898.

†H. Linenthal, M. D., *ibid.*, p. 907.

empty into air-shafts connected with exhaust fans. Of the laws then in effect the writer cited the Michigan law of 1899 as the best example of regulation of this character.

The inspection service also covered heating and lighting of workshops in New Jersey and Ohio, overcrowding in New Jersey and New York, and the "sweating system" in Massachusetts, New Jersey, New York, Pennsylvania and Illinois. In eight states factories were subject to inspection in regard to sanitary conditions, including toilet facilities. In 22 states the inspection covered safety apparatus for mine-shafts, safety lamps, and the like.

Progress of Factory Legislation from 1890–1920. All of the states now have some form of legislation for the protection of children. In 26 states there is a provision for the exclusion of children under sixteen years from dangerous trades, and three other states besides 12 of the 26 specify other dangerous trades in which persons under 18 may not be employed. Fourteen states prohibit the employment of persons under 21, or minors, in a few other trades injurious to morals as well as to health, or in trades affecting the safety of others.

But in most cases the statutes are vague and lacking in uniformity.

Where one state specifies simply mines and quarries as dangerous, the other gives a long list of carefully defined processes or occupations dangerous to health or morals, leaving the definition of such occupation to the enforcing officials. Almost invariably when a state has such a loose statute, the machinery for its administration is so weak that the law is practically a dead letter. The only attempt at uniformity in such legislation in the United States is the "Uniform Child Labor Law," drafted by the National Child Labor Committee in 1911 and later endorsed by the American Bar Association.

Forty-five states have laws relating to the hours of female labor, and 52 states and territories require seats for women in certain occupations.

It is gratifying to report that in 1920, 50 states had laws providing for inspection of factories and workshops, and 36 states required inspection of mines; 21 states inspection of bakeries; and 30 states inspection of steam-boilers.

Thirty-four states require fire-escapes, ready egress by outward-swinging doors and other methods of fire protection.

Thirty-six states require guards for dangerous machinery. Twenty-eight states make reports of accidents in factories obligatory; and 34 states make reports of accidents in mines obligatory. Forty-three states have laws relating to railroad safety, and 39 states demand reports of railroad accidents. Twenty-six states have laws providing for the protection (in the way of safety scaffolds and the like) of employees on buildings.

Thirty-five states have laws on sanitation of factories and workshops, including laws on ventilation, many of which require the removal of injurious dust and fumes by mechanical devices and exhaust ventilation.

Forty-three states have laws referring to toilet rooms and washing facilities.

The following states have laws relating to the manufacture and storage of explosives: Iowa, Maryland, Massachusetts, Missouri, New Jersey, Ohio, and Oklahoma.

Fifty-four states have laws relating to liability of employers for injuries to employees. Forty-five of these states and 3 territories have abandoned the older idea of employers' liability and adopted the principles of compensation for accidents.

The following states have enacted laws providing for mothers' pensions: California, Colorado, Idaho, Illinois, Iowa, Massachusetts, Michigan, Minnesota, Missouri, Nebraska, Nevada, New Hampshire, New Jersey, Ohio, Oklahoma, Oregon, Pennsylvania, South Dakota, Utah, Washington, and Wisconsin.

The following states have laws providing seats for street railway employees: Connecticut, Louisiana, Missouri, New Jersey, Oregon and Vermont.

The following states have laws relating to meal hours: California, Delaware, Indiana, Louisiana, Massachusetts, New Jersey, New York, Ohio, Oregon, and Pennsylvania.

The following states require vaccination in certain occupations: Connecticut, Maine and Virginia.

The following states prohibit the employment of women within two weeks before or four weeks after childbirth: Connecticut, Massachusetts, New York and Vermont.

By an Act of March 14, 1881, a hospital for miners was established in the state of California, where indigent miners are charged at actual cost for medical attendance, surgical operations, board and nursing, while pay-patients, whose friends can pay their expenses, and who are not chargeable upon townships and counties, pay according to the terms decided by the trustees of the State Miners' Hospital and Asylum.

In 1887, by Acts 264 and 265, the state of Pennsylvania established state hospitals for the middle coal-fields, the hospitals to be devoted to the reception, care and treatment of persons injured in or about the mines, workshops and railroads, or any other laboring men.

New Mexico, in Section 2337 of the compiled laws of 1897, has a provision that whenever any employee in smelting works contracts lead poisoning, the employer becomes responsible for the medical care and treatment of the victim. The same territory, under Chapter 2, Act of 1903, established a state hospital for the treatment and care of resident miners of the territory of New Mexico, who may become sick or injured in the pursuit of their occupation, care and treatment to be free, unless the patient is possessed of property and means sufficient to pay the actual costs and charges incurred.

Arkansas, by Act 299 of 1909, compelled railway companies who have heretofore collected or received hospital fees from their employees to provide hospital facilities in this state of such capacity and equipment as will be sufficient for the care, needs and accommodations of their sick and injured employees who are residents of the state. Any such employees injured while in the service of any such railroad shall not be taken or sent out of the state for treatment.

Workmen's Compensation in the United States. The Fourth Special Report of the Commissioner of Labor, issued in 1893 under the title of *Compulsory Insurance in Germany,* was the first publication in this country devoted to the subject of workmen's insurance. Before that time compensation for industrial accidents had been established in Germany in 1884, and in Austria in 1887. Norway did not follow until 1894. The present report, Bulletin Number 126, entitled *Workmen's Compensation Laws of the United States and Foreign Countries,* dated December 23, 1913, shows that 41 foreign countries (including all European countries except Turkey) have introduced some form of workmen's compensation for industrial accidents. All of these forms, while showing great variations in the industries covered, the amount of compensation provided, and the methods by which compensation payments are secured, recognize the principles of compensation as distinguished from the older ideas of employers' liability previously accepted in the civil law of Continental Europe, as well as in English and American law.

It is interesting to learn that the state of Maryland in 1902 provided legislation for stated benefits payable without suit in the form of a coöperative insurance law, and applicable to certain occupations, such as mining, quarrying, steam and street railways, and public work. This law was declared unconstitutional.

In 1905 the United States Philippine Commission authorized the continuance of wages for a period during disability, but not exceeding 90 days, in case of injury to employees of the insular government in line of duty. In 1908 the Federal Government enacted a law "granting to certain employees the right to receive from it compensation for injuries sustained in the source of employment."

On March 4, 1909, Montana enacted a statute to take effect October 1, 1910, providing for the maintenance of a state coöperative insurance fund for miners and laborers in or about the coal mines of the state. Contribution to the fund was compulsory in the case of both of employers and employees.

According to Clark, in the United States the period of investigation and education began somewhat late (1909), as compared with European countries. The first American state commissions were appointed in New York, Wisconsin and Minnesota in 1909, and legislation followed in New York in 1910, in Wisconsin in 1911 and in Minnesota in 1913. Within the period between 1909 and 1913, 27 commissions (not including one federal commission) had been appointed to consider the subject, and compensation laws were enacted in 23 states. Following 1914 progress in compensation legislation has been very rapid, 45 states and 3 territories having enacted laws. (See Table I).

The laws in the majority of states provide for compensation for industrial accident only, but the following 16 states since 1911 have enacted laws requiring the notification of certain occupational maladies and also provide for compensation in these diseases, viz: California, Connecticut, Illinois, Maine, Maryland, Massachusetts, Michigan, Minnesota, Missouri, New Hampshire, New Jersey, New York, Ohio, Pennsylvania, Rhode Island and Wisconsin.

According to Commons and Andrews, the earliest of these laws called for reports on all cases of anthrax, compressed air illness, and poisoning from lead, phosphorus, arsenic, mercury or their compounds, to which were later added brass and wood alcohol poisoning. The most recent tendency, however, is to make the laws include any ailment or disease contracted as a result of the nature of the patient's employment, in which form the laws will probably be productive of more important results. The duty of reporting falls upon the physician in charge of the case, who makes his report either to the state labor department or to the board of health.

Great Britain under the Workmen's Compensation Acts has a schedule of 30 occupational diseases. The Occupational Disease Compensation law of the state of New York, in effect May 5, 1920, covers 23 diseases. The Ohio Act, passed April 20, 1921, covers 15 maladies.

Other Forms of Health Insurance. A brief reference should be made to the excellent health work carried on by the Metropolitan Life Insurance Company and other insurance companies engaged in industrial insurance work. Much good has also been done by the so-called "Group Insurance" system, and the numerous Employees' Mutual Benefit Associations, of which there are over 500 in this country.

TABLE I

State or Territory	Age Limit for Children 1890	Age Limit for Children 1920	Seats for Women 1890	Seats for Women 1920	Inspection of Factories, Workshops, etc. 1894	Inspection of Factories, Workshops, etc. 1920	Inspection of Mines 1890	Inspection of Mines 1920	Inspection of Steam Boilers 1890	Inspection of Steam Boilers 1920	Fire Escapes 1890	Fire Escapes 1920	Guards for Dangerous Machinery 1890	Guards for Dangerous Machinery 1920	Health of Employees; Ventilation and Sanitation of Factories 1890	Health of Employees; Ventilation and Sanitation of Factories 1920	Toilet Rooms 1890	Toilet Rooms 1920	Report of Accidents in Factories 1890	Report of Accidents in Factories 1920	Report of Accidents in Mines 1890	Report of Accidents in Mines 1920	Liability of Employers for Injuries to Employees 1920	Date of Workmen's Compensation Legislation	Labor Bureau Prior to 1900	Labor Bureau After 1920
Alabama		*		*		*		*				*				*		*				*	*	1919		
Alaska		*				*		*		*								*				*	*	1915		
Arizona		*		*		*		*				*		*		*		*				*	*	1912		*
Arkansas	*	*				*		*				*										*	*		1883	
California		*		*		*		*		*		*		*		*		*		*		*	*	1911	1887	*
Colorado		*		*		*		*		*		*		*		*		*		*		*	*	1915	1873	*
Connecticut	*	*		*		*				*		*		*		*		*		*			*	1913		*
Delaware	*	*				*						*											*	1917		
Dist. of Columbia	*	*		*		*						*						*		*			*	1919		
Florida	*	*				*												*					*			
Georgia	*	*				*																	*	1916	1890	*
Hawaii		*		*		*		*		*		*		*		*		*		*		*	*	1915	1879	*
Idaho	*	*		*		*		*		*		*		*		*		*		*		*	*	1917	1879	*
Illinois	*	*		*		*		*		*		*		*		*		*		*		*	*	1911	1884	*
Indiana	*	*		*	*	*		*		*		*		*		*		*		*		*	*	1915	1885	*
Iowa	*	*		*		*		*		*		*		*		*		*		*		*	*	1913	1876	*
Kansas		*		*		*						*				*		*		*		*	*	1911	1900	*
Kentucky	*	*		*		*		*		*		*		*		*		*		*		*	*	1915	1887	*
Louisiana	*	*		*		*		*				*				*		*				*	*	1914	1884	*
Maine	*	*		*		*				*		*		*		*		*		*			*	1915	1869	*
Maryland		*		*	*	*		*		*		*		*		*		*		*		*	*	1914	1883	*
Massachusetts	*	*		*	*	*		*		*		*		*		*		*		*		*	*	1911	1887	*
Michigan	*	*		*		*				*		*		*		*		*		*			*	1912	1883	*
Minnesota		*		*		*		*		*		*		*		*		*		*		*	*	1913		
Mississippi	*	*		*		*		*		*				*		*		*		*		*	*		1876	
Missouri	*	*		*		*		*		*						*		*		*		*	*	1919	1893	
Montana	*	*				*		*		*		*				*		*		*		*	*	1915	1887	
Nebraska	*	*		*		*				*		*		*				*		*			*	1913		

State or Territory	Age Limit for Children (1890 1920)	Seats for Women (1890 1920)	Inspection of Factories, Workshops, etc. (1894 1920)	Inspection of Mines (1890 1920)	Inspection of Steam Boilers (1890 1920)	Fire Escapes (1890 1920)	Guards for Dangerous Machinery (1890 1920)	Health of Employees; Ventilation and Sanitation of Factories (1890 1920)	Toilet Rooms (1890 1920)	Report of Accidents in Factories (1920 1920)	Report of Accidents in Mines (1890 1920)	Liability of Employers for Injuries to Employees (1890 1920)	Date of Workmen's Compensation Legislation	Labor Bureau Prior to 1900	Labor Bureau After 1920
Nevada		*		*							*	*	1911		
New Mexico	*		*	*	*	*	*					*	1917		*
New Hampshire	*	*	*		*	*	*	*	*	*		*	1911	1893	*
New Jersey	*	*	*	*	*	*	*	*	*	*	*	*	1911	1878	*
New York	*	*	*	*	*	*	*	*	*	*	*	*	1913	1883	*
North Carolina	*			*	*	*	*	*		*	*	*		1887	*
North Dakota	*	*	*									*	1919	1890	*
Ohio	*	*	*	*	*	*	*	*	*	*	*	*	1911	1877	*
Oklahoma	*			*			*			*	*	*	1915		*
Oregon	*	*	*									*	1913	1872	*
Pennsylvania	*		*	*	*	*	*					*	1915		*
Philippine Isl.	*														*
Porto Rico	*	*	*										1915		*
Rhode Island	*	*	*			*		*	*	*		*	1912	1887	*
South Carolina	*	*	*	*	*		*	*	*	*		*			*
South Dakota	*	*	*	*								*	1917		*
Tennessee	*	*	*									*	1919	1891	*
Texas	*	*	*				*			*		*	1913		*
Utah	*	*	*	*	*	*	*	*	*	*		*	1917		*
Vermont	*	*	*	*	*		*	*	*		*	*	1915		*
Virginia	*	*	*	*	*	*	*	*	*	*	*	*	1918	1898	*
Washington	*	*	*	*	*	*	*	*	*	*	*	*	1911	1897	*
W. Virginia	*	*	*									*	1913	1889	*
Wisconsin	*	*	*	*	*	*	*	*	*	*	*	*	1911	1883	*
Wyoming	*	*	*	*	*		*	*	*	*	*	*	1915		*
United States													{1908 1916}	1884	*
Totals	34	52	19 52	14 50	22 36	23 30	13 34	13 36	21 35	13 43	14 28	22 32	51 54	48	32 40

FEDERAL AND STATE ACTIVITIES IN LABOR PROTECTION

Establishment of Bureaus and Departments of Labor in the United States. According to Carroll D. Wright, in consequence of some agitation started in Massachusetts by the Order of the Knights of St. Crispin, in 1869, and as a direct result of the rejection of the petition of this Order for an act of incorporation, a bill creating the Bureau of Statistics of Labor was suddenly introduced by some shrewd politician and received the Governor's approval June 22, 1869. "Thus was created by the act of the Legislature one of the first offices in the world whose function was the collection of information relating to social and industrial conditions."

The functions of that bureau were defined by law as follows:

The duties shall be to collect, assort, systematize and present in annual reports to the Legislature, on or before the first day of March in each year, statistical detail relating to all departments of labor in the Commonwealth, especially in its relations to commercial, social, educational and sanitary conditions of the laboring classes and to the permanent prosperity of the productive industry of the Commonwealth.

The substance of this language finds a place in nearly every law creating a state bureau in this country, and also in the federal law organizing the United States Bureau of Labor and subsequently the Department of Labor.

Efforts pointing toward the establishment of a federal office date from April 10, 1871, but in spite of repeated attempts nothing was accomplished until out of the various bills previously introduced an act establishing a Bureau of Labor in the Department of the Interior was framed, and was signed by the President June 27, 1884.

The act provided that the Commissioner of Labor shall collect information upon the subject of labor, its relation to capital, the hours of labor, and the earnings of laboring men and women, and also upon the means of promoting their material, social, intellectual and moral prosperity.

Dr. Carroll D. Wright, a scholar, was appointed the first Commissioner of Labor and the office was organized in January, 1885.

After the Bureau of Labor had been in existence three years and had shown the character of its work, which had been largely educational, the "Knights of Labor" demanded the creation of a Department of Labor, to be independent of any of the general departments. This was done by an Act approved June 13, 1888, without, however changing its function. In 1903 when an executive Department of Commerce and Labor was established, the Department became a Bureau of Labor Statistics of said Department, and in 1913, when a separate Department of Labor was created it was transferred to that department.

The Bureau, since its creation in 1885, has had but four bureau chiefs — Carroll D. Wright, who resigned in 1905; Charles P. Neill, who held office until May, 1913; Royal Meeker, who resigned July 31, 1920, and the present commissioner, Ethelbert Stewart, whose appointment took effect August 1, 1920.

The publications of the United States Bureau of Labor Statistics from 1886 to June 15, 1921, consist of 25 *Annual Reports* (discontinued after 1910); 12 special reports; 38 miscellaneous reports; 291 *Bulletins;* 13 special publications, and 12 volumes of the *Monthly Labor Review.* All of these contained items of great educational value, and a large number are of special interest to the student of industrial hygiene.

Bureau of Mines. The Bureau of Mines was created by Chapter 240 of the Acts of 1909–1910 as amended by Acts of February 25, 1913. The object of the Bureau is stated as follows:

It shall be the province and duty of the Bureau of Mines, subject to the approval of the Secretary of the Interior, to conduct inquiries and scientific technologic investigations concerning mining, and the preparation, treatment and utilization of mineral substances with a view to improving health conditions and increasing safety, efficiency, economic development . . . . to investigate explosives . . . . and to disseminate information concerning these subjects in such a manner as will best carry out the purposes of this act. . . .

The Bureau has issued 196 valuable *Bulletins,* among them a number of high grade contributions relating to accident prevention, health and sanitation. Space will not permit many details. It may, however, be said that the creation of the Bureau has been more than justified, as is shown by the following facts. Whereas in 1907, among 680,492 miners employed, 3,242 men, or 6.19 per 1,000 day workers were killed by accidents; in 1918, among 762,426 miners, only 2,580, or 3.94 per 1,000 workers, were killed.

Children's Bureau. Chapter 73 of the Acts of 1911–12 established in the Department of Commerce and Labor a bureau to be known as the Children's Bureau.

The said bureau shall investigate and report to said department upon all matter pertaining to the welfare of children and child-life among all classes of our people, and shall especially investigate the questions of infant mortality, the birth-rate, orphanages, juvenile courts, defectives, dangerous occupations, accidents and diseases of children, employment, legislation affecting children in several states and territories. . . . . The chief of said Bureau may from time to time publish the results of these investigations in such a manner and to such extent as may be presented.

This Bureau was transferred in 1913 to the Department of Labor. It has done useful work for the benefit of present and future genera- tions of American citizens of every class, but more especially for the wage-earning community.

The Bureau has published since its establishment to 1921, 80 special bulletins, 10 child-welfare dodgers, 20 leaflets and 2 charts — one on "State Child Labor Standards," January 1, 1921, and one on "State Compulsory School Attendance Standards Affecting the Em- ployment of Minors."

United States Public Health Service. By an act approved August 14, 1902, the name of the Public Health and Marine Hospital Service was changed to the "Public Health Service," and this branch was authorized to "study and investigate the diseases of man and spread thereof, and to publish information for the public."

Up to this time this service had been chiefly occupied with the study and prevention of communicable diseases and epidemics and the care of seamen of the Merchant Marine, although several important investigations relating to industrial hygiene were made in 1914. In 1915 a division of Industrial Hygiene and Sanitation was organized under the direction of Surgeon J. W. Schereschewsky, now Assistant Surgeon General. The office with a research laboratory was estab- lished in the Marine Hospital, Pittsburgh, Pennsylvania, under the name of "Office of Field Investigations into Occupational Diseases." In April, 1917, the name was changed to the "Office of Field Investigations in Industrial Sanitation." In August, 1918, the Bureau approved a plan signed by the Secretary of the Department of Labor and the Secretary of the Treasury, whereby the Service, through the Office of Field Investigation in Industrial Sanitation, would coöperate with the "Working Conditions Service" of the Department of Labor.

Following Dr. Schereschewsky's transfer to Washington, D. C., to assume charge of the Division of Scientific Research in the Bureau, Dr. A. J. Lanza (then *passed* assistant surgeon in the service) became the incumbent of the office.

In October, 1918, the office and laboratory work was transferred from Pittsburgh to Washington, D. C., and the personnel detailed to the Working Conditions Service was known as the Division of Industrial Hygiene and Medicine. This coöperative work was discontinued June 30, 1919, in view of the fact that no funds were appropriated to continue the work of the Working Conditions Service, and the Division of Industrial Hygiene and Medicine on July 1, 1919, automatically became the "Office of Industrial Hygiene and Sanitation," in charge of Surgeon L. R. Thompson.

Dr. Lanza resigned from the Service in January, 1920, and Dr. Bernard J. Newman, then sanitarian in the Reserve Corps of the Service, took charge. Dr. Newman tendered his resignation from active duty with the Service and is at present a consultant.

The laboratory work is now carried on at the Hygienic Laboratory of the Public Health Service at Washington, D. C., and also in coöperation with a laboratory under Professor Winslow, in which is being made a study of factory ventilation and the industrial dust hazards. The Public Health Service has done excellent work in scientific investigations in a number of occupations and dangerous processes. In March, 1914, the first publication by the division emanated from the pen of Dr. Schereschewsky, on *Trachoma in Steel Mill Workers.* Since this time sixty-seven other contributions have appeared.

The following is the program of the Public Health Service, intended especially to meet after-the-war needs in industrial hygiene:

(a) Continuing and extending health surveys in industry with a view to determining precisely the nature of the health hazards and the measures needed to correct them.

(b)　Securing adequate reports of the prevalence of disease among employees and the sanitary conditions in industrial establishments and communities.

(c)　National development of adequate systems of medical and surgical supervision of employees in places of employment.

(d)　Establishment by the Public Health Service, in coöperation with the Department of Labor, of minimum standards of industrial hygiene and the prevention of occupational diseases.

(e)　Improvement of the sanitation of industrial communities by officers of the Public Health Service, and coöperation with state and local health authorities and other agencies.

(f)　Medical and sanitary supervision by the Public Health Service of civil industrial establishments owned or operated by the Federal Government.

Exhibit of Safety Devices in Washington, D. C.　In 1915 and 1916 the United States Government assembled an excellent exhibit of safety devices in the National Museum in Washington. This exhibit was opened in February 21, 1916, and continued for a week. It had been the hope of those in charge of the exhibit to use it at the end of this period as a railway traveling exhibit in the important industrial cities in the United States. This plan, however, had to be abandoned for lack of funds. It was also hoped that the collection would become the nucleus of a permanent exhibit in the Museum, but this hope has only been partly realized. The exhibit was first suggested by the Bureau of Mines. It was participated in by nineteen government bureaus, the American Red Cross and the Metropolitan Police Department. Many illustrated lectures and addresses explanatory of the exhibit were given, and it is remembered as one of the most remarkable and interesting government exhibitions ever brought together, proving in every respect most effective and satisfactory. The attendance of visitors for the week was 35,447. The governors of the various states had been notified of the national aspect of the exposition, and one of the results of such notification was the meeting of the State Mine Inspectors in the Museum, to which manufacturers and operators from all parts of the country were invited to be present.

COMMUNITY ACTIVITIES IN LABOR PROTECTION

American Association for Labor Legislation.　This Association was organized in New York City, February 15, 1906. The objects of the Association are stated as follows: 1. To serve as the American branch of the International Association for Labor Legislation. 2. To promote uniformity of labor legislation in the United States. 3. To encourage the study of labor conditions in the United States with a view to promoting desirable labor legislation. With only twenty-one charter members, the Association's growth in membership has been most gratifying; the roster at the close of 1920 containing 3,124 names.

In consequence of this growth it became possible to increase the staff of workers and to extend the scope of the Association's activities, so that by 1912 the program of work covered the following divisions: 1. Organization. 2. Investigation. 3. Education. 4. Legislation. The Association has been active in the promotion of conferences on special phases of its work, such as the Conferences on Industrial Diseases in June, 1910 and 1912, and the first National Conference on Social Insurance in June, 1913.

The Association has published over fifty-two editions of the *American Labor Legislation Review*, and has done more for the promotion of labor legislation than any other agency in this country.

Much credit for the success of the Association is due to the zeal and the devotion of the secretary, Dr. John B. Andrews and the assistant secretary, Irene Osgood Andrews, who have been true to the Association's motto, "The fundamental purpose of labor legislation is the conservation of the human resources of the nation."

American Museum of Safety. This meritorious institution was incorporated by Chapter 152 of the Acts of 1911 of the State of New York. The objects are: "To study and promote means and methods of safety and sanitation and the application thereof to any and all public or private occupations . . . . to establish and maintain a museum, library and laboratories and their branches, wherein all matters, methods and means for improving the general condition of the people as to their safety and health may be studied, tested and promoted, with a view of lessening the number of casualties and avoiding the causes of physical suffering and premature death; and to disseminate the results of such study, researches and tests, by lectures, exhibitions and other publications."

Dr. William H. Tolman was the first director of the Museum, and he, as well as Dr. N. E. Ditman, who had charge of the department of Industrial Hygiene, has rendered a very important service to the country.

Mr. Albert A. Hopkins, the present acting director, writes me that the Museum of Safety is now known as the "Safety Institute of America." For lack of suitable quarters the Museum was closed January 1, 1920, but it is the intention to resume this activity in the fall. During the past two years the Institute has conducted, under the auspices of the Metropolitan Safety Council (a combination of the National Safety Council and the Safety Institute of America for the Metropolitan District), lecture courses for safety supervisors and foremen in New York City, Long Island City and Newark, New Jersey. The purpose of these lectures has been to stimulate and render more efficient the safety work in the industries in the Metropolitan District. The safety movement is making rapid strides and contributing fundamental values to industry. The courses have been well attended, and proved of great interest to "safety-men."

The Institute has published, in book form, the lectures on *Safety Fundamentals*, and also the magazine, *Safety*, which is a high grade periodical. The Institute maintains an excellent library, and has a collection of lantern slides, which are loaned to schools and for safety rallies.

The American Museum of Safety had obtained a lease from the city of New York for the occupation of the Arsenal in Central Park, but the matter was contested in the courts and was decided by the Court of Appeals in favor of the Parks and Playgrounds Association. It is to be hoped that the great metropolis of New York may soon erect and maintain at least as good a museum for wage earners as Berlin provided as early as 1904 and Vienna in 1909. At the present writing there is only one museum of the kind in operation in this country, and this one is located in Jersey City, New Jersey.

The Institute has authority to award six different medals:

1. The *Scientific American* Medal, awarded eight times for the most efficient safety device invented within a certain number of years and exhibited at the Museum.

2. The Traveller's Insurance Company's Medal, awarded seven times to the American employer who has done notable work in protecting the lives and limbs of workers.

3. The Louis Livingston Seaman Medal, awarded six times for progress and achievement in the promotion of hygiene and the mitigation of occupational disease. (Dr. Alvah H. Doty of New York was the recipient of the medal in 1911 and Surgeon General William C. Gorgas in 1914.)

4. The Rathenau Medal, awarded twice for the best device or process in the electrical industry, safeguarding life and health.

5. The E. H. Harriman Memorial Medal awarded five times to the American steam railroad which during the year has been the most successful in protecting the lives and health of its employees and of the public.

6. The Anthony N. Brady Memorial Medal, awarded three times to that American electric railway company which for the year of the award has done most to conserve the safety and health of its employees and of the public.

Organization of the Section on Industrial Hygiene in the American Public Health Association. In 1914 the writer was invited by the president of the American Public Health Association to deliver an address on the "History and Development of Industrial Hygiene in the United States," at one of the general sessions of the meeting of the Association at Jacksonville, Florida, November 30 to December 4, 1914.

The other contributors to the symposium were Dr. E. R. Hayhurst, chief of the Survey of Occupational Diseases, State Board of Health of Ohio, who discussed "The Prevalence of Occupational Factors in Disease and Suggestion for their Elimination," Dr. John B. Andrews, secretary, American Association of Labor Legislation, who presented the subject of "Health Insurance," and Dr. C. T. Graham-Rogers, of the New York Department of Labor, who read a paper on "Industrial Hygiene the Basis of Industrial Efficiency."

At the meeting of the executive committee of the Association, Secretary Gunn strongly urged the organization of a Section on Industrial Hygiene, and upon the petition of ten or more signers, including the names of Drs. W. A. Evans, E. L. Fisk, Alice Hamilton, E. R. Hayhurst, B. S. Warren and others, the Executive Committee recommended that the section be organized. At a later period the Executive Committee appointed the following officers of the section; President, Dr. George M. Kober, Washington; Vice President, Dr. Alice Hamilton, Chicago; Secretary, Dr. E. R. Hayhurst, Columbus, Ohio. The section met for the first time at the Rochester meeting, September 6-10, 1915.

EDUCATIONAL INSTITUTIONS OFFERING COURSES IN INDUSTRIAL
MEDICINE

It is reasonable to assume that all medical schools in this country which have courses in hygiene and public health also have eight to ten lectures on industrial hygiene and the more dangerous occupations. American text-books on hygiene, like Harrington's, Rosenau's and Park's, devote special chapters to this subject.

The writer has pursued this plan of special lectures since 1890, with a view to stimulating the interest of his students in one of the most beneficent subdivisions of hygiene. He is of the opinion that this is about all that can be undertaken in the undergraduate courses of medical schools and was therefore greatly pleased when opportunities were afforded for postgraduate work.

Massachusetts Institute of Technology. Prof. C. E. Turner writes: "It appears that instruction in industrial hygiene in the Department of Biology and Public Health at the Massachusetts Institute of Technology began about 1905, when C.-E. A. Winslow began giving instruction in this subject. In 1908 Professor Gunn came back to the 'Tech' to teach and continued instruction in industrial hygiene until he left the 'Tech' during the period of the war. I have been giving this course only since my post-war return to the 'Tech' in 1919."

The *Harvard Medical School* established in 1910 courses in public health in connection with the Massachusetts Institute of Technology, in which considerable attention was given to industrial hygiene. In June, 1918, Harvard University was the first institution in the world to establish a course of instruction and research leading to degrees in industrial hygiene. Work was begun in the session of 1918–1919 and instruction has been offered for each of the subsequent years. Courses leading to the certificate on public health in industrial hygiene include: applied physiology of industry; methods of air analysis; industrial toxicology; vital statistics; industrial sanitation; preventive medicine and hygiene; industrial health administration; employment management; workmen's compensation and the legal aspects of industrial disease; nutrition; industrial surgery, orthopedic surgery and industrial medicine. These subjects also form the work of the first year for candidates for the degree of doctor of public health in industrial hygiene, the second year being devoted to an investigation upon some phase of industrial health. Work in the occupational disease clinic at the Massachusetts General Hospital is required of all students of industrial medicine who hold the medical degree. The staff of the division of industrial hygiene of this school has published 38 noteworthy contributions to industrial hygiene from November, 1917, to May, 1921, many of which are based on laboratory research. Among the noteworthy investigations are the following: the dust content of air in various industries; new apparatus for dust collection and dust measurement; effects of mineral dusts; chronic manganese poisoning; poisoning by lead, ether, tetrachlorethane and trinitrotoluene; a study of oil folliculitis; health in mercantile establishments, etc. It publishes the *Journal of Industrial Hygiene*.

The College of Medicine of the Ohio State University in 1915 offered in its department of public health and sanitation elective courses in industrial hygiene and preventive medicine to undergraduate medical students. Students in the graduate schools have been permitted to specialize in industrial hygiene and preventive medicine. These courses were dropped during the war, but during 1920–21 a few students, candidates for the degree of master of science were specializing in this subject. Dr. E. R. Hayhurst, who has been an ardent advocate of special courses in industrial hygiene for a number of years says: "I have had over 100 students for each year for the past two years in our undergraduate two-hour course entitled 'Industrial Hygiene.' The present industrial slump is not propitious for activity in advanced training in this line, but I believe this is only temporary."

Johns Hopkins University. The School of Hygiene and Public Health was opened in October, 1918, under the direction of Dr. Wm. H. Welch, and considerable attention is given to industrial hygiene. Important studies of fatigue by Spaeth were published in 1919–20, and a method for determining the finer dust particles in air (Meyer) Journal of Industrial Hygiene, June, 1921.

The Rush Medical College of the University of Chicago offers to senior medical students a 48-hour clinical and conference course. Another course in the department of hygiene and bacteriology is offered on dangerous trades, industrial health hazards, and occupational diseases, to which also sociological students are admitted.

The Medical Department of the University of Pennsylvania as early as 1906 in connection with courses in public health leading to the degree of doctor of public health, placed considerable emphasis upon industrial hygiene, including inspection of industrial plants; service in first-aid stations and emergency hospitals in some of the larger plants, and the occupational disease clinic of the University Hospital. This school of hygiene has made studies of: (1) health hazards of cigar manufacturing; (2) dust hazards in certain industries; (3) anilin fumes in the air; (4) anthrax problem in horsehair; (5) CO_2 and CO content of air in a felt-hat factory; (6) conditions in an organic color mixing plant; (7) oil grinders' furunculosis in a steel ball-bearing factory; (8) condition of the lungs of workers in stove foundries. Numbers 1, 2, 7, and 8 were made in collaboration with the clinic for occupational diseases of the University Hospital.

The Medical School of Yale University offers to its students in the public health courses (begun 1917) opportunities to specialize in industrial hygiene and to carry on research work. The University, in connection with the United States Public Health Service, has an experimental laboratory for the study of factory ventilation and the industrial dust hazards (Shuford). Professor C.-E. A. Winslow and his associates Greenburg and Angermeyer have carried on some of these studies in the abrasive industry, polishing shops, grinding shops of an ax factory, among sandblasters, etc.; a number of studies of the katathermometer, and miscellaneous factory inspections have also been made.

The Medical School of the University of Cincinnati in October, 1919, established courses of one year, open to graduates in medicine and leading to a certificate of public health in industrial medicine. The program includes the training of students in industrial medicine and public health, and field work among the industries, also coöperation of the department with the National Safety Council. The training of students in the clinical aspects of industrial medicine is provided by an occupational disease clinic and the medical departments in local industrial plants.

The University of Cincinnati is not listed on page 538 of the Journal of the American Medical Association August 13, 1921 which in addition to the schools already mentioned enumerates the following as having graduate courses in public health. The *University of Wisconsin* began in 1910; the *University of Michigan*, in 1913; *Detroit College of Medicine and Surgery*, 1913; the *University of California*, 1915; *University and Bellevue Hospital Medical College*, 1916; *Albany Medical College*, 1920. Two other institutions, the University of Colorado and Tulane University, suspended their courses in 1918.

The *Ohio State Department of Health* has maintained a very efficient division of industrial hygiene under the supervision of E. R. Hayhurst which includes the investigation of occupational disease complaints, gives advice to individual plants, commissions, and employees, and also does special research work.

Recently an *Industrial Health Service Bureau* has been established in Chicago under competent leadership, which offers its services in furnishing sources of information concerning the organization of the health work in industries, schools and institutions. The Bureau also offers two postgraduate courses in industrial medicine and surgery, beginning July 6, 1921: a three weeks' course of lectures and demonstrations and work in clinics and industrial establishments in Chicago; an additional three weeks' course of demonstration and observation in industrial plants may be taken by those who have completed the first three weeks' course.

Dr. Hayhurst has furnished me with an elaborate table of medical schools which offer courses in public health leading to degrees and which presumably give attention likewise to industrial hygiene. Apart from those already referred to are the following: University of Iowa; Minnesota; Missouri; Chicago; Leland Stanford; Columbia; University of Louisville; McGill University, Montreal; Queen's University, Kingston, Ontario; University of Toronto; Wellesley College; American Institute of Medicine. A list given by Eugene C. Howe, *American Journal of Public Health*, Aug., 1918, pp. 600-607, includes Chicago Hospital College of Medicine.

According to Thompson, of the medical schools not already referred to in detail, the following have done or are carrying on research work: *University of California,* Department of Hygiene: investigations in progress on "packers' itch," a skin disease found among packers using infected straw, and on a peculiar infection of the fingers of dried fig packers. *The College of Physicians and Surgeons of Columbia University,* New York, Department of Physiology, under the able direction of Professor Frederic S. Lee, has made a number of important studies of industrial fatigue. *The College of Medicine, University of Iowa,* Division of Hygiene, published in 1920 a study of health hazards in the pearl button industry, made by Birge and Havens. *Leland Stanford Junior University,* Department of Physiology, has published "Strength Tests in Industry" (Martin) and "Studies of the Effects of Tobacco on Mental and Physical Work." In addition to these medical schools, the *Henry Phipps Institute* of Philadelphia has made studies on factors affecting the health of garment workers, and various effects of dust inhalation, etc. This Institute coöperates with the University of Pennsylvania in industrial hygiene surveys in Philadelphia. *The William H. Singer Memorial Research Laboratory,* Pittsburgh, has made industrial studies on the prevention of epidemic influenza, based on about 50,000 steel workers and railroad employees; unresolved pneumonia, associated with severe anthracosis; trinitrotoluene poisoning. *The Mellon Institute of Pittsburgh* has likewise carried on important researches in industrial medicine. *The Nela Research Laboratory* of the National Lamp Works, General Electric Company, Cleveland, Ohio, has published results of experimental investigations on the physiology and psychology of illumination, glasses for protecting the eyes in industrial processes, injurious effects of ultra-violet rays, etc.

The Psychological Laboratory of Bryn Mawr College has made similar studies. *The Nutrition Laboratory* of the *Carnegie Institution* has made and published studies on the influence of various factors upon metabolism, such as variations of temperature, muscular work, etc.; on the effect of under-nutrition, ingestion of alcohol as affecting skilled muscular performance, etc. *The Houghton Research Staff* (E. F. Houghton & Co.), Philadelphia, has made investigations and published in 1920, "Investigations of the Causes of Skin Sores and Boils Among Metal Workers." *The Cleveland Hospital Council* made an elaborate hospital and health survey of Cleveland, including an industrial survey (1920). *The National Industrial Conference Board* has issued a series of research reports on "Hours of Work as Related to Output and Health of Workers" in various industries; also a research report on "Health Service in Industry." *The Cabot Fund* has made investigations of the present condition of the steel and iron industry with reference to the eight-hour day in Great Britain and the twelve-hour day and the seven day week in the United States (1921). *The Carnegie Foundation* (Americanization Studies) has issued a "Study of the Special Medical Sanitary and Health Problems Due to Immigrant Employees" (1921).

OCCUPATIONAL DISEASE CLINICS

1910. The first occupational disease clinic in this country was established by Dr. W. Gilman Thompson in connection with the Cornell University Medical College in New York City in 1910. This clinic was discontinued when Dr. Thompson resigned from that institution in 1916.

1911. In July, 1911, the Sprague Memorial Institute of the University of Chicago established a special clinic for occupational diseases in connection with the Rush Medical College. It is now operated as an evening clinic. This Institute in 1913–14 supported special investigations (by Bassoe) of compressed air disease, and occupational brass and lead poisoning (by Hayhurst). During the world war it supported investigations on the toxicity of various explosives or chemicals used in munition plants. (Thompson).

1913. According to Dr. Wade Wright, the first attempt to study industrial disease in the Massachusetts General Hospital was made in 1913 when a social worker began work in the out-patient department to whom were referred by the visiting physicians such cases as they considered of industrial interest or importance. In March, 1916, a regular industrial clinic was operated, the staff eventually consisting of one full-time salaried physician, a full-time industrial social worker, a secretary, and a number of volunteer social workers. The importance of careful study of industrial poisoning is shown by the fact that during the first year after the establishment of this clinic, 148 cases of lead poisoning were diagnosed while in the previous five years only 147 cases were reported in the various departments of the hospital. There were 54 cases of industrial dermatosis, exclusive of anthrax, of which there were 18 cases; 19 persons were affected by naphtha fumes, usually in the chronic form. There were 12 cases of caisson disease, none very acute, and 46 cases in the group of miscellaneous diagnoses.

1914. The hospital of the University of Pennsylvania organized an occupational disease clinic more as a center for consultation and investigation than as a place for treatment. Apart from the investigations already mentioned in connection with the department of hygiene, special studies have been made of pulmonary diseases in potters and cement workers; women employees in the textile industry; and comparative investigations of dust within and without the buildings.

1915. In 1915 Dr. S. S. Goldwater, the health commissioner of New York City, established a clinic exclusively devoted to occupational diseases in connection with the Health Department. Since then the Department has established an occupational clinic in each borough of the city.

In 1915 the Medical College of the Ohio State University inaugurated an occupational disease clinic.

The School of Medicine of Washington University held each week an industrial clinic in its out-patient department.

The Cincinnati General Hospital established an occupational disease clinic in which all the services of the hospital participate.

1920. The American Hospital, Chicago, established an industrial department. The Delray Industrial Hospital, Detroit, has for a number of years also operated an out-door department.

The Joint Board of Sanitary Control of the Cloak and Suit Industry, New York City, has established a clinic for workers in that industry which is supported by joint contributions from employees and employers.

A RETROSPECT OF AMERICAN LITERATURE

The growth of interest in the United States in the subject of general and industrial hygiene and occupational diseases since the birth of the American Public Health Association may be judged by the following facts:

The index catalogue of the library of the Surgeon General's Office shows that prior to 1880 there were but 80 subjects indexed by American authors, including 5 books and monographs, and 75 journal articles, against 166 contributions by English authors, of which 16 were books and monographs.

Among the earliest American contributions should be mentioned Dr. B. W. McCready's "On the Influence of Trades, Professions and Occupations," the prize dissertation for 1837 of the New York State Medical Society. Dr. F. A. Walker, of Boston, in 1869 published a monograph on "Occupation of the People." Dr. J. T. Wilson delivered an address on "Diseases Incident to Some Occupations," which was published in the *Transactions of the Medical Society of Youngstown, Ohio,* 1879–1880.

During the period between 1880 and 1900 English authors made 39 contributions to the literature and American authors but 22.

Among the American contributions should be mentioned an article on the "Hygiene of the Laboring Classes," by William J. Scott, and one written by Dr. George H. Rohé on the "Hygiene of Occupations," (1884) followed in 1886 by Dr. J. H. Ireland's essay on "The Preventable Causes of Disease, Injury and Death in American Manufacture and Workshops and the Best Means for Preventing and Avoiding Them," the Lomb Prize essay.

In 1895 Dr. J. H. Lloyd wrote an excellent article on "Diseases of Occupations." In 1896 a striking editorial on industrial hygiene appeared in the *Transactions* of the American Public Health Association. The editorial discussed the report of a parliamentary committee which embraced 134 works or factories in Great Britain. The occupations included bronzing, steam locomotives, India rubber works, the use of inflammable paint, dry cleaning, and aerated waters.

From 1900, and more especially from 1908 contributions from American authors have increased with wonderful rapidity so that by June 30, 1921, 702 subjects had been indexed in the library of the Surgeon General's Office as compared with 169 by English authors. These subjects are indexed under the following headings: occupation accidents; occupation, diseases incident to; occupation diseases, jurisprudence; occupation diseases, legislature; occupation diseases, notification; occupation diseases, prevention of; occupation, hygiene of; occupations, hygiene exhibits; occupations, statistics; occupation therapy.

Reference has already been made to the early publications of the Bureau and Department of Labor, which have been of great educational value in stimulating the enactment of labor and factory laws. In 1902 Dr. Kober, upon request of the Hon. Carroll D. Wright, commissioner of the Department of Labor, recommended his former student, Dr. C. F. W. Doehring, for the purpose of making an investigation of the manufacture of white lead, paint, etc., and of the manufacture of linseed oil, varnishes, oil cloth and linoleum, tallow, fertilizers, etc. The results of this investigation, the first of its kind in this country, were published under the title of "Factory Sanitation and Labor Protection" in *Bulletin 44*, January, 1903. In 1905 the State

Board of Health of Massachusetts submitted a brief report on the conditions affecting the health and safety of employees in factories and other establishments. This report was supplemented in 1907 by a more exhaustive report. In 1906, according to Dr. Mock, Dr. Frank Fulton of Providence, R. I., began a physical examination of employees among the workers in a large saw factory. This he did free of charge for the purpose of discovering tuberculous workmen. Dr. Mock undertook the examination of the employees of Sears, Roebuck & Co., Chicago, in 1909, and refers to reports setting forth the benefits of this practice, by Dr. Irving Clark, of the Norton Grinding Co., Worcester, Mass.; Dr. Otto Geier, of the Cincinnati Milling Machine Co.; Wilbur Post, of the Peoples Gas Co., Chicago; Dr. C. G. Farnum, of the Avery Company, Peoria, Illinois; Dr. S. M. McCurdy, of the Youngstown Sheet and Tube Co., Dr. Lowe, of the Goodrich Rubber Co. A splendid symposium was presented before the National Tuberculosis Association in 1914, and at present writing physical examination of employees, in spite of considerable opposition at first, has been found most beneficent to workers afflicted with all forms of diseases, which when discovered in their incipiency can be checked.*

In September, 1907, during the International Congress on Hygiene at Berlin, the writer met Dr. E. J. Neisser, who had just completed an *International Review of Industrial Hygiene* covering a volume of 352 pages. Dr. Neisser deplored his inability to present an extended review of the work accomplished in the United States, since with the exception of the Department of Labor and one or two states, no data concerning factory sanitation were available. Realizing the importance of the subject, not only to wage-earners, but to all interested in the conditions under which our fellow men live and work, he returned with the determination to do what he could for the promotion of industrial hygiene. Fortunately an excellent opportunity was afforded by his appointment as secretary of President Roosevelt's Homes Commission. In February, 1908, he submitted as chairman of the Committee on Social and Industrial Betterment a "Report on Industrial

---

*Mock, Harry A. "Industrial Medicine and Surgery, a Résumé of Its Development and Scope." *Journal of Industrial Hygiene*, May 3, 1919.

and Personal Hygiene," covering 175 pages. This was followed in December, 1908, by a "Report of the Committee on Social Betterment," covering 281 pages. It was hoped that this somewhat hasty study of the causes of sickness, and the means of promoting industrial efficiency and earning power would direct attention to the need of a more critical study and of remedial legislation in the country. This hope, thanks to the general publicity given these publications by the lay and medical press and the interest aroused among officials, social workers and thoughtful employers, has been fully realized, as shown not only by doubling the amount of protective legislation since 1907, but also by the gratifying increase in American literature on the subject.

In November, 1908, and May, 1909, Dr. Frederick L. Hoffman's valuable monographs on "The Mortality from Consumption in the Dusty Trades" were published by the United States Bureau of Labor. Dr. George M. Price, a pioneer in public health work and author of a *Handbook on Sanitation* (1901), wrote in 1908 an 80,000-word article on "Occupational Hygiene" for Wood's *Reference Handbook of Medical Sciences*. In January, 1910, the epoch-making report of Dr. John B. Andrews on "Phosphorus Poisoning in the Match Industry in the United States" appeared in *Bulletin 86 of the United States Bureau of Labor Statistics*.

On June 10, 1910, the First National Conference on Industrial Diseases met at Chicago at the call of the American Association for Labor Legislation. "The present situation of our Association," said Prof. Henry W. Farnam of Yale University, then president, in his opening address, "is like that of a watchman on a high tower. He does not know exactly how the attack is to be made but he knows enough to justify him in giving the alarm and in advising that scouts be sent out to ascertain more precisely the strength and position of the foe. In this warfare against industrial diseases we need the operation of many different people. This is a warfare in which science, labor, business enterprise and government must all unite."

At this meeting a committee was appointed to present a memorial to President Taft on the magnitude and importance of the subject.

Although hampered by lack of official American statistics on sickness, the committee estimated that among 33,500,000 occupied persons in this country, there were lost every year 284,750,000 days through illness, at an economic loss of $772,892,860. Assuming that at least one quarter of the sickness was due to strictly preventable causes, it was estimated that by deliberate efforts no less than $193,000,000 could be saved to the nation annually. Plans were presented for further study of the question by a commission of experts representing preventive medicine, sanitary engineering, and industrial chemistry.

In 1910, Dr. W. Gilman Thompson, professor of medicine in the Cornell University Medical College, organized an informal committee for studying occupational diseases, which was composed of experts in industrial chemistry, medicine, economics, social service, insurance, and labor legislation. The committee was absorbed in 1914 by the American Association for Labor Legislation, which created a committee on industrial hygiene, of which Dr. Thompson was made the chairman.

In 1910 the Illinois State Commission on Occupational Diseases began its labors and in 1911 published a large number of specific instances of industrial poisoning contracted by wage-earners in the discharge of their employment. In July, 1911, the Bureau of Labor Statistics published in *Bulletin 95* the result of an extensive study by Dr. Alice Hamilton, which disclosed 388 cases of lead posioning, of which 16 were fatal in the white lead and lead oxide industries in the United States from January, 1910, to April 30, 1911. The same bulletin also contained a report by Dr. John B. Andrews on 60 deaths from industrial lead poisoning actually reported in New York in 1909 and 1910.

The report on lead poisoning in potteries, tile works and in porcelain and enameled sanitary ware factories, by Dr. Alice Hamilton, and her admirable monograph on the hygiene of painters, were published by the Bureau of Labor Statistics in 1912 and 1913. These were followed by a report on lead poisoning in the smelting and refining industry, 1914. Since then Dr. Hamilton has made special investigations and reports on other industrial posions. Dr. William C. Hanson's monograph on the dangers to workers from dust and fumes and methods of protection, illustrated with 62 photographs, was published by the Bureau in 1913.

Much excellent work of a highly educational character has been accomplished by the special commissions for the study and prevention of occupational diseases and numerous official and private investigators.

In 1911 the National Safety Council was organized and later created a section on health service, which held its first session in connection with the Fourth Annual Congress of the National Safety Council at Philadelphia in October, 1915. Excellent work has been done in the past, and a committee is now investigating the best modes of preventing and controlling occupational skin diseases. This organization was the result of joint action by the Association of Iron and Steel Electrical Engineers and the Coöperative Safety Congress, and took the name of "National Council for Industrial Safety," the fundamental purpose of the organization being the promotion of safety to human life in the industries of the United States.

In September, 1912, the Fifteenth International Congress on Hygiene and Demography was held in the city of Washington. Section IV of this Congress, devoted to the hygiene of occupation, was presided over by the writer. The transactions of this section covered 986 printed pages consisting of 8 English, 2 French, 2 Italian, 8 German, 1 Belgian, 1 Japanese, 1 Austrian, and 41 American contributions. This Congress, as also the Sixth International Congress for the prevention of Tuberculosis, held in the same city in 1908, with their excellent exhibits illustrating the dangers of numerous occupations, stimulated a profound interest in the subject of industrial hygiene.

It is doubtless true that the 64 contributions from distinguished experts covering all phases of the subject laid the foundation for a scientific literature on industrial medicine in this country. Much credit is also due to the Section of Industrial Chemistry of the American Chemical Society and other national societies mentioned previously.

In 1912, as already stated, the United States Public Health Service created a Division on Industrial Hygiene with Dr. J. W. Schereschewsky in charge. In the same year Miss Josephine Goldmark of New York published a very comprehensive study of fatigue in its industrial aspects.

In June, 1914, Dr. W. Gilman Thompson's treatise on *Occupational Diseases* was published. Dr. Thompson, as already pointed out, was one of the first among American physicians to appreciate the importance of occupational diseases from the medical, social and economic point of view. He has made a number of valuable contributions to the literature on this subject and his writings and activities have been exceedingly fruitful. In the same year, Dr. George M. Price of New York, having presented an excellent address on "Medical Factory Inspection" before the Congress for the Prevention of Tuberculosis, followed up his good work by a splendid book of 574 pages, entitled *The Modern Factory*. In the same year the American Public Health Association created its Section on Industrial Hygiene.

In 1915 Dr. Otto P. Geier, the chairman of the Section on Hygiene and Preventive Medicine of the American Medical Association, and one of the most ardent pioneers in industrial hygiene and medicine, prepared a splendid symposium for the San Francisco meeting, Since then these subjects have found a place on every program of that Section.

In 1915 and 1916 the United States government assembled an excellent exhibit on safety devices in the National Museum in Washington, which was opened in February, 1916. In 1915 a "survey of industrial health hazards and occupational diseases" was made in Ohio, under the direction of Dr. E. R. Hayhurst. The report containing the results of the investigation, published by the Ohio State Board of Health, constitutes one of the most valuable American contributions on the subject to date.

In 1916 a book entitled *Diseases of Occupations and Vocational Hygiene*, covering 918 pages, was published by P. Blakiston's Son & Company. The book was written by 29 experts and edited by the writer and Dr. William C. Hanson. In justice to the publishers, it should be stated that the senior editor (the writer of this article) declined their request to write or edit a book in the early part of 1911, because the scarcity of statistical and other data in reference to disease and accident hazards in the various occupations of this country had compelled him in his former writings, especially for his monograph in 1908, to gather most of his facts from European sources. He entertained the hope that with a general awakening in this country and the publication of the transactions of Section IV of the Congress on Hygiene (the program for which he was then preparing) and Dr. Hayhurst's report, above referred to, valuable material on diseases of occupations as they occur in the various states of the Union and in foreign lands would be available. This hope has not been idle.

On June 28, 1917, Mr. Samuel Gompers of the American Federation of Labor and a member of the Council of National Defense, called in Washington a conference of experts to aid him in the formulation of recommendations for the promotion of health and efficiency among the industrial workers in the United States. This conference resulted in the appointment of various committees and the preparation of reports on lighting of industrial establishments, dust hazards, sanitation of rural workmen's areas, and general welfare work. Most of these reports were republished by the United States Public Health Service.

In October, 1917, Dr. Franklin Martin, chairman of the medical section of the Council on National Defense organized a subsection on industrial medicine. According to Dr. Mock, "This committee proposed elaborate plans for the supervision of the health of all workers engaged in essential war occupations. Few of those in authority were familiar with this new field in medicine, and it took weeks and weeks of patient endeavor to sell the idea." On May 27, 1918, Dr. Otto P. Geier, who was the director of the committee, submitted an excellent report on "Industrial Medicine and Surgery as a War Measure."

On July 1, 1918, the President issued an executive order that "All sanitary or public health activities carried on by any executive bureau, agency or office, specially created for or concerned in the prosecution of the existing war, shall be exercised under the supervision and control of the Secretary of the Treasury." The order did not include the Medical Departments of the Army and Navy, but designated the United States Public Health Service as the Bureau of the Treasury Department responsible for the work. This program could not fail to have a beneficent effect on our war-workers.

26

The fundamental principles of Dr. Geier's report should be applied at all times, and a careful study of it will convince every thoughtful person that much remains to be done to prevent the terrific human waste in industry.

In May, 1919, the *Journal of Industrial Hygiene* was established and the founders and supporters of this excellent journal may well feel rewarded by its glorious achievements in the last two years and a half. It is under the editorship of David L. Edsall, a well-known American pioneer in industrial medicine. He enjoys the support of an able staff of associate editors both in this country and in Great Britain, Australia and South Africa, with Dr. Cecil K. Drinker as managing editor.

In the same year *Modern Medicine*, now *The Nation's Health*, a monthly journal, was established in Chicago, and it can be confidently predicted that these two publications will set the pace for all others in the subject of industrial hygiene, medicine and surgery.

In the spring of 1919, the president of the American Federation of Labor invited a number of experts to a conference to assist him in the consideration of a number of important agenda likely to be presented at the International Labor Congress to be held in Washington in October, 1919. It is gratifying to report that at all these conferences the American Public Health Association was largely represented.

In 1919 Dr. Harry A. Mock of Chicago wrote a very timely and creditable volume, entitled *Industrial Medicine and Surgery*, covering 785 pages, published by the Wm. B. Saunders Company of Philadelphia.

Garrison says:

In America the investigations and reports of George M. Kober (1908–16), Frederick L. Hoffmann (1909–16), John B. Andrews (1910–16), and Alice Hamilton (1911–14) on industrial poisons, and of William C. Hanson on dust and fumes (1913) have proved of great value. Important monographs are those of Josephine Goldmark on industrial fatigue (1912), George M. Price on the manufactory (1914), W. Gilman Thompson on occupation diseases (1914) and the coöperative treatise on the same subject edited by George M. Kober and William C. Hanson. . . . .

The best pioneer work was done by the United States Department of Labor, and much was accomplished through the labors of George M. Kober, W. Gilman Thompson, John B. Andrews, Alice Hamilton, J. W. Schereschewsky, S. S. Goldwater, and others.*

*Garrison, Fielding H., *History of Medicine*, 2d Edition, 1917, Wm. B. Saunders Co., Philadelphia.

INDUSTRIAL SURGERY

Progress has not been confined to industrial hygiene and medicine, for it must be recalled that equally great advances have been made in industrial surgery, largely due, as stated by Dr. Mock, to the studies and contributions of such surgeons as Moorhead, Clark, Farnum, Corwin, Harvey, Lauffer, Shoudy, Cotton, Bloodgood, Edward Martin, Lounsbury, Warnshius, Mock, and others.

In 1914 a "Conference Board of Physicians in Industrial Practice" was organized, with headquarters in New York City, and Dr. Magnus as secretary. Its activities were largely focused in the Eastern states. Many of the leaders in industrial medicine and surgery were numbered among its members, some of the greatest contributions to this specialty having been made by this group. In the same year great advances were also made in the mining and lumber regions of the far west, largely due to the efforts of Doctors Corwin, of Colorado, Tucker, Philip King Brown, and R. T. Legge, of California and Dr. Yokom, of Washington.

In 1916 the American Association of Industrial Physicians and Surgeons was organized in Detroit. The objects of this Association are to "stimulate scientific study and research in all branches of industrial medicine, to stimulate industries to adopt a comprehensive health service and to raise the standards of the physicians engaged in industrial practice." Much credit is due to Dr. Harry A. Mock and Dr. Francis D. Patterson and 125 other charter members for inaugurating this movement. The Association has now about 600 members, and we quite agree with Dr. Mock that the combined efforts of this body have undoubtedly done more to increase the benefits from this work to both employees and employers than any other one agency which has entered the field.

PHYSICAL RECONSTRUCTION OF DISABLED WORKERS IN THE INDUSTRIES

According to Mock, several industries with comprehensive systems of industrial medicine and surgery have been practising the best forms of reconstruction of the disabled for many years, although their work was not so designated. In fact the medical staffs of these concerns have developed a more practical coördinated system of reconstruction than any yet devised by our government or any of the other nations in this war. The terms conservation and reclamation more clearly define the scope of their efforts in industry than do the terms physical reconstruction and rehabilitation.

But whatever terms are used to designate this work the desired results can only be attained by a completely rounded-out plan similar to that developed in these industries. It includes: 1. Prevention of disease and accident. 2. Constant health supervision. 3. Adequate medical and surgical care for all disabled. 4. Proper selection of work according to the physical qualifications of each individual, including properly chosen work for the handicapped men upon recovery. 5. Practical vocational training in the plant for men in new occupations when the disability prevents return to the old job. 6. Sufficient compensation for the disabled man and his dependents to live on while he is undergoing reconstruction."

On July 18, 1918, Dr. W. Gilman Thompson established a clinic for functional reëducation of disabled soldiers in New York City, but it has also from the first dealt with civilian cripples. During the first year of the clinic's work 1150 cases were treated of which about 50 per cent were civilians. The clinic conducts departments of electrotherapy and thermotherapy, hydrotherapy, mechanotherapy, and a social science department. Dr. Thompson writes that the clinic since February 15, 1921, is known as the "Reconstruction Hospital" and has treated more than 3500 patients. It must be gratifying to Drs. Mock, Thompson, and others that their ideals are being rapidly realized, since we are told by one of the leading advocates, Dr. John B. Andrews, secretary of the American Association for Labor Legislation, that Congress has provided for federal-state coöperation in the work of rehabilitating injured workmen, and nearly half of the states have already taken advantage of this provision.

THE PROBLEM OF ECONOMIC LOSS AND WASTE IN INDUSTRY ARISING FROM LOWERED HEALTH CONDITIONS, SICKNESS AND ACCIDENT AMONG THE WORKING POPULATION

Dr. Eugene Lyman Fisk, medical director of the Life Extension Institute, has recently rendered an excellent report with the above title to the Hoover Commission, the perusal of which is urgently recommended. Dr. Fisk has kindly placed at my disposal his manuscript from which I shall offer extracts. Before doing so it may not be amiss to quote the following from my report of President Roosevelt's Homes Commission written in 1908:*

Industrial disease and accidents are everywhere assuming more and more importance and our knowledge should be based upon accurate data. In countries like Great Britain, where reports of certain diseases are compulsory, it is quite possible to secure for example reliable data as to the number of cases of lead poisoning, and other specific industrial diseases. The same may be said of the facilities afforded by the statistics of the German industrial insurance institutes, which furnish not only the number of deaths, but also the number of cases treated, together with the age period and the duration of the disease. Similar facts should be collected in this country. This is all the more important when it is remembered that even with the most complete statistics, it is extremely difficult to determine all the factors which influence the health and longevity of operatives. Great differences are found in the conditions under which the work is performed, some of which are entirely avoidable, while others are not, and it is hardly fair to characterize certain occupations as dangerous when experience has shown that no harm results when proper safeguards have been taken. In the consideration of this question, the personal element of the workmen, their habits, mode of life, food, home environments, etc., cannot be ignored.

Progress has crowned the efforts of those interested in the prevention of human waste in the industries, but much more remains to be done before we can claim that victory is in sight. It is one thing to enact laws for the protection of labor, but it is infinitely more important to see to it that existing laws are enforced, and if inadequate to secure the enactment of better laws. Even now state laws lack uniformity and proper standards for correct ventilation, illumination and sanitation of factories, mills, mercantile establishments and other work places, and much of the criticism the writer offered in his report of President Roosevelt's Homes Commission in 1908 is to a great extent even true to-day. Dr. E. R. Hayhurst and Messrs. W. H. Dittoe and W. C. Groeniger of the Ohio State Board of Health have prepared standards for the text-book on *Diseases of Occupation and Vocational Hygiene,* now undergoing revision.

It is less than 15 years since serious attention has been paid to industrial hygiene in this country, but fortunately the effects of legislation and factory sanitation, together with the gospel of personal

*Senate Document No. 644, 60th Congress, 1909.

hygiene and higher standards of living conditions are already strikingly shown by a most marked decrease in the mortality from tuberculosis in eight of the most dangerous trades in the state of New Jersey.

Dr. F. S. Crum, assistant statistician of the Prudential Insurance Co., has kindly furnished me with tables showing that the percentage of mortality from tuberculosis in *hatters* has been reduced from 29.7 in the period of 1909–1913 to 23.6 in the period of 1914–1918; the pneumonia rate during the same period has been reduced from 8.5 to 7, and other respiratory diseases from 4.9 to 2.3. In *stone cutters* the percentage of deaths from tuberculosis during the same period has been reduced from 26.3 to 19.7; in *metal grinders*, from 39.2 to 29.1; in *molders, founders, and casters*, from 19.7 to 17.4; in *other iron and steel workers*, from 24 to 17.2, and in *plumbers*, from 32.5 to 22.6. There was no decrease in the *textile industry*, the rate in the period 1909–1913 being 21.3, and in 1914–1918 21.7 per cent.

In *potters* there was an increase in the percentage of tuberculosis from 32.4 (1907–1913) to 36.6 during the period from 1914–1918. This increase, fortunately, does not indicate an increased hazard, for by reference to the tables it will be noted that there was a distinct decrease at ages between 10 and 39, showing that the protective measures are really effective in all newcomers, but that they could not avert the damage inflicted in the older workers before the adoption of the present safeguards.*

LOSSES FROM PREVENTABLE SICKNESS AMONG WAGE-EARNERS AND OTHERS

Dr. Eugene L. Fisk, in his report already referred to, cites Professor Irving Fisher's report on *National Vitality* for the National Conservation Committee appointed by President Roosevelt in 1909, estimating that there were about 3,000,000 persons seriously ill at all times in the United States, and that 42 per cent of this illness was preventable with a resulting extension of life of over 15 years.

The investigations of the U. S. Commission on Industrial Relations in 1913–1915 which cover a survey of the sickness prevalent among approximately a million workers of representative occupations, revealed an average loss to more than 30,000,000 American wage-earners of about 9 days per year.

The data collected during 1915–1917 by the Metropolitan Life Insurance Company covering 637,038 white and colored persons show an average loss from sickness of 5.8 days for males and 6.9 days for females.

---

*Tables omitted for lack of space.

The general death-rate in the United States registration area has fallen from 17.6 per 1,000 in 1900 to 12.9 per 1,000 in 1919, so that since Professor Fisher's report was issued, according to Dr. Fisk,

. . . . a considerable measure of his prediction has been fulfilled. The duration of life has probably been extended a period of five years and the estimate of 13 days annual loss from illness must now be reduced to approximately seven. Changes that have taken place in the death-rates from some of the principal diseases that contributed to the morbidity rate when the "Report on National Vitality" was issued, furnish consistent and confirmatory evidence of the facts suggested by the morbidity surveys herein quoted that there is now less disability and sickness present, than there was even 15 years ago. He also points out the significant fact, that the death-rate from organic diseases is greater in this country than in England and Wales and that the death-rate in the middle age of life is now likewise greater, although not formerly so, and that there is evident need to combat the chronic maladies like diseases of the heart, arteries, etc., that limit the work span and are not now systematically attacked as are typhoid, tuberculosis and venereal diseases.

The general death-rate among those employed at ages 15 to 65 as estimated (by Dr. Louis I. Dublin, cited by Fisk) on the basis of the industrial insurance mortality experience for the year 1920 was 11.46 per 1000 living. An estimate of 42,000,000 persons gainfully employed in 1920 is considered conservative. The application of this death-rate to such a group would give a total loss for the year 1920 of 483,000 lives and a probable loss in 1921 of 500,000 lives.

The sickness rates actually determined in recent studies, according to Dr. Fisk, show that 2¼ per cent of wage earners are constantly ill to an extent to be incapacitated. This would justify an estimate of approximately 2,400,000 people continually ill instead of Professor Fisher's estimate in 1909 of 3,000,000. Dr. Fisk estimates that by supervision and periodic physical examination a still further reduction amounting to a mortality gain of four lives, and the elimination of eight cases of chronic illness, or a reduction of 2,920 days of illness, with a net profit of $29,000 to the state or community per 1,000 of population could be secured.

Dr. Fisk also estimates that the cost of periodic examinations applied to the entire population would amount to $525,000,000, and assuming that one-third of the substandard cases or about 10,000,000 revealed by these examinations required medical, surgical or dental treatment at a cost of $100 per case, the cost of this repair work would aggregate $1,000,000,000.

Dr. Fisk cites the losses from the following diseases which he considers all theoretically wholly preventable, and at least 75 per cent practically preventable.

Tuberculosis: $500,000,000 annually from death alone, $26,000,000,000 in this generation from diminished longevity. *Typhoid fever:* $135,000,000 annually. *Malaria:* $100,000,000 annually. *Hookworm:* Dowling estimates the loss from this disease at least $250,000,000 annually; 33 per cent increase in industrial efficiency has resulted from hookworm prevention in certain sections (Ferrell). Ashford, based on his experience in Porto Rico, writes, "It can be truthfully said that treatment and education alone have raised the laboring efficiency of the working class by nearly 68 per cent."

Influenza: Dr. Fisk gives further interesting data and informs us that influenza and pneumonia in non-epidemic years claim about 35,000 lives in the working ages (20–60) and thus accounts for at least 350,000 cases of illness. *Focal Infection:* More than 60 per cent of workers show definite focal infection of some degree. This has been confirmed by X-ray examination of over 5,000 people by the Life Extension Institute. There are more than 130,000 deaths annually in the working age from the organic conditions largely due to focal infection and there are not less than 14,000,000 people in industry showing signs of organic impairment of some degree.

Venereal Infection: Dr. Fisk in discussing this subject says: "It is impossible to give definite figures. Drawing conclusions from the draft figures, 5.6 per cent would be an outside estimate for ages 21 to 31. It may be roughly estimated that 1,500,000 workers are affected. The Life Extension Institute found less than 1 per cent of syphilis in industry and about 3 per cent in a mixed population. The Mayo Clinic found 4.6 per cent of syphilis in mixed classes and 10 per cent among railway men."

Eye Strain: Among over 10,000 employees in factories and commercial houses examined by the Life Extension Institute 53 per cent had uncorrected faulty vision. The Institute in its examination of 675 employees in the Underwood Typewriter Company — individuals engaged in close work — found 58 per cent in need of correction by glasses. Fisk reports the condition of lighting in 446 plants as follows: excellent, 8.7 per cent; good, 32.0 per cent; fair, 29.1 per cent; poor, 18.8 per cent; very poor, 3.5 per cent; partly good and partly poor, 7.8 per cent. He states that the Industrial Commission of Pennsylvania reported that last year 18 persons lost both eyes in industrial accidents, the compensation totalling $63,731; 652 workmen lost one eye, the compensation totalling $826,674.

Dr. Fisk adduces statistics to show how corrected eyesight increased the productivity 28 per cent in the Whiting-Davis Company, where a large amount of close, fine work is done; he also points out the need of providing adequate illumination for the entire industry, and shows how by the use of safety goggles the eye accidents in the American Locomotive Company have been reduced from 38.9 per 1,000 of full-time men per year during 1910–13 to 15.7 in 1915 and the number of eyes lost during the same period from 10.5 to 2.

Fatigue: Dr. Fisk discusses this subject in a very able manner, and very properly suggests that in a survey of fatigue it is first necessary to inquire: Does the output fall because the worker is tired or because he is physically deficient? Is the worker ill because he is tired or tired because he is ill? To which we may add another important factor, viz., the subject of fear, anxiety, worry, and the personal habits of the individual such as vice, dissipation, loss of sleep, etc.

ECONOMIC LOSS FROM ACCIDENTAL INJURY

According to the United States Department of Labor, 875,000 people are annually disabled four weeks or more by industrial accidents. If we assume that the cost of turnover or replacement of these people is $35, it would mean a direct waste in turnover alone of $30,625,000. If we added for those killed, $980,000, the increased production cost due to industrial accidents amounts to $31,605,000 annually.

Crum estimated the total economic annual loss from public accidents in the general population as $2,229,156,000, based on the value of human life at various ages and the accident fatalities at those ages. This takes into account 45,000 fatal accidents in 1917 and an estimate of 5,625,000 non-fatal injuries by public accidents.

At least 75 per cent of the accident rate is preventable. Even greater reduction has been made in some plants by safety measures and education. The economic value of these lives on the lowest basis of computation is $8,000 each and the saving of 20,000 of them (75 per cent) would mean an economic gain in industry of $160,000,000. If we apply this rate to the general population on the basis figured by Crum, it would mean a saving of $1,671,867,000.

Dr. Fisk also presents a table taken from the National Industrial Conference Board in its Research Report No. 37, of which the following is a digest of important medical work in industry now being carried on. Total number of plants reporting, 207; total number of workers, 764,827; total new injuries, 1,034,807; new injuries per worker, 1.35; redressings, 2,083,662; redressings per new injury, 2.01; total number of medical cases, 1,073,731; medical cases per worker, 1.40; total number of physical examinations, 525,818.

REMEDIAL RECOMMENDATIONS

In order to remedy the unfavorable conditions, Dr. Fisk says:

There is need to develop among the people at large a higher sense of responsibility for the care of their bodies, in other words, higher ideals of personal hygiene, as well as in citizenship generally. In order practically to apply these ideals, organization and certain governmental and social machinery is necessary. The possible lines of organization may be grouped as follows: federal, state, community, industrial, national, state and local extra-governmental health agencies. He then devotes considerable space to each of these topics, all of which are well worthy of close consideration.

It is most gratifying to the writer that Dr. Fisk has outlined such an excellent plan of attack which in the main accords with his own views previously cited. The writer has felt for years that the question of personal hygiene, physical education, and periodic medical examination with correction of defects for the prevention of permanent disabilities was of fundamental importance. He realized that many of the physical defects, such as defective vision and hearing not only handicapped the child in school but also in its subsequent struggle for existence. He was also convinced from his sociological studies of physically and mentally defective persons, who contribute such a large contingent to our charitable institutions, that many of these partial and complete disabilities could have been corrected by proper care and treatment in childhood.

The reports of the United States draft boards show that "47 per cent of the men examined were found to have certain defects, and that 53 per cent were accepted as fully meeting the physical standard with no defects recorded." The percentage of rejections varied from 14.13 in South Dakota to 46.67 in Pennsylvania. The draft boards rejected 209,304 men for rupture alone. O. A. Lauffer (*Journal of Industrial Hygiene*, 1920) says that hernia is the greatest single frailty of the American worker. Three per cent of the men offering themselves in the industries have hernia and 14 per cent have incipient hernia. There is every reason why this defect should receive prompt attention in childhood.

In view of the foregoing facts, the writer in May, 1920 strongly urged before the United States Senate Committee on Labor and Education, federal aid for the promotion of physical education. No system of education can be considered complete that does not provide for the promotion of physical education, including medical inspection and the correction of all remedial physical defects. Children are the most valuable assets of the nation, and every movement which makes for better health, a temperate, untainted, and virile race, will be the best safeguard in the prevention of disease, and greatly promote the efficiency and happiness of present and future generations. He also advanced military training between the ages of 18 and 20, because of its physical, hygienic and moral benefits, during which all physical defects of a remediable character could receive proper treatment.

Until this is accomplished no opportunity should be lost in the school health crusade to emphasize the importance of personal hygiene and general sanitation. When we supply our children with healthful school rooms and teach them the value of periodic medical inspection, of pure air, sanitary homes, proper and sufficient food, physical culture, baths and suitable clothing, and the importance of pure, clean lives, the lessons taught will be applied in the homes and workshops of the nation, and a very important advance in the conservation of life and efficiency in the industries will be the consequence.

A FIFTY YEAR SKETCH HISTORY OF MEDICAL
ENTOMOLOGY AND ITS RELATION TO PUBLIC HEALTH

L. O. HOWARD, M. D., PH. D., LL. D.

Chief, Bureau of Entomology, Washington, D. C.

A REAL history of medical entomology would require a year or more in its preparation and should be done perhaps by two men, the one a medical man (a pathologist), and the other an entomologist, since a complete history, written by one or the other, would unconsciously emphasize the importance of one side. But the time has come for the preparation of a consecutive account of the main features of the extraordinary development that has taken place in the past few decades and this article, however faulty and however hasty, is an attempt to give such an account. In any history there is always a balancing of the advantages and the disadvantages of a too near or a too distant view of events, and if the present view is too near it may at least contain suggestions for the consideration of the future historian.

In 1871 the idea that any specific disease might be insect-borne was not mentioned in any of the standard medical treatises. In this direction the world was as ignorant as it was three hundred years earlier when Mercurialis suggested the idea of food contamination by flies coming from the excretions of those dying from the "black death" to visit exposed food supplies. Even this perfectly obvious conclusion of the old Italian physician made little impression, and although occasionally repeated from time to time through the years by one observer or another, mainly in reference to Asiatic cholera, flies generally were regarded as harmless nuisances, perhaps, indeed, even as beneficial, in their maggot stage, as destroyers of offal.

We can hardly blame the workers in medical sciences before the days of microbiology for indifference or for lack of vision in this direction, in spite of the fact that here and there, in different parts of the world, there existed among the people popular beliefs which connected certain insects with disease. It was so in India, in Africa, in South America, and even on the Roman Campagna, a home of malaria, the poor peasants long ago connecting the idea of mosquitoes with the idea of fevers.

But there were a few men, before Pasteur's discovery of pathogenic bacteria and long before any one had dreamed of disease-carrying protozoa with alternate hosts, who had imagined in a way the connection between mosquitoes and yellow fever. Louis D. Beauperthuy, a French physician long resident in the West Indies, as early as 1853 elaborately argued that yellow fever is conveyed to man by mosquitoes, but he supposed that the insects carried the virus from decomposing matter which they had visited. Even earlier, 1848, Dr. Josiah Nott, of Mobile, had contended in a published article that the specific cause of yellow fever exists in some form of insect life.

The first decade of our fifty years was almost passed when the first great discovery in medical entomology was made, a discovery which, although it had no connection with bacteria or protozoa, led directly to others, and in fact opened the way to the vast field of discovery in which many men of many countries have worked and are now working. This was the discovery by Dr. Patrick Manson of the full life round of certain filarial worms, in which certain mosquitoes play a vital part. This work seemed revolutionary and its results unimaginable, even to intelligent practitioners; indeed, the late medical inspector, J. S. Ames, of the United States Navy, has told me how the navy surgeons of different nations who came together by chance at a China station "used to chaff crazy Pat Manson about his mosquito filaria ideas." Manson's discovery was brilliant and revolutionary. It was the result of long work under trying conditions and in the face of a discouraging lack of interest; in fact, serious doubts were entertained on the part of his colleagues as to his perfect sanity. He deserves even greater honor than was given to him, although he has been hailed as a pioneer and a great leader by the medical profession and the scientific world at large. His work led directly to the great achievement of Ross in regard to malaria.

But before we take up Ross's wonderful work, we must for an instant refer to an extraordinary paper by A. F. A. King, a Washington physician with a speculative mind, who published in 1883 an extended argument to prove that malaria is carried by mosquitoes. As a closely reasoned argument, this paper was as nearly conclusive as would be possible without actual experimental evidence. But the time was not ripe for the acceptance of this idea, and laboratory technique and microbiological science were not far enough advanced to allow even promising confirmatory experimentation. I am inclined to pity myself when I remember my incredulous frame of mind as Dr. King broached his theory to the late C. V. Riley and me before he read his very notable paper before the Philosophical Society of Washington in the early eighties. It is worthy of note that although several prominent medical men were present at the meeting, including the late Drs. J. S. Billings and Robert Fletcher, the paper fell utterly flat as to encouraging discussion. When published, a number of months later, in the old *Popular Science Monthly* for 1883, the article attracted little attention and, so far as I know, received none of the favorable comment it deserved until George Nuttall recognized its remarkable character sixteen years later and reviewed it at some length in his admirable summary, "The Role of Insects, Arachnids and Myriapods as Carriers in the Spread of Bacterial and Parasitic Diseases of Man and Animals," in Volume VIII of the *Johns Hopkins Hospital Reports* (1899). It is certain that at the time King formulated his mosquito-malaria theory, he had no knowledge of Laveran's discovery, in 1880, of the causative organism of the disease, or of Manson's discoveries regarding the carriage of filariasis by mosquitoes, since he would undoubtedly have added another strong argument to the twelve he so admirably formulated had he possessed this information.

But here we must leave malaria temporarily in order to discuss briefly, in chronological order, the extraordinary and basic discoveries of Theobald Smith with regard to the Texas fever of cattle.

The so-called Texas or Southern cattle fever had long been known as a disease transmitted to northern cattle by cattle coming from the southern regions of the United States. The region from which infected cattle came was large and well defined, including most of the Southern states. Southern cattle themselves, as a rule, were free from any signs of disease. Cattle coming from the south in the winter were harmless but when they were brought north during the summer, the disease came with them. Curiously enough, it did not seem to be an infection which was communicated directly from southern cattle to northern cattle; the southern cattle infected the ground over which they passed and the northern cattle, when grazing over this same ground, caught the fever.

It had long been the belief among certain cattle raisers in the West that ticks were the cause of this fever and that they were carried and scattered everywhere by southern cattle. Many, however, disbelieved this theory. Observations confirmatory of the tick theory, however, had been made. For example, it was noticed that when southern cattle had been driven for a considerable distance, after a time they lost their power to infect pastures. Moreover, it was noticed that after southern cattle had passed, the disease did not appear among northern cattle grazing on their trail until thirty days or thereabouts had elapsed.

Our knowledge was in this condition when the investigation of the disease was taken up seriously by the Bureau of Animal Industry of the United States Department of Agriculture. Dr. Theobald Smith was a young man who had graduated at Cornell University in 1880 and had afterwards received his degree in medicine at Albany. He had taken special studies which admirably fitted him for this work and became connected with the Service at Washington. In 1889 he succeeded in discovering a peculiar micröorganism in the red blood corpuscles of an infected cow which corresponded in every respect with what one would expect as the true cause of the disease. Dr. Smith was associated at that time with Dr. F. L. Kilborne, who had charge of the field experiments connected with this work and who soon succeeded in showing that the cattle tick was somehow necessary to the transmission of the disease. These observations were fully confirmed in 1890. In the autumn of that year it was found that when young ticks which had been artificially hatched were placed on cattle there was a sudden astonishing loss of red blood corpuscles which could by no means be explained by the simple abstraction of the blood. Additional experiments showed that the fever was caused by putting recently hatched cattle ticks on susceptible cattle. These results were confirmed in the summer of 1891 and 1892.

Here again results confirmed an idea current among the people, but these results were not indorsed, and, indeed, were even derided, by scientific men. In 1868 Dr. John Gamgee, who had been brought over from England to study the plague for the United States Government, wrote: "The tick theory has gained quite a hold during the past summer, but a little thought should have satisfied anyone of the absurdity of this idea."

The great importance of Smith's work consists in the demonstration that the infection is carried from the adult ticks into the eggs, from them to the young, which later introduce the virus. The first thing that occurred to the discoverer was that the tick drew out the causative organism from the blood of the cattle and distributed it on the pasture, the cattle eating this organism with their food; but it was not until 1891, when he accidentally found that he could obtain eggs from the ticks in confinement, that it was possible to begin experiments to prove the transmission by the bite. His discovery of the causative organism had enabled him to recognize mild cases of the disease produced experimentally, since only by an examination of the blood microscopically and with the blood counter could such a diagnosis be made.

The remarkable benefits to the people of the United States which have resulted from this discovery are of course well known. Southern cattle, after having been "dipped" to free them from ticks, can now be carried north beyond the "tick line" without the slightest danger that the Southern fever will be transmitted to northern cattle. And moreover, the Southern country is being rapidly freed from the cattle tick, while by rotation of pasturage and by dipping, county after county has been retrieved from quarantine, and now a vast area, formerly dangerous, is fever-free. Curiously enough, the old fever quarantine line corresponded closely to the dividing line between the upper and lower austral life zones on Merriam's early life zone maps of the United States. Theoretically, therefore, the cattle tick is a lower austral form and can more easily be exterminated from its more northward range. But cattle culture can now be carried on with profit in many regions of the South where diversified agriculture has become a necessity.

This in itself is a noteworthy result of Smith's discovery, but biologically it is of the very greatest importance as the pioneer discovery of a blood-inhabiting protozoan in its dual relation between an articulate and a mammalian host. It is true that the cattle tick is not, strictly speaking, an insect, but it is closely related to the insects and is popularly called one, so that this demonstration, first described in full in 1893, ranks as the second great discovery in medical entomology.

While Smith was completing his college course at Cornell, Dr. A. Laveran, a French army surgeon, was studying malaria in Algeria. The latter succeeded in 1880 in demonstrating an amoeboid organism in the blood of malarial patients. This he studied at length and showed to be the causative organism of the disease, which thus became established as a parasitic malady. The details of the life cycle of this organism as it occurs in man were traced by Laveran after the discovery that it was the true cause of the disease, and there was much speculation as to the manner in which it is transferred to healthy people. The drinking of contaminated water was an early suggestion, and there were others, but experimental work failed to prove their truth. Laveran himself eventually suggested that the parasitic organism might be carried by mosquitoes, but Manson, after his success with filaria, insisted upon the necessity for experimentation with these insects, and formulated the hypothesis that they might be the necessary secondary hosts. It was, in fact, largely due to Manson's suggestions that Ronald Ross, then a surgeon in the Indian Medical Service, began his studies.

The details of Ross's work have now become well known among the medical profession and those engaged in sanitary work. Starting with nothing but a theory and a knowledge of the appearance of the parasite after it appears in the blood of man, and with no knowledge whatever of how the parasite might look in another stage of its development or whether it might be found in one kind of mosquito and not in another kind, Ross spent two years and a half of the most strenuous work before he solved the question and found the parasites among the cells of the stomach of what he termed "dapple-winged mosquitoes." This result was reached in August, 1897. After its announcement, many workers attacked the problem and confirmation rapidly followed. The complete life-history of the parasite was worked out and the mosquitoes of the genus *Anopheles* were definitely shown to be the sole means by which malaria is transmitted from man to man. The Italian workers, Grassi, Bignami, and Bastianelli, began to work along the same lines shortly after Ross had begun his investigation, and for a long time contended that the credit for the establishment of the relation between *Anopheles* and human malaria belonged to them, since Ross's first work was done with mosquitoes of the genus *Culex* and a malarial disease of sparrows. The Nobel Prize, however, was awarded to Ross in 1902, after a careful examination of the matter of priority, and of late the Italians have advanced no claim. In fact, when talking with Angelo Celli in 1910, I jocularly referred to his "old friend Ross" (Ross had been particularly harsh in his criticism of the claims of the Italian school), and Celli replied to the effect that it was "all smoothed over," and that he had contributed a chapter to Ross's big book on malaria, which had then just been published. It seems that Ross knew nothing of Theobald Smith's discovery of the blood-inhabiting protozoan of the Texas fever of cattle and of its established vital relation with the cattle tick, so that his work with malaria was absolutely original with him and, so far as he knew, was the first accomplishment of this nature in respect to protozoan parasites. The importance of his work cannot be over-estimated. It was one of the great discoveries in biological science applied to medicine and will eventually mean more for the health and happiness of mankind than almost any discovery that has ever been made. Ross, like Manson, was knighted and has lived to enjoy many honors, as well as to see in many directions the vast fruits of his discovery.

Practical work based on Ross's discovery was immediately begun in different parts of the world. He himself headed an expedition to Lagos on the west coast of Africa, and by putting anti malaria measures into effect greatly reduced the malaria incidence. Elsewhere the same thing was done. The governors of the British colonies, especially the authorities of the crown colonies, did not act with sufficient rapidity and enthusiasm to satisfy Ross, who felt, with his crusader's spirit, that they should have accomplished more. In 1901 he published a little book called *Mosquito Brigades*, in which he gave explicit directions, as a result of his field work, as to the best means of organizing and operating anti malaria campaigns, especially in the tropics. In this book he said severe things about the dilatoriness of British "officialism" in sanitary matters. Three years previously, I had published a bulletin on mosquitoes and anti-mosquito work, in which I referred to Ross's discovery and described the best measures for fighting mosquitoes. A number of bits of experimental work were done in several parts of the United States, details regarding which were given in the book entitled *Mosquitoes; How They Live, How They Carry Disease, and How They May Be Destroyed*, which was published in 1901.

It is astonishing how rapidly conviction followed this great discovery and how wide-spread the belief in its soundness soon became. The leaders of the medical profession adopted it at once and doubters were astonishingly few and were soon silenced. Certain state health officers in this country took it up and preached it. As early as 1898 I was invited to address the Section on Medicine of the American Medical Association at its annual convention at Atlantic City on the subject of the malarial mosquito, and no serious objections to the so called "theory" were in evidence. The only note of protest which I remember was at New Orleans in December, 1905, at a meeting of the section of Physiology and Experimental Medicine of the American Association for the Advancement of Science, during a symposium of insect-borne diseases. No one present will ever forget the dramatic manner in which the late Dr. Chaillé crushed the unfortunate speaker.

As always, the center in this country of early adoption and dissemination of this wonderful discovery was Johns Hopkins University. Dr. William S. Thayer went to Italy and studied the work on the Roman Campagna and in the laboratories of Grassi and Celli. He returned to Baltimore and began an enthusiastic campaign of education. Dr. Walter Reed, of the United States Army, Dr. Jesse W. Lazear and Dr. James Carroll, all with Johns Hopkins affiliations, absorbed the new ideas with interest, and from this group of men came the next great discovery in medical entomology.

The war with Spain had just been completed. The American Army of Occupation was in Cuba. The Surgeon General of the Army, Dr. George M. Sternberg, was a bacteriologist and had been a student of yellow fever. Sanitary conditions in Cuba were extremely bad. The possibility of an epidemic of yellow fever among the American troops was very great, and malaria was rife on the island. Therefore, General Sternberg formed a commission, composed of Doctors Reed, Carroll, and Lazear, and added to their number, Dr. Aristides Agramonte, a Cuban physician educated in the United States, instructing them to investigate sanitary conditions in Cuba in as thorough a manner as possible, and to pay special attention to yellow fever.

Now it happens that as early as 1880 a Cuban physician of a speculative turn of mind, a man of imagination (of the A. F. A. King type) named Carlos J. Finlay had been filled with the idea that yellow fever was carried by mosquitoes. Not content with theorizing, he put his ideas to the test; but, working single-handed and in defiance of accepted views, knowing nothing of protozoology and little of bacteriology and laboratory methods, he failed to bring forward any convincing proof, although his experiments were in a high degree suggestive. He had, however, selected the exact species of mosquito which was eventually proved by the United States Army Commission to be the true vector of the disease, namely, *Culex fasciatus*, as it was then called — the most abundant of the household mosquitoes of Cuba. Sternberg, who had been a member of an American commission to study yellow fever in Cuba at that time, had met Finlay and was familiar with his experiments, but neither at that time nor at any other after the Reed Commission results were gained is there any evidence to show that Sternberg was at all favorably impressed by Finlay's theory. The fact, however, that Finlay's ideas were ultimately proved to be true, that his experiments failed only in detail, and that he selected the exact species of mosquito as the probable carrier of the disease entitled him to great credit, and he is to-day acclaimed throughout all Latin America as the real hero of the "mosquito-yellow fever discovery." With this, however, North America and most of the rest of the world does not agree, since he did not prove his case.

Reed, knowing Finlay's theory and filled with enthusiasm over the results of Ross's investigation, and those of the Italians, went to Cuba with the determination to give the mosquito idea a thorough test. Lazear, I knew from calls which he had made at my office with Thayer to find out what I knew about the malaria mosquitoes. Reed and Carroll, before they went to Cuba on this mission, spent some time in the Bureau of Entomology studying *Culex fasciatus*, learning to differentiate it from other mosquitoes which they were likely to find in Havana.

The story of their work for the next two years is known to all the world. By a series of most carefully guarded experiments on volunteering American soldiers, experiments which the physicians of Havana, experienced in every phase of yellow fever, were invited to view and to criticize, Reed and Carroll succeeded in showing that the current idea that the fever is carried by infected clothing, bedding and other articles was utterly wrong, and that it is carried solely by the bite of the common house mosquito of tropical America, *Stegomyia fasciata*.* Announcements of their results were made in two papers at intervals of a year, and while the first was received with some doubt by the London *Lancet*, the second was so conclusive, although wonderfully modest and matter-of-fact, that the acceptance of the result was general and enthusiastic. Later work by others only confirmed the conclusions reached by Reed and his colleagues, and

---

*Now known as *Ædes calopus* or *Ædes argentus*.

to-day the world is in a fair way to be completely rid of yellow fever—one of the greatest scourges of mankind in warm countries.

All through the progress of this work Dr. Reed was in constant correspondence with Washington. He returned to the States in October, 1900, to read before the annual meeting of the American Public Health Association the first announcement of the results gained from his first series of experiments, later returning to Cuba to carry out the second and conclusive series. He wrote to me frequently and of course corresponded regularly with Surgeon General Sternberg. The Surgeon General and I used to meet at the Cosmos Club after office hours to compare notes and read to each other the letters we had received from Cuba. One of my most highly treasured possessions is a final letter from Reed written January 13, 1901, when he was confident that he had proved his case beyond cavil. He said:

Of course you have already heard from General Sternberg of our complete success in repeating our former observations. The mosquito theory for the propagation of yellow fever is no longer a *theory*, but an established *fact*. Isn't it enough to make a fellow feel happy? *Anopheles* and *Culex* are a gay old pair! What havoc they have wrought on our species during the last three centuries!

He finished by stating that with the aid of anti-mosquito measures, which he was good enough to say that I had developed, yellow fever would be wiped off the earth.

The control of yellow fever by anti-mosquito work was soon demonstrated in a very big way. The Army of Occupation in Cuba took up at once the task of ridding Habana from the disease and incidentally from malaria. How well this was done all the world knows, and the active director of the work, Dr. Gorgas, stepped at once into the light of fame.

Only a few years later, the United States staged a very conclusive demonstration. In the early summer of 1905 yellow fever broke out in a certain quarter of New Orleans. The number of cases rapidly increased and an epidemic apparently comparable with the disastrous one of 1878 had begun to spread. The United States Public Health Service took command of the situation early in June, and under the direction of Dr. J. H. White carried on a thorough anti-mosquito campaign. The results were striking. The fever stopped spreading.

Very few new cases developed, and, comparing the number of deaths in that year with those of 1878, there was a clear saving of four thousand lives, due to the discovery of Reed and his colleagues.

It will be unnecessary to carry the story of yellow fever demonstrations further. Rio de Janeiro was soon rid of the plague by the intelligent and energetic efforts of Oswaldo Cruz and his colleagues. Admirable work was done in Mexico under the direction of Eduardo Licéaga. It was not long, however, before all of this was overshadowed by the magnificent results gained by Gorgas in his administration of the sanitary affairs in the building of the Panama Canal. The results of Gorgas' work proved that the tropics may be inhabited by the white race — a fact of tremendously far-reaching importance to the future of the world.

Unlike Sir Patrick Manson and Sir Ronald Ross, on whom honors have been showered, and who are still living to enjoy the fame that has come to them, the three American members of the Commission are dead. Lazear succumbed to the fever during the progress of the investigation. Reed died not long afterwards, and Carroll a year or so later, both indirectly as the result of their Cuban work.

Reed died too early to receive the Nobel Prize, which probably would have been awarded to him, and I happen to know, from a conversation with Sir Ronald Ross and Sir Rupert Boyce in Liverpool in 1905, that Carroll's name was under consideration for this prize just before his death.

The actual causative organism of yellow fever was not found by the Reed Commission nor was its development in the mosquito ascertained. They found that the blood serum of a patient retained its toxicity after passing through a Berkefeld filter and concluded that the causative organism must be ultramicroscopic. Recently Noguchi, of the Rockefeller Institute, has isolated a spirochete which he considers to be probably the true cause of the disease. This opinion is shared by Simon Flexner and other prominent pathologists. However, the well-known authority on yellow fever, Juan Guitéras, of Habana, has just analyzed the results and shows that there is still some room for doubt. At any rate, just what happens to the organism in the body of the mosquito remains to be determined.

The next most important discovery in this direction related to dengue, or breakbone fever, a disease common in semitropical and tropical countries, in the West Indies, and in the southern United States. It is also found in southern Asia, in the Philippines, in the South Sea Islands and in the countries about the eastern end of the Mediterranean. In 1902 Dr. Graham, working in Beirut, Syria, showed that the disease was not contagious in the absence of mosquitoes but that isolated persons contracted the disease when bitten by mosquitoes which had bitten dengue patients. Later, Ashburn and Craig of the United States Army, who were working in the Philippines, showed with mosquitoes bred in the laboratories and fed upon dengue patients that the insects will transmit the disease after a period of three days. The mosquitoes used by Graham in Syria were the cosmopolitan water-barrel mosquitoes of the tropics, *Culex fatigans* (now called *C. quinquefasciatus*), while the yellow fever mosquito, *Ædes calopus* (or better, *argenteus*), carries the disease in the Australasian life zone. In Formosa, Koizumi has inculpated *Desvoidea obturbans* in the same relation.

The spirochetes, protozoal organisms of wide distribution, have, however, been shown to be the cause of other diseases of man and animals and to be insect-borne, but in nearly all of these the arthropod carrier is a tick rather than a true insect, and it is interesting to note that with at least one of these the infected tick transmits the disease to its offspring just as Theobald Smith found to be the case many years earlier with the Texas fever of cattle.

The series of discoveries of spirochete-tick diseases began shortly after the establishment of the yellow fever-mosquito relation, by the findings of Ross and Milne in Uganda, and Dutton and Todd in the Congo, in 1904, of the spirochete cause of the so-called "African relapsing fever" and its tick vector, *Ornithodoros moubata*. That this fever resulted from the bite of a special tick had long been known to the natives of Africa, but as in the case of the *nagana* disease of cattle, which will shortly be referred to, the fever was supposed to be due to some special virulence of the tick. In this case the carrier occurs abundantly in native huts, feeds upon birds and mammals as well as upon man, and resembles the bedbug in that it works by night.

Another spirochete disease is the "European relapsing fever." As early as 1897 Tictin infected monkeys with this disease by inoculating them with bedbugs which had fed upon a diseased patient 48 hours earlier. Therefore, bedbugs are supposed to be the carriers of this disease, although the evidence is not complete.

In 1903, however, Marchoux and Salimbeni, working in Brazil under the auspices of the Pasteur Institute of France, secured conclusive evidence of the transference of another spirochete disease, known as the spirochætosis of domestic fowls, by a tick known as *Argas persicus.* Still another proved relation of the kind is that of the spirochætosis of cattle in the Transvaal, where the disease is carried by a tick known as *Margaropus decolaratus.*

Even antedating the work of the Yellow Fever Commission was the extremely important work of Colonel David Bruce, of the British Army, with the so-called "nagana" or tsetse-fly disease of cattle in Africa. In this case the causative organism was found to be another type of protozoan of the genus *Trypanosoma*, and it was this organism, transmitted by the bite of a tsetse-fly from sick cattle to healthy cattle, which caused the disease, which had previously, just as in the case of the "African relapsing fever," been attributed solely to the virulence of the bite, "fly sickness" of cattle having been known to all African explorers. Here, then, is another group of micro-organisms which cause disease in warm-blooded animals and are transmitted by insect bites. In this case it was long a matter of doubt whether the fly was simply a mechanical carrier of the pathogenic organism or whether it was a necessary secondary host. This point was partly cleared by Koch, who discovered what he considered to be sexual forms of the trypanosome in the intestine of the fly, but Kleine in 1909 succeeded in finding the different stages of the parasite in the intestine of the insect and proved that part of the life-cycle of the insect must occur in this secondary host.

Bruce's discovery and the work of others who followed him in the study of the nagana disease led directly to the discovery of the cause of the terrible sleeping sickness of man in Africa, by Dutton, in 1902, which was confirmed by Castellani a little later. When this discovery was announced, the Frenchman, Brumpt, and Sambon, in England, advanced at once the theory that this disease is also transmitted by a tsetse-fly. Their argument was based upon Bruce's discovery with nagana, and also upon the geographic distribution and epidemiology of the disease. Their theory was abundantly demonstrated not long afterwards by practical experimentation. In this case Sambon was much more fortunate than he was some years later when he advanced the theory that pellagra is carried by the black flies of the genus *Simulium*, which was afterwards abundantly disproved.

The serious and fatal disease called "sleeping sickness" had been known among the natives of parts of Africa for many years. The earliest published account that has been found was by a naval surgeon, John Atkins, in a book entitled *Physical Observations on the Coast of Guiney*, published in 1741. For a long time the disease seemed to be limited to West Africa, but with the opening up of the interior it found its way into Uganda with terrible results. In 1901 it was reported by Dr. Albert Cook, of a missionary society, that two hundred natives had died and that thousands appeared to be infected on Buvuma Island. The disease spread with dreadful rapidity and the government became intensely alarmed. A commission was sent out from England under the auspices of the Royal Society, and such men as Low, Christie, Castellani and Sir David Bruce began an immediate investigation which has continued without interruption (except for the period of the Great War) until the present time. An International Sleeping Sickness Congress was held in London in 1907, which was attended by the most eminent pathologists and parasitologists of many nations, including especially those having African colonies.

During all the early stages of the investigation, and for a number of years after it was discovered that the disease was carried by the tsetse-flies, field investigations were carried on exclusively by medical men. E. E. Austen, of the British Museum, a well-known entomologist, especially skilled in the *Diptera* (the order to which tsetse-flies belong) was consulted as to the taxonomy of the insects and as to their probable biology. Professor Newstead, of the Liverpool School of Tropical Medicine, another competent entomologist, was also consulted. A new element was added to the investigation when W. F. Fiske, a former expert of the United States Bureau of Entomology, was employed by the Tropical Diseases Bureau of London in 1911, and proceeded with a competent expedition to Uganda, where he studied the problem from the viewpoint of his broad experience in field entomology, until the outbreak of the Great War. In 1919 he returned to Africa, where he is at present. His preliminary reports have been published and are of great interest from a broad biological point of view as well as in their practical suggestions. It will be impossible to dwell at further length upon Fiske's work, in view of the interesting and important investigations that have been carried on by an army of other observers. His work is especially mentioned here because he is the first American, broadly trained in economic zoology, to give his entire attention to this problem.

The problem of the control of sleeping sickness by the control of the breeding places of the fly, or perhaps of its other hosts in the shape of wild animals, has not yet been settled, but it is hoped that the numbers of the flies may be greatly reduced by the destruction, or the alteration in the character, of its present breeding-places, or by the preparation of attractive breeding-places where it may be exterminated in the pupa condition. It still remains one of the problems in medical entomology.

We must now return chronologically to another tick-disease, namely, the Rocky Mountain spotted fever of man. For the past forty-eight years a disease which has come to be known as Rocky Mountain spotted fever has been found in portions of Montana and Idaho, and cases have also been reported from a number of other western states, including Washington, Wyoming, Utah, Nevada, Colorado, California and Oregon. It is characterized by chills and fever and a characteristic skin eruption. The mortality differs widely in different localities, ranging from four per cent in Idaho to as high as seventy-five per cent in the Bitter Root Valley of Montana. The credit for the full establishment of the relation between the disease and certain ticks is given to Dr. H. T. Ricketts, who conducted carefully guarded experiments in 1906 which indisputably proved the relationship. Ricketts himself, however, gives the credit for the first experimental evidence in support of the tick hypothesis to McCalla and Brereton, who conducted two positive experiments a year earlier. As early as 1902 Wilson and Chowning had reported the causative organism of the fever to be related to the organism which causes the Texas fever of cattle, but Stiles, after carefully working on the problem in 1905, failed to confirm this conclusion. Much more recently Wolbach (1919) has found an organism, which he has described as *Dermacentroxenus rickettsi*, which he considers the cause of the disease. He finds that it is intracellular in mammals and ticks but intranuclear only in ticks. It is reasonably certain that some of the native small animals furnish the reservoir of the disease, and the destruction of ground squirrels and the dipping of domestic animals to destroy ticks have been tried with good results in the Bitter Root Valley. The tick most closely associated with this disease is *Dermacentor andersoni* Stiles (*D. venustus Banks*), but it has been experimentally shown by Maver that the disease may be transmitted by several species of ticks.

The investigation of Rocky Mountain spotted fever has been marked by the martyrdom of several of the investigators. Dr. F. B. McClintock, of the United States Public Health Service, died while engaged in studying this disease. Later Dr. A. H. McCray died of the same disease while working for the Montana State Board of Health. Dr. Ricketts himself, to whom the confirmation of the tick relation in this disease is due, while he passed successfully through his work with spotted fever, died later of typhus fever in Mexico, while studying the relation of lice and typhus.

There has been no systematic arrangement of the accounts so far given of the discoveries in regard to the carriage of disease by insects, but I have considered them rather chronologically, one account of a discovery being followed by the story of the next one. Arriving now at approximately the middle of the first decade of the present century, the work in this direction all over the world has been so intense and discoveries have been so various, or have followed one another so rapidly, that any strict chronological sequence must be abandoned; in fact, it will be possible to touch only briefly upon a few of the principal ones.

Antedating the investigations described in the last few paragraphs were the experiments in the transmission of bubonic plague by fleas, carried out successfully by Simond in 1898. This terrible disease, which from time to time has ravaged the old world in epidemic form, is supposed to have caused the death of 25,000,000 people on the continent of Europe in the fourteenth century. In modern times it has raged in oriental countries, causing, for example, for many years in India, an average of nearly 1,000,000 deaths annually. The causative organism of the plague is *Bacillus pestis*, described simultaneously by Kitasato, the famous Japanese investigator, and Yersin, a Frenchman. The establishment of the identity of the disease with the one which occurs in rats had been established by Yersin in 1894, and Simond's transmission of the disease by means of rat-fleas was confirmed by Verjbitski in 1903 and by Liston in 1904. The British Plague Commission in India proved most conclusively that the rat-flea is the principal means of transmission of the bubonic form of the plague. No less than eight species of fleas have been shown by various workers to be carriers of the plague bacillus, but the rat-flea, known as *Xenophylla cheopsis*, is the principal carrier in great epidemics. The Indian Plague Commission, finding the bacilli only in the alimentary tract of the fleas and not in the salivary glands, concluded that the bacilli are present in the excreta of the flea and are inoculated into the human host by scratching. Experiments by Bacot and Martin, however, indicate that the plague can be transmitted by the bite of fleas when a temporary obstruction of the proventriculus of the insect causes the blood laden with bacilli to be regurgitated into the bite puncture.

This is the first of the diseases which we have mentioned in which the insect seems to be simply the mechanical carrier of the disease organism. In this case, as in many others, some of which we shall briefly mention, there is obviously no development of the disease-germ in the body of the insect, which is therefore not a necessary secondary host, but simply a carrier, and the inordinate spread of disease is caused by the presence of the insect in great numbers. There are a number of insect-borne diseases in which the causative organism has not yet been discovered in which this point has not clearly been ascertained. When Reed, Carroll, and Lazear failed to find the cause of yellow fever and yet were able to produce the disease from the blood serum which had been filtered, they were nevertheless of the opinion that there must be a causative organism too small to be seen by the highest power of the microscope, and which undergoes a part of its development in the body of the yellow fever mosquito, since a certain definite period must elapse between the infection of the mosquito and the time when its bite transmits the infection to a non-immune, just as is the case with malaria, where the organism and its full life-history are so well known and so easily demonstrable.

But we must return to Ricketts and his second great discovery. This excellent investigator at the beginning of his career was with the Public Health Service, but at the time of his work on the Rocky Mountain spotted fever, he was connected with the Medical Department of the University of Chicago. Upon the conclusion of his work in Montana his attention was attracted to typhus fever.

Typhus fever, a serious disease formerly prevalent under unsanitary conditions in most civilized countries when people were crowded together in camps, hospitals or jails, and which a hundred years and more ago was known as "jail fever" in England — the disease which nearly killed the "Vicar of Wakefield" in his life of many tribulations, — while practically non-existent in the United States for many years, was still rife in the prisons and densely populated portions of the principal cities of Mexico. Therefore Ricketts and his colleague Wilder went to the City of Mexico and carried on their experiments, which resulted in the establishment of the fact that typhus is communicated by the body-louse, the results being published in 1910. The Frenchmen, Nicolle, Comte and Conseil, working in Tunis, had reached similar results the year previously, and the discovery was confirmed soon afterwards by Anderson and Goldberger of the United States Public Health Service.

The causative organism of typhus is still unknown. Several different micro-organisms have been found both in typhus patients and in lice, but that anyone of these micro-organisms is the actual cause of the disease is still disputed. That the disease is transmitted by the bites of lice is now thoroughly accepted, but with the micro-organism still in doubt the question of its partial development in the bodies of the lice is also still in doubt. Several workers have claimed that the disease is transmitted hereditarily by lice, while this has been disputed by other equally competent authorities. That the absolute destruction or prevention of lice will ward off typhus is beyond doubt.

Never in the history of the world have there been such opportunities for the demonstration of the value of a prophylactic measure as the Great War afforded in connection with this disease. The epidemic which began in Serbia in January, 1915, spread all over the country. The necessary sanitary measures with regard to cleanliness and louse-destruction and prevention were apparently unknown in that country, and the majority of the native physicians were soon taken with the disease and died. The American Red Cross then stepped in. American physicians were sent to Serbia, and although by April of 1915 people were dying at the rate of 9,000 a day, the epidemic was measurably controlled. In this great work the French and the English participated. After the Russian armies mobilized typhus appeared and the dread disease was more or less prevalent all along the eastern front. Russian prisoners in German detention camps spread the disease and its obvious prophylaxis was put into effect by German physicians, while the life-history of the body-louse was carefully studied by Haase, a competent entomologist. By strenuous efforts the disease was prevented from making inroads in the armies of the Allies, although it was impossible to keep the troops at the front free from lice. This brings us, although chronologically out of order, to the subject of another louse-borne disease, namely trench fever.

In the early part of the war, a young American physician, Dr. Plotz, had been studying a fever in New York City known as "Brill's disease," and had supposedly isolated the causative organism. Symptomatically this disease is closely related to typhus fever, resembling a mild form of that malady, and being louse-borne. The fever which developed among the troops in the trenches resembled the disease studied by Plotz in New York. American and English physicians. soon decided that it also was louse-borne, and measures were at once instituted to control lice in camps and entrenchments. Toward the close of the war an enormous amount of experimentation was carried on, and successfully, as to the best means of destroying lice, not only on the person but in temporarily discarded clothing. Troops moving from country to country or returning from the front were deloused, their clothing was steamed or fumigated, and all American troops returning from Europe were subjected to similar processes.

Without the slightest doubt in the world, there are many species of insects which act as carriers of disease in a purely mechanical way. There are many species which are attracted to exposed foods which are also attracted to excreta, to sputum, and to other substances carrying disease germs. This fact has, however, only recently become a matter of general information. The carriage of Asiatic cholera by flies was considered most probable by a number of earlier writers, but nothing seems to have been placed on record with regard to the very certain carriage of typhoid fever by the house-fly until the late 90's. Kober, in a report of the Health Department of the District of Columbia on an investigation of a small epidemic of typhoid, suggested the contamination of milk by the house-fly, which had previously visited the excreta of typhoid patients. The subject was brought prominently before the public during the Spanish-American War. Although the Surgeon General of the Army, Dr. Sternberg, gave careful instructions regarding the disposal of the excreta in concentration camps, his orders were not well carried out, and typhoid became epidemic at many points. A commission of army surgeons, consisting of Drs. Reed, Shakespeare and Vaughan, was appointed, and their report indicated that under concentration camp conditions the terrible spread of typhoid was due almost entirely to the common house-fly. During that brief war, more than eighty per cent of the total deaths were caused by typhoid fever.

From that time on, the control of the house-fly became a very important subject, and many volumes and hundreds of pamphlets have been written giving the results of careful studies of the biology of the house-fly in all its aspects as well as methods of control. Later, vaccination against typhoid was discovered and proved to be so effective that control of flies in camps became less important. The house-fly is nevertheless a very dangerous insect, being an important factor in the spread of infantile diarrhea during the summer months, and in other ways a constant menace to health. The necessity for laboratory proof of carriage by the house-fly of typhoid and other diseases of the same general nature, which has been insisted upon by Graham-Smith and other writers, while scientifically sound, does not especially appeal to the writer from the practical point of view. The case is altogether too obvious.

It is so obvious, in fact, as amply to justify the general crusade against the house-fly that began in this country about 1908 or 1909. Boards of health, both state and local, women's clubs, civic bodies, including the American Civic Association, and many newspapers have pushed the campaign against the house-fly with great vigor. The destruction of the house-fly has been taught in the schools and prizes have been awarded to the child killing the greatest number of flies. It should be noted that a few members of the Society for Prevention of Cruelty to Animals have objected to such teachings; but it is also true that there are people who are opposed to vaccination against smallpox, and still others who object to well-planned vivisection. While this tremendous crusade is doing a great deal of good educationally, a lot of energy is being misdirected in a way. Crushing a few hundred or a few thousand or a few hundreds of thousands of flies with a paddle will do little good if their breeding-places are left undistrubed.

We have now briefly described many of the principal discoveries of the relation of certain insects to certain diseases. A great many more discoveries have been made and doubtless many more are yet to be made. Many trained workers are investigating sanitary problems with the idea of possible insect-carriage constantly in mind.

28

Some poor guesses have been made on insufficient grounds, which have been widely heralded before thorough laboratory investigation and transmission experiments, but all plausible guesses must be carefully considered, and the men trained in investigation work of this kind are rapidly increasing in number.   Already Pierce has tabulated in his recent work on *Sanitary Entomology* more than two hundred diseases that have been shown to be carried by insects, and the bibliographical journals and reviews devoted to such subjects announce new discoveries almost every month.

Most of the important discoveries have been made by pathologists, bacteriologists and protozoologists, or by a class of workers calling themselves by the general term "parasitologists."   But, transmission of a disease by an insect or a group of insects once established, the trained entomologist makes his contribution, giving his knowledge of the insect vector and investigating every phase of its biology and behavior.   An admirable estimate of what medical entomology to-day means, or should mean, is given by Colonel Alcock, assistant director of the Tropical Diseases Bureau of London, himself an investigator of note, in the following words:

Medical entomology, too, during the last decade has become more critical and more formal.   We are not now suddenly afraid of an insect merely because it has been caught in the act of sucking blood; nor even when dealing with an arthropod of unquestioned pathogenic significance do we now think that we have done with it once for all by a command that its breeding-places shall be blotted out, or its natural enemies be let loose upon it.   The business of medical entomology, as now understood, is, in the case of any species convicted on pathological evidence of being a standing danger to the public health, to unriddle its biology in every detail, and to investigate all the varying circumstances that influence its acquisition and retention of pathogenic capacity. The biological inquest must comprehend every stage of the creature's existence, from the egg to the engendering adult, and must include not only its affinities and its structure, but also its bionomy and its relations to environment.   The bionomic inquiry must embrace the geographical distribution and seasonal incidence; the habits and the hours of activity; the powers and range of locomotion and the propensity to spread; the food preferences, meteorological influences, and power of resisting vicissitudes of season and climate; the sexual instincts and fecundity; the mode of reproduction, breeding-places and seasons, and the provision for larvæ; and the duration of life in every stage of development.   If it be not a specific parasite the bionomic investigation must also include the relations of the species to its environment, organic and inorganic, such as the physiographical and hydrographical featues of the habitat, natural shelters, help-givers, parasites, enemies and rivals.   An excellent example of the range of the inquiry is furnished by Swynnerton's "Examination of the Tsetse Problem." published in the *Bulletin of Entomological Research* for March 1921 (page 22). With the accumulation of exact information on all these points and the rational inferences drawn from it, medical entomology claims to be a science of practical application in preventive medicine — in short, a branch of hygiene, and a branch which, although it finds its fullest and most constant application in those tropical countries where sanitary arrangements are still crude and imperfect, cannot in the mutability of human affairs be neglected in any country.*

In this article we have considered in a far too summary way a dozen of the great discoveries in medical entomology, practically all of them made within the space of five and twenty years. Even to list the others would fill far more space than can be given here. Scientific laboratories were teeming with work of this kind down to the outbreak of the Great War in 1914. For the next four years many investigations were stopped. The men working on the sleeping sickness problem in Africa, for example, had to abandon this work and join the military forces. Men from the laboratories in all the countries at war were sent to the front, or to concentration camps to help in the care of the health of the troops. Many a promising investigator was killed. Printing facilities and postal facilities were so hampered that there was almost no news of the progress of investigations sent out from one country to another as in times of peace. None of the scientific men of the Allied nations knew for several years what was being done by the trained investigators of the Central Powers. Nevertheless the War gave a tremendous impetus to the study of medical entomology. Typhus in the Balkans and in Poland and Russia and in camps containing prisoners from those countries, the trench fever which soon developed alarmingly on the western front, and the spread of malaria in non-malarious regions of Germany, France, and even England, due to the infection of native *Anopheles* by malaria-carrying soldiers returning from the fever-stricken fields of southeastern Europe, intensified the importance of the most careful and continued study of insect vectors of disease.

During the past twenty years the scientific world has thrown itself with ever-increasing activity into the great field opened by the initial discoveries. The greater importance of insect-borne diseases

---

Tropical Diseases Bulletin, vol. 18, no. 1, 1921, pp. 1, 2,

in the tropics was immediately recognized, and England's great colonial possessions justified, and in fact necessitated, the founding of the great Schools of Tropical Medicine at Liverpool and London. A similar school was founded later at Hamburg by the German Government, but the loss of her tropical possessions has minimized the later work at this institution. Too much praise can hardly be given to the wonderful work done by the Oswaldo Cruz Institute at Rio de Janeiro. The corps of admirable investigators there has been increased from time to time, and important discoveries have been made in the lines of medical entomology, which the limited space allotted to this article prevents us from considering.

Medical entomology, however, is only a branch of tropical medicine, but it is a branch which absolutely requires the help, not only in investigation but also in teaching, of entomologists. A medical man who is a trained pathologist can hardly, after devoting years of research to other lines, become a skilled entomologist, since the field of entomology is so vast that to become skilled in any one of its many aspects requires a lifetime of work. This is coming to be realized. Not only must the taxonomy of insects engaged in the carriage of disease be critically studied, but their behavior under all possible conditions, their complete biology and ecology, their physiology, and many other things must be studied; and the man trained in so-called economic entomology is the one who must be called upon to suggest the best and most economical methods of suppressing these carriers.

Thus there have grown up in many of our colleges and universities departments of medical entomology conducted jointly by entomologists and by medical men. At the Harvard Medical College a thoroughly competent entomologist gives instruction in medical entomology. At Cornell University, where there exists one of the strongest teaching corps of entomologists, especial instruction is given in this direction. The same may be said for the University of Cailfornia, for the University of Wisconsin, and other institutions.

Excellent and comprehensive books on the subject of medical entomology have already been published, aside from numerous special books, such as those of the writer on mosquitoes and on the house-fly, those of the late Gordon Hewitt and Graham-Smith on the house-fly and other flies, and the excellent volume by LePrince and Orenstein on *Mosquito Control in Panama.* As early as 1910 Prof. R. W. Doane, of Leland Stanford Junior University, published a book entitled *Insects and Disease.* This was followed by the excellent volume entitled *Handbook of Medical Entomology* published by Professors Riley and Johannsen of Cornell University in 1915, and by the excellent compendium, *Medical and Veterinary Entomology,* by Dr. W. B. Herms, of the University of California, in the same year. Later there appeared the admirable volume of Dr. A. C. Chandler, of the Oregon Agricultural College, *Annual Parasites and Human Disease,* in 1918, and the excellent work, *Entomology for Medical Officers,* by Lieut. Col. A. Alcock, published in London in 1920; and in the present year has been published the very up-to-date volume entitled, *Sanitary Entomology,* edited by Dr. W. D. Pierce, formerly of the Bureau of Entomology at Washington. All of these works contain full bibliographies, and it will perhaps not be necessary to add a bibliographical list to this sketch.*

A number of periodicals have also been started which are largely, and in some cases entirely, devoted to medical entomology.

The enormous and promising field is rapidly being exploited, and the more it is being worked the more obvious it becomes that a tremendous fight is on between the human species and the class of insects which not only destroy man's crops and damage most of his valued possessions, but threaten his bodily health in a host of different ways.

The effect of these discoveries on the public health is already very apparent. Thousands upon thousands of lives have already

---

*An excellent review of recent progress in medical zoology, covering the past six or seven years, will be found in *Tropical Diseases Bulletin,* vol. 18, no. 1, 1921, pp. 1-14, prepared by Lieutenant Colonel Alcock, assistant director of the Tropical Diseases Bureau of London.

A historical "Scientific Record" of the Liverpool School of Tropical Medicine is published in vol. XV, no. 1, pp. 1-47, of the *Annals of Tropical Medicine and Parasitology* (April 27, 1921). It was compiled by Dorothy Allmand, librarian of the school.

A summary of the efforts in mosquito control in different parts of the world during the past ten years, prepared by the writer of this article, will be found in the *Proceedings of the New Jersey Mosquito Extermination Association,* Seventh Annual Meeting, 1920.

been saved as a result. The intensity of many great world scourges has been relieved. One of them, yellow fever, has measurably become a thing of the past. Gorgas' magnificent demonstration at Panama has shown that, so far as disease is concerned, the tropics may be inhabited by the white race, and what that means for the future of the world no one can now estimate. All over the United States even, a country which is fortunately for the most part situated in the healthiest of climates, life on the average is longer and happier because of the knowledge that has been gained regarding insect-borne diseases. The American Public Health Association has borne its important part as an exploiter of these discoveries, as a publicist, as an influential evangelist in the preaching of the new crusade.

In glancing through the fifty or more volumes of the publications of this society one is very greatly impressed by their high character. The whole series serves as an accurate record of the advance of preventive medicine in the United States, in Canada on the north and in Mexico and the West Indies on the south. It is interesting to note, for example, the multitude of articles and reports on yellow fever in the earlier volumes, these beginning with an admirable address in Volume 1 by my old friend, Dr. J. M. Toner, now dead for many years. On reading this address I find many suggestive statements, suggestive in the light of later discoveries. But perhaps the most interesting article in the volumes, from the historical point of view, is the revolutionary paper read by Walter Reed in October, 1900, modestly entitled, "A Note on the Etiology of Yellow Fever." Lazear had just died (September 25), and Reed, when calling upon me in passing through Washington on his way to the meeting, told me that he was making his first announcement before this Association on account of its great activity in matters relative to the dread disease.

The list of investigators who have died for the public good in the course of the investigations we have been considering is already large. I have mentioned Lazear, Ricketts, McClintock and McCray, and have shown that the deaths of Reed and Carroll occurred most prematurely shortly after their monumental discovery was announced. As a fairly complete list of these martyrs of science is given in another chapter of this volume, they need not be repeated here.

THE HISTORY OF PUBLIC HEALTH NURSING

LAVINIA L. DOCK, R. N.
Secretary, International Council of Nurses

PUBLIC health nursing, as it is to-day, in its still incomplete phase of development, has expanded slowly and naturally from that neighborly office of visiting and attending the sick which has been an age-old custom. Springing from spontaneous goodwill and the gentler emotions, visiting nursing has always been impressed to some extent by the stamp of the special ideals or altruism peculiar to its age, and has also measurably strengthened and disseminated those ideals. When religion held a predominant place in thought, visiting nurse orders or sisterhoods saw, beyond the patient's suffering, a soul to be saved. When humanistic or rationalistic views were entertained, nursing orders became animated by a more freely ranging thought.

As modern science has transformed the medical art, visiting nurses have become infused with a hopeful zeal for a corresponding transformation in the crude adjustments of our physical and social mechanism of living, such as may set free the higher spiritual forces. There has been throughout the ages a certain unconscious democracy of outlook and purpose among those men and women who were the pioneers of public health nursing. It shows clearly in Francis of Assisi; in that revered man, the founder of the Sisters of Charity, Vincent de Paul; and it is unmistakable in the leaders as well as in the rank and file of visiting nurses to-day.

Florence Nightingale, whose many remarkable writings are too little known, had all through her life the vision and ardor of spirit befitting the first and most eminent public health nurse, though it is as a hospital nurse that she is usually regarded. The phrase "health nursing" was hers, and recurs over and over on many a page in her trenchant printed criticisms and comments on conditions in her day. That phrase was not then understood except by a select few. Preventive medicine was then only beginning to be thought of, and preventive nursing was even more unimaginable. In her long years of work for sanitary reforms in India she impressed the idea of the "health missioner" on the mind of the public, and continued to dwell on the theme in her coöperation with William Rathbone, the philanthropist who founded in Liverpool the first district nursing association on modern lines (1859-1862); in her articles on "Village Sanitation" and "District Nursing," and in her efforts to train an order of "health missioners" as such, in 1890. Her biographer says, "She was possessed by the idea of the district nurse as health missioner."

While many European countries had systems of visiting nursing in the nineteenth century, sometimes carried out under the religious motive, as the Kaiserwerth and other orders of deaconesses, and the Sisters of Charity, sometimes as an expression of humanity in the spirit of the modern Red Cross, England was the first to organize "district nursing," as it was then called, on comprehensive lines, with principles endorsed by modern social reformers. The East London Nursing Society (1868) raised the whole plane of district nursing by requiring that nurses should be educated gentlewomen. Queen Victoria's Jubilee Institute for Nurses, endowed and incorporated by royal charter (1889), created a great national institution for "improved means for nursing the sick poor," lifted district nursing from individual hands, and stands to-day an eminent model of organization for good nursing in the homes of people. From the initiative of a queen's nurse, Miss Amy Hughes, responding to the appeal of a teacher in an English school, the whole modern development of public school nursing has grown up. A touch of caste, however, clung to the English models in their suggestion of charity. Mr. Charles Booth wrote, "Of all the forms that charity takes, there is hardly one that is so directly successful as district nursing." Another weak point was the accepted affiliation with country nursing associations employing "village nurses," who were certified midwives with three months' teaching in district nursing. The best features of the English model were copied by the dominions: the Victorian Order (1897) covers Canada, and similar societies are at work in Australia and New Zealand.

THE GROWTH OF PUBLIC HEALTH NURSING IN THE UNITED STATES

The phrase "health nursing" used by Miss Nightingale was expanded to "public health nursing" at the time the National Organization for Public Health Nursing was established.

From 1877 to 1890 district nursing in the United States has been developing in various centers. The Women's Branch of the New York City Mission (1877) worked with denominational limitations. The New York Ethical Society (1879) also sent trained nurses into the homes of the poor, coöperating with the free dispensary movement, Boston first organized on the basis of educational health propaganda combined with bedside care, in the Boston Instructive District Nursing Association (1886). Philadephia, in 1866, and Chicago, in 1889, discarded the word "district" as meaningless in our cities, and took the name "Visiting Nurse Society" or "Association," as being at once more descriptive and more friendly.

In 1893, Miss Wald and Miss Brewster founded the Nurses' Settlement, as it was at first called, going into the East Side of New York City to live among the people of almost wholly foreign birth. It was the untrammeled and spontaneous character of their enterprise that gave it the inspirational power it has had and still displays. From the first, Miss Wald directed her work and study by the light of a rare feeling for genuine democracy, a determination to bring the best of everything to the service of all.

But she was not alone in this position. Visiting nurses over the country seemed to receive similar impressions, spontaneously and irresistibly, as they pushed farther into paths so different from their hospital work, and as they perceived the conditions that had sent their hospital patients into their care. Poverty must be recognized as a social maladjustment capable of being abolished by intelligent coöperation. It was perceived as the fruitful cause, rather than the result of, illness and misery, though there was often a vicious circle.

The teachings of science, so plain, clear, and simple, must be accepted as guiding principles. The services of nurse and physician must be as easily attainable by the poor as by the rich, and there must be no exclusion. From this point of view arose the conception of the guardianship of the public health as one of the chief functions of the muncipality, the community, the state, the federal government.

Impelled by these vital forces, the nurses of the country often found themselves unequipped for the new fields of service they were entering. The anti-tuberculosis crusade was pressing them to join it as teachers and investigators. It has been said that the leaders of this crusade were the first to recognize the value of the nurse as a teacher of hygiene and sanitation. The public school nursing movement, begun in this country as an experiement by the Henry Street Settlement (1902), spread rapidly over the country and made extreme demands on the knowledge and qualities of nurses. Big employers had begun to engage nurses as early as 1895. The Proctor Marble Company, of Proctor, Vermont, was the first to employ nurses to conserve the health of their employees and familes, followed in 1897 by John Wanamaker, of New York and Philadelphia, with his large mercantile establishments. This was another field of unknown social dimensions. The Metropolitan Life Insurance Company began, in 1909, a system of home nursing for its industrial policy-holders which has grown to vast dimensions. In this service, nurses first learned, and with difficulty, how to keep absolutely accurate but complex records.

In 1910, a course in public health nursing was established under the direction of Professor M. Adelaide Nutting at Teachers' College, Columbia University.

In 1912, the National Organization for Public Health Nursing was formed. At the request of some of the leaders in visiting nursing who realized the imperative need of organizing themselves for concerted effort, the American Nurses' Association, formed in 1896 as the Associated Alumnæ of Training Schools for Nurses, and the League for Nursing Education, formed earlier as the Society of Superintendents of Training Schools for Nurses, had called a joint committee (1911) to consider the question of standardization for public health work.

All existing organizations employing public health nurses, then numbering 1,092, were asked to send delegates to form a national organization. The response was enthusiastic, and the purpose of the new society was thus expressed:

> To stimulate responsibility for the health of the community by the establishment and extension of public health nursing; to facilitate efficient coöperation between nurses, physicians, boards of trustees, and other persons interested in public health measures, to develop standards and technique in public health nursing service; to establish a central bureau for information, reference, and assistance in matters pertaining to such service; and to publish periodicals or issue bulletins from time to time in the accomplishment of the general purpose of this organization.

The new organization, while remaining an integral part of the American Nurses' Association, admits lay membership, and has had a most important share in the development of public health nursing. To the energy and devoted service of the first executive secretary, Ella Phillips Crandall, who served from 1912 to 1920, is due much of the effective energy of the organization.

Coincident with the rise of this group came the most potential practical demonstration of public health nursing yet shown, in the resolution of the American Red Cross to found a system of rural nursing (1912). At first begun under the name "Red Cross Rural Nursing Service," it expanded within a year to the "Red Cross Town and Country Nursing Service," and is now the "Bureau of Public Health Nursing." The work thus begun has grown to striking proportions, covering the entire country and involving intricate yet harmonious relations with public health bodies from the smallest to the largest. During the first five years of its existence, made difficult by the cataclysm of war, the Red Cross Town and Country Nursing Service was directed by Fannie F. Clement, whose sympathies and intelligence were exerted to the full in its upbuilding. Her successors, Mary S. Gardner and Elizabeth G. Fox, brought unusual gifts to the service. This Bureau now represents one of the most extensive activities of the American Red Cross.

It may be of interest and importance to note that, as the Red Cross includes on its national committee on nursing the *pro tempore* presidents of the three national nursing associations and other nurses who are prominent in the National Organization for Public Health Nursing, the work of the two bodies may be regarded as largely unified by the guiding influence of the same women on both councils and both lists of elected officers. With this in mind, the functions and accomplishments of these two powerful societies may be regarded as complementary, embodying both the theory and practice of public health nursing.

When to this outline of national groups, it is added that many individual societies, such as the visiting nurse associations, and state or municipal boards of health, such as that of Los Angeles, are consciously and purposely carrying out experimental policies with a view to continuous advance in constructive work, and that ever-increasing numbers of educational institutions are opening the way for qualified nurses to receive a special higher education fitting them for the new demands, we shall have said all that the limits of our article will allow on this point.

THE SPECIAL BRANCHES OF PUBLIC HEALTH NURSING

In the earlier and simpler days, one and the same visiting nurse encountered and dealt with, as best she might, every form of illness and emergency. But the progress of medical science and, no doubt too, to some extent the rising emphasis laid upon prevention, have brought forward many specialties, whose number seems to increase rather than diminish. The first was tuberculosis. Then followed public school work, child welfare, infant welfare, prenatal nursing, maternal nursing. The usual infectious and contagious diseases form a special problem. To these have now been added the preventive and educational propaganda in regard to venereal diseases. Mental hygiene is a recent specialization whose first primer is just being learned. Industrial nursing is an older specialty, which has not yet, however, become as well standardized and supervised as other branches of public health work. It must involve some acquaintance with industrial philosophies and with labor legislation, which is, in some countries, as Australia, Germany and England, much in advance of ours, though our different states are not without certain codes. Medical social service (formerly called hospital social service) is yet another highly specialized branch of public health work. Dental clinics, especially in connection with public school service, are extending, and every year sees the introduction of one or more specialized lines.

In this multiplication of the specialist nurse, one of the most per-plexing administrative questions arises. It is discussed with great clarity and temperateness by Mary S. Gardner in her book *Public Health Nursing* (pp. 70-73), and able arguments are advanced on both sides. It would seem, however, that when left free to develop their work, nurses themselves have experienced a practical compulsion to specialization, and this in considerable degree. The tendency must not, of course, proceed to extremes. It appears, moreover, that the specialist is a leader, or torch-bearer. Where she has first worked alone, her successors can utilize her results in a more generalized type of service. Miss Gardner "feels that to reach the highest possibilities in special lines of nursing, there must be women giving their entire time to these lines, and by so doing becoming experts in them, able to lead others, able to contribute to the literature which is so greatly needed; able, in short, to do for the nursing profession what the specialist in medicine is so successfully doing for the medical profession." While this function of the specialist will always exist, the trend is steadily toward general service of staff nurses, adequately supported by highly trained and experienced experts as consultants or supervisors.

The question of privately administered versus public control is also a controversial one. Here it would seem that the mission of the privately managed society for public health nursing is much like that of the expert specialist, as related to the all-round or general nurse, i.e., it is that of a pathbreaker. In its freedom to experiment and initiate it has a valuable contribution to give, in the object lessons and demonstrations it may make, from which public bodies of more routine character can draw fresh advantages. On this point Miss Gardner says:

From one point of view it is felt that until public health nursing is placed on the same basis as our free educational system, we shall never be really successful in providing adequately for the health of the American people. Others feel that a dual responsibility for the work will always be more desirable, that municipalities or states will never be likely to take the lead in new endeavor, and that unless private bodies still exist to make experiments and bring to bear upon public bodies the weight of a public opinion stimulated by the example of enlightened private enterprise, we shall be in danger of losing a much needed impetus now common where private organizations and a municipality divide the responsibility of the public health nursing of a city between them.

The Special Training of the Public Health Nurse

In the stress of trying to meet the public demands, the individual nurses themselves made the first pleas for a more complete preparation for their work. But few understood whence it should come, and hospital training schools were deluged with insistant claims to have such and such specialties included in their three years' time. Miss Gardner says on this point: "A woman who is poorly prepared for the work does more harm than good. Mere hospital training does not fit a nurse for the complexities of public health nursing, and it has become plain that every nurse undertaking unsupervised work should have had either sufficient experience of the right kind, or special training." Such training is now (1920-21) given in the form of post graduate courses, of which there are twenty-two offered by universities in various parts of the country extending from New York to California.

The first of these, we have said, was offered by Teachers College, where a course in hospital economics was already in existence under Miss Nutting's direction. It was the generosity of Mrs. Helen Hartley Jenkins that, in 1910, made it possible to enlarge that department to the department of nursing and health. In a very large measure the success of this university work, boasting the first endowment in America for nursing education, has been mainly due to the vision and creative energy of Miss Adelaide Nutting and her assistant, Miss Isabel Stewart. Other universities and colleges where nurses are given opportunity for higher training are: University of Pennsylvania, Simmons College, University of Minnesota, University of California, Western Reserve University, University of Iowa, University of Oregon, St. Louis School of Social Economy, Richmond (Va.) School of Social Work and Public Health Nursing, University of Michigan, Yale University, in connection with the New Haven Visiting Nurse Association, and Washington University.   This list is not complete, nor is it likely to remain stationary.

But postgraduate schools represent only half the problem.   It is even more important that a very considerable reorganization of the entire system of nursing education should be brought about in the interest of all practice of nursing, but very especially to better prepare women for public health nursing.   A most searching and scientific study of this fundamental question has been under way for nearly two years by a committee on nursing education, under the direction of Miss Josephine Goldmark.   This work is financed by the Rockefeller Foundation, and the report is expected within the current year.

THE GROWTH OF PUBLIC HEALTH NURSING

Within twenty years' time (up to January, 1920), the organizations engaged in public health nursing have increased in number from 58 to approximately 4,000, and the number of nurses employed by them from 130 to approximately 11,000.   These represent, besides voluntary agencies, departments of health and of education, city, county and state, and great industrial corporations.

Perhaps the most significant single factor in the development of public health nursing at the present time is the rapid extension of state direction and control.   This is due in considerable measure to the influence of the war and the epidemics of 1918-19, and especially to the peace program of the American Red Cross.   The latter has given great impetus to the movement through its offers of financial and administrative coöperation until the states were able to assume full charge.   There are now in the various state health departments the following:

Divisions or Bureaus of Public Health Nursing 10
Divisions or Bureaus of Public Health Nursing and Child Hygiene 10
State Supervising Nurses (without Bureaus) 4
State Supervising Nurses, financed privately 2

The first, and perhaps the most notable, law providing for a state public health nursing service is that of New York, enacted in 1913.

PRESENT STATUS OF THE NATIONAL ORGANIZATION FOR PUBLIC HEALTH NURSING

During 1920 and 1921 this organization became one of the constituent members of the National Health Council and of the National Child Health Council. This latter connection offers almost unlimited opportunities, not only for more efficient and economical administration (this being true of all members of the Council), but for expansion and increasing effectiveness of service.

Its staff includes the following positions: executive secretary, assistant to the executive, educational secretary, librarian, assistant librarian, eligibility secretary, membership secretary, statistical secretary, assistant statistician, editor, assistant editor.

It publishes a monthly magazine, *Public Health Nurse.* It maintains a library department, the plan of which is to place literature on public health nursing in a selected library in each state and to circulate "packet libraries." Forty-three such centers have been established, the libraries selected being usually state libraries or those of universities. The library department keeps current publications on classified subjects in the field of public health. The library also maintains an active advisory service through correspondence.

The organization has standing committees on the following: Public Health Nursing Education; Organization and Administration; Legislation, Records and Reports.

Four sections have been created for the development of the following special subjects: Tuberculosis Nursing; Child Hygiene Nursing; School Nursing; Industrial Nursing.

The War Service of the Organization was of considerable import-ance. A Washington office was maintained during the war. The executive secretary was loaned to the Council of National Defense, where she served as secretary to the three committees on nursing of the Council. The associate secretary, Miss Mary E. Lent, was loaned to the United States Public Health Service to organize the nursing service in twenty-two zones. Of her work, Surgeon General Blue said:

For the first time in its history, the United States Public Health Service, during the recent war, organized a division of public health nursing. The work which these nurses performed was of inestimable value. It is not too much to say that without their aid our success in keeping down sickness in the extra-cantonment zones and in making the venereal disease rate in our army lower than that of any other army in modern times, could not have been achieved.

Of special importance also was the war work of the Sub-Committee on Public Health Nursing under the chairmanship of Miss Mary Beard. This committee secured special Red Cross enrollment of public health nurses, exclusively for public health work. It served, through the secretary, on a special advisory committee to the Red Cross Department of Nursing. It was largely instrumental in securing special service chevrons for Red Cross nurses, public health nurses and others, who stayed at home as a patriotic duty. It prepared a series of lectures on the historical, social, economic, and clinical aspects of venereal diseases for the use of training schools, of public health nurses and social workers in venereal disease clinics. It shared with the National Organization the responsibility for the construction of a complete plan for an emergency preparation for public health nurses to meet the demands created by the Children's Year program.

The activities of the Committee on Home Nursing, of which Lillian D. Wald was chairman, were as follows: It prepared for the Committee on Labor a report on the extent of industrial nursing in the United States and of the industries in which nursing care is especially desirable. It placed at the disposal of all industries, especially those engaged in war work, information concerning the location of existing public health nursing agencies whose services could be utilized in case of emergencies or other need. It interested the United States Shipping Board and the National Emergency Housing Commission in the importance of providing accommodations for public health nurses in their plans for housing units. It prepared and circulated 42,000 letters setting forth the increased importance of health protection of industrial workers and the value thereto of public health nursing care. These were sent accompanied by letters of transmittal, written by Mr. Gompers, to all trade and labor unions and to all employers' associations in the United States.

The activities of the General Committee on Nursing during the war, M. Adelaide Nutting, chairman, were too numerous to be mentioned in full, and pertained only indirectly to public health nursing.

Soon after the war, the National Organization for Public Health Nursing entered into working agreement with the National Tuberculosis Association and the American Red Cross, which offered an admirable opportunity for combined service in the standardization and extension of public health nursing.

PRINCIPLES OF WORK

With all the variation in types of public health nursing and despite conflicting practical conditions, certain fundamental principles which have been tested by experience are quite universally accepted. These we may briefly summarize as follows:

The training and preparation of the nurse has been spoken of. Another general principle is that the nurse should not work under a charitable organization. If she does, her services are limited to those below the poverty line, and others are unwilling to ask for her. If she dispenses material relief, patients learn to look for and value such assistance rather than her own gifts of nursing skill and wise advice. Miss Gardner says:

A nurse should stand upon her public health nursing ability alone, meeting the material needs of her patients through coöperation, and she should be available to all who may need her services. The work should be on as sound a financial basis as possible. All who can afford to make payment for services of the nurse should do so. This usually is arranged on a sliding scale, the maximum being the cost price of the visit, and the minimum, the amount possible for the poorest patients, a range usually covering from five cents to fifty or sixty. In every city there are many who can save nothing from an inadequate income for the rainy day of illness (this is equally true of country dwellers, who often have almost no money, though they may be able to live from the products of their garden), and there are others who because of ill health, age, widowhood or some other handicap never rise to the level of self-support at all. These groups must receive free care, yet the general rule should nevertheless obtain, that wherever possible, payment for visits should be made. This is now generally accepted where bedside care is given.

Referring to Miss Gardner's statement of fifty or sixty cents as a maximum fee, it should be said that a considerable number of Associations now offer a so-called hourly nursing service at full cost or more, amounting to seventy-five cents or a dollar. This is increasingly sought by families of ample means. The burning question of the day is to find a means of bringing education and curative nursing to the great wage-earning and middle-class population at a cost which they can afford.

Record-keeping is a most important part of public health nursing. Records should be kept in such a way as to supply a perfect picture of the volume and type of work done in reference to its cost, and should furnish data from which information can be obtained concerning the various aspects (i. e., social, economic, status of public sanitation and hygiene, effects of industry, rural problems) of sickness and health. They should also permit of simple and convenient reference to individual cases.

One of the earliest principles adopted in modern visiting nursing was that of non-interference in religious belief. Miss Gardner says:

The wisdom of this general principle has only been emphasized with succeeding years. It has also been found that it is wiser for public health work not to be carried on by a church. A certain limitation of usefulness then becomes inevitable, for it is difficult to avoid the appearance, at least, of sectarianism. It is far better for the churches to contribute to the support of an association which will care for the whole of the community without geographical or other limitations. We have, however, not said all when we say that the nurse shall not interfere. From her position in the home, she can often give positive help in strengthening already existing church connections. The question is not a difficult one if the public health nurse remembers that she is not representing her own religious faith, but the spirit of helpfulness which expresses itself in the effort on her part to strengthen all bonds, making for the better life of the patient.

The art of coöperation has become the keystone of good public health nursing work. Alone, the nurse is powerless to change conditions for her patients. To attain her best usefulness she must know every source to tap for help in meeting the conditions caused by the complexity of modern life. Yet this side of coöperation has perhaps been dwelt upon to excess. What, on the other hand, is the well-trained public health nurse to do, when in a flourishing town of, let us say, 12,000 to 20,000 inhabitants, she finds a local health board so negligent and casual as to be practically non-existent; no truant officers; no active groups of civic-minded men and women; no segregation of the feeble-minded; no hospital provision for the isolation of contagious cases; no civic interest in housing problems;   not even a charity organization society?

In the bedside care of the patient the best private-duty standards are aimed at, so far as possible. On professional relationships with physicians, Miss Gardner says:

The public health nurse should not diagnose, should not prescribe, should not recommend a particular doctor or a change of doctors, should not suggest a hospital to a patient without the concurrence of the doctor, and should never criticize by word or unspoken action any member of the medical profession.

But on this statement, Athel Campbell Burnham, M. D., makes this statement:—

These rules appear to me too severe, and I believe that in time they may be modified so that a nurse will not be compelled to serve under a physician who is palpably ignorant or dangerously careless.*

*The Community Health Problem, p. 43.

INDEX

INDEX

Accidents, economic loss from, 409.
Activated sludge process, 186–188.
Air, analysis, 78; bacteriology, 77–79; flow, 343–344; humidity, 341–342, 345, 348–349, 356, 358–359; recirculation, 350–351; temperature, 341–342, 345, 348, 358, 360; vitiated, 337–341. *See also* Ventilation.
Adulteration of food, 210–213.
Agriculture, Department of, 318.
Alberta, 63–64.
Algæ in water, 170–172.
American Association for Labor Legislation, 386–387.
American Child Hygiene Association, 292, 320–321.
American experience table, 106.
American Museum of Safety. *See* Safety Institute of America.
American Public Health Association, Committee on bacteriological analysis of milk, 83; on refuse disposal, 190–191; on trades waste disposal, 202; on water analysis, 82–83; effect on food control, 210; finances, 27; future, 26–29; headquarters moved, 26; history, 13–55; *Journal*, 20–23, 24, 26; *News Letter*, 24, 26; organization, 3, 10–11; platform, 27; presidents, historical sketches, 30–55; publications, 20–23, 26; resolution on federal bureau of health, 17; section on industrial hygiene, 389; sections, 18–19; standards, 19, 25–26, for testing milk, 83, 241, 283–284, of water analysis, 83.
American Society for Study and Prevention of Infant Mortality. *See* American Child Hygiene Association.
Anthrax, 16.

Antiscorbutic vitamine, 263.
Antiscorbutics, 223.

Babcock test, 238, 282.
Baby week, 314.
Bacteriologists, early American, 72–76.
Bacteriology, air, 77–79; course in, first, 72; early technique, 70–71; journals, 92–93; literature, 74, 77–78; milk, 83, 239, 242–243, 282–285; progress in U. S., 76; relation to preservation of food, 228, to public health, 16–17, 66–93, 76; societies, 92; water, 79–83.
Beriberi, 261.
Big Brothers, 296.
Big Sisters, 296.
Billings life tables, 106.
Birth registration area, 14, 293.
Boer war, 224.
Bomb-calorimeter, invention, 256.
Bovine tuberculosis, 250–253; and human, 251; old laws regarding, 251; per cent of cattle infected, 252; tuberculin test, 251.
Boy Scouts, 305.
Breakbone fever, 424.
British Columbia, 63.
Bubonic plague, 85, 429.
Bureau of Chemistry, Office of Coöperation, 217.
Bureau of Education, 317–318.
Bureau of Labor Statistics, history, 382–383.
Bureau of Mines, history, 373–384.
By-products in industry, value, 200.

Calorie, 256.
Camp Fire Girls, 305.